W9-ACD-221

Trauma and Health

Physical Health Consequences of Exposure to

Extreme Stress

Trauma and Health

Physical Health Consequences

of Exposure to

Extreme Stress

Edited by

Paula P. Schnurr and Bonnie L. Green

American Psychological Association • Washington, DC

First Printing, November 2003
Second Printing, November 2005

Published by
American Psychological Association
750 First Street, NE
Washington, DC 20002
www.apa.org

To order
APA Order Department
P.O. Box 92984
Washington, DC 20090-2984
Tel: (800) 374-2721
Direct: (202) 336-5510
Fax: (202) 336-5502
TDD/TTY: (202) 336-6123
Online: www.apa.org/books/
E-mail: order@apa.org

In the U.K., Europe, Africa, and the Middle East, copies may be ordered from
American Psychological Association
3 Henrietta Street
Covent Garden, London
WC2E 8LU England

Typeset in Goudy by World Composition Services, Inc., Sterling, VA

Printer: Port City Press, Baltimore, MD
Cover Designer: Naylor Design, Washington, DC
Technical/Production Editor: Kristen S. Boye

Library of Congress Cataloging-in-Publication Data
Trauma and health : physical health consequences of exposure to extreme stress / edited by Paula P. Schnurr and Bonnie L. Green.
    p. cm.
        Includes bibliographical references and index.
        ISBN 1-59147-066-8 (alk. paper)
        1. Stress (Psychology)—Physiological aspects. 2. Stress (Physiology)—Health aspects. 3. Psychic trauma. 4. Post-traumatic stress disorder. 5. Traumatic neuroses. 6. Psychoneuroimmunology. 7. Health—Psychological aspects. I. Schnurr, Paula P. II. Green, Bonnie L.

    RC455.4.S87T735   2003
    616.85′21—dc22   2003016818

British Library Cataloguing-in-Publication Data
A CIP record is available from the British Library.

Printed in the United States of America

CONTENTS

CONTRIBUTORS

Ron Acierno, PhD, National Crime Victims Research and Treatment Center, Medical University of South Carolina, Charleston

Carolyn M. Aldwin, PhD, Department of Human and Community Development, University of California, Davis

Andrew Baum, PhD, Departments of Psychology and Psychiatry, University of Pittsburgh, PA

Angela Liegey Dougall, PhD, Department of Psychology, University of Pittsburgh, PA

Charles C. Engel, Jr., MD, MPH, Department of Psychiatry, Uniformed Services University of the Health Sciences, Bethesda, MD; Department of Defense Deployment Health Clinical Center at Walter Reed, Washington, DC

Daniel E. Ford, MD, MPH, Departments of Medicine, Psychiatry, Epidemiology, Health Policy, and Management, Johns Hopkins University, Baltimore, MD

Matthew J. Friedman, MD, PhD, National Center for Posttraumatic Stress Disorder, Department of Veterans Affairs Medical and Regional Office Center, White River Junction, VT; Departments of Psychiatry and Pharmacology, Dartmouth Medical School, Hanover, NH

Bonnie L. Green, PhD, Department of Psychiatry, Georgetown University Medical School, Washington, DC

Rachel Kimerling, PhD, Department of Psychiatry, University of California at San Francisco Medical Center

Mary P. Koss, PhD, Department of Family and Community Medicine, University of Arizona Prevention Center, Tucson

Bruce S. McEwen, PhD, Harold and Margaret Milliken Hatch Laboratory of Neuroendocrinology, Rockefeller University, New York

Elana Newman, PhD, Department of Psychology, University of Tulsa, Tulsa, OK

Heidi S. Resnick, PhD, National Crime Victims Research and Treatment Center, Medical University of South Carolina, Charleston

Alyssa A. Rheingold, PhD, National Crime Victims Research and Treatment Center, Medical University of South Carolina, Charleston

Paula P. Schnurr, PhD, National Center for Posttraumatic Stress Disorder, Department of Veterans Affairs Medical and Regional Office Center, White River Junction, VT; Department of Psychiatry, Dartmouth Medical School, Hanover, NH

Edward A. Walker, MD, Departments of Psychiatry and Behavioral Sciences and Obstetrics and Gynecology, University of Washington Medical Center, Seattle

Loriena A. Yancura, PhD candidate, Department of Human and Community Development, University of California, Davis

PREFACE

Since the publication of Selye's (1956) seminal book, *The Stress of Life*,[1] a great deal of research has attempted to further our understanding of the relationship between stress and physical health. Most of this research has focused on stressors such as divorce, bereavement, and job loss. However, a number of studies have examined the health effects associated with extreme stressors, including war-zone exposure, sexual and other criminal victimization, natural and human-made disasters, and serious accidents. We bring these findings together in this edited volume in which contributors comprehensively summarize the findings on how such stressors relate to physical health.

This book is designed for academic and clinical audiences. The consolidation and integration of findings provides a framework to support future research on the topic by scholars from both the stress and the traumatic stress fields. The emphasis on clinical relevance provides guidance for mental health clinicians whose patients may be struggling with medical illnesses and for clinicians in primary and specialty care settings, who often are confronted with trauma-related health or mental health problems in their patients. Contributors first present an overview of their topic, then show appropriate empirical findings, and, finally, discuss the clinical relevance of their subject matter, making concrete suggestions for clinical practice if possible. The book is appropriate for a graduate seminar on the health effects of traumatic stress or as part of a broader seminar on stress or trauma. Chapters can be read independently of one another yet are organized around a theoretical model, presented in the last chapter, that posits a central

---

[1] Selye, H. (1956). *The stress of life*. New York: McGraw-Hill.

role for distress reactions in mediating the relationship between traumatic exposure and physical health.

Our interest in the health outcomes associated with psychological trauma arose from a series of fortunate and complementary experiences that illustrate the development of this field of study. In 1992, Paula P. Schnurr was approached by Jessica Wolfe, of the Women's Health Sciences Division of the National Center for Posttraumatic Stress Disorder, to review a dataset on female Vietnam War veterans. These women had served primarily as nurses and, through their experiences, were confronted with the serious injury or death of male combatants. Many of the women also were exposed to traditional war stressors, and some were sexually assaulted while in the service. Initial analyses had shown that war-zone trauma was associated with poor perceptions of health and reports of numerous illnesses. Schnurr suggested that the investigators examine the effects of posttraumatic stress disorder (PTSD) as a mediator of the trauma–health relationship, hypothesizing that one's reaction to a trauma would be an important determinant of subsequent outcomes. She reanalyzed the data to test this hypothesis, which was supported.[2]

The literature review for Wolfe and colleagues' (1994) article revealed an interesting pattern. By the early 1990s, a number of studies had examined the physical health effects of psychological trauma, but, with few exceptions,[3] virtually no studies had examined the health effects of PTSD. Schnurr therefore began a series of investigations aimed at elucidating the processes by which exposure to a traumatic event could lead to poor health, focusing on PTSD as a primary mediator.

Bonnie L. Green's interest in the physical health outcomes of traumatic events started when she began studying "contamination stressors," including a study of a community that learned that the feed-processing plant with the checkered tower in their neighborhood was a nuclear weapons facility, not a Purina plant, and that nuclear waste was being released into the local groundwater for several years before it was discovered.[4] This study, and similar investigations by other colleagues, indicated that individuals in these types of disasters had low rates of PTSD but seemed especially preoccupied with their physical health and scored relatively high on somatization indices.

---

[2] Wolfe, J., Schnurr, P. P., Brown, P. J., & Furey, J. (1994). PTSD and war-zone exposure as correlates of perceived health in female Vietnam veterans. *Journal of Consulting and Clinical Psychology, 62*, 1235–1240.

[3] For example, see Litz, B. T., Keane, T. M., Fisher, L., Marx, B., & Monaco, V. (1992). Physical health complaints in combat-related post-traumatic stress disorder: A preliminary report. *Journal of Traumatic Stress, 5*, 131–141.

[4] Green, B. L., Lindy, J. D., & Grace, M. C. (1994). Psychological effects of toxic contamination. In R. Ursano, B. McCaughey, & C. Fullerton (Eds.), *Individual and community responses to trauma and disaster* (pp. 154–176). Cambridge, England: Cambridge University Press.

A similar phenomenon was observed in breast cancer survivors,[5] who indeed had PTSD symptoms in the form of intrusion and denial but whose hypervigilance was focused on their bodies and their health rather than on the external world. These reactions were quite logical in the context of the particular traumatic events and fears of cancer or its recurrence, but they also focused attention on the importance of the relationship between mental and physical health.

Another angle on physical health and trauma for Green is her more recent interest in the study and treatment of trauma in primary care settings, especially among poor women in public medical care. With a focus on primary care as the setting in which trauma-related problems are most likely to be present, it seemed critical to consider the nature of presenting complaints that would arise in this non-mental health setting. This new work introduced her to a series of studies, conducted by investigators researching mental health services in medical settings, that linked histories of childhood abuse to certain types of medical conditions or complications and to higher levels of service use. Continued work on several grants in this research area keeps in the forefront the question of how trauma-related problems are presented, and best addressed, in medical settings, particularly primary care.

We came together as collaborators in an investigation focused on acute exposure to mustard gas as a traumatic stressor with the properties of both traditional and contamination stressors.[6] The study sample was a group of veterans who had participated in secret military tests of mustard gas during World War II. Posttraumatic stress disorder, which was present in one third of the sample, was associated with adverse health outcomes (perceptions, impairment, illness, and disability), independent of the effects of amount of mustard gas exposure, smoking, alcohol abuse, and age. These results provided further evidence for the role of PTSD as a mediator in the relationship between trauma exposure and physical health.

This book would not have been possible without the help of a number of people. Susan Reynolds and Rebecca Richters at the American Psychological Association have been excellent editors. Jessica Wolfe provided the first opportunity for Paula Schnurr to explore hypotheses about the role of PTSD in mediating the relationship between trauma and physical health. Ron Spiro and Matt Friedman at the National Center for PTSD have been key collaborators in the work that followed. Friedman in particular engaged in hours of discussion that have been essential to the evolution of the ideas

---

[5]Green, B. L., Rowland, J. H., Krupnick, J. L., Epstein, S. A., Stockton, P., Stern, N. M., et al. (1998). Prevalence of posttraumatic stress disorder (PTSD) in women with breast cancer. *Psychosomatics, 39,* 102–111.

[6]Schnurr, P. P., Ford, J. D., Friedman, M. J., Green, B. L., Dain, B. J., & Sengupta, A. (2000). Predictors and outcomes of posttraumatic stress disorder in World War II veterans exposed to mustard gas. *Journal of Consulting and Clinical Psychology, 68,* 258–268.

presented here and has been a source of support throughout. Jack Lindy and Mary Grace at the University of Cincinnati played key roles in the conceptualization of contamination stressors with Green. Julia Rowland, Janice Krupnick, and Steve Epstein at Georgetown University helped to shape the understanding of PTSD symptoms in breast cancer survivors and introduced Green to addressing mental health issues in medical settings. Jeanne Miranda, Ed Walker, and colleagues at Georgetown have mentored and supported ongoing work addressing trauma in primary care settings. And last, but not least, the contributors to this book have worked hard to align their chapters with our vision to make this book a true collaborative effort.

Trauma and Health

Physical Health Consequences of Exposure to

Extreme Stress

1

A CONTEXT FOR UNDERSTANDING THE PHYSICAL HEALTH CONSEQUENCES OF EXPOSURE TO EXTREME STRESS

PAULA P. SCHNURR AND BONNIE L. GREEN

Accounts of psychological syndromes among combat veterans and survivors of life-threatening accidents have appeared in the medical literature at least as far back as the late 1600s (Babington, 1997; Trimble, 1981). These accounts have varied in terms of the labels used to describe the syndromes: for example, "railway spine," "shell shock," and "traumatic neurosis." The accounts have varied also in terms of the presumed etiology, ranging from injury and infection to psychological factors. Nevertheless, there has been a consistent recognition that extreme events can induce profound emotional and physical symptoms in previously healthy individuals.

Posttraumatic stress disorder (PTSD) was first formally introduced by the American Psychiatric Association in 1980 as a diagnosis that described

This chapter was coauthored by an employee of the United States government as part of official duty and is considered to be in the public domain. Any views expressed herein do not necessarily represent the views of the United States government, and the author's participation in the work is not meant to serve as an official endorsement.

the serious and enduring consequences of exposure to events such as war, disaster, sexual and physical abuse, and serious accidents. Posttraumatic stress disorder is distinct from most psychiatric disorders in that there is an explicit etiologic stimulus: a traumatic event. Traumatic events were initially characterized as being "generally outside the range of usual human experience" (American Psychiatric Association, 1980, p. 236), but in fact they are surprisingly common. According to the National Comorbidity Survey, approximately 60% of men and 50% of women in the United States have been exposed to at least one traumatic event during the course of their lives (Kessler, Sonnega, Bromet, Hughes, & Nelson, 1995). Indeed, epidemiological studies in the early 1990s documented so much trauma in the general population (up to 75%; e.g., Breslau, Davis, Andreski, & Peterson, 1991; Norris, 1992) that the conceptualization of a traumatic event as unusual could no longer stand. In the current diagnostic criteria, a traumatic event is defined as involving "actual or threatened death or serious injury, or a threat to the physical integrity of self or others" (American Psychiatric Association, 1994, p. 424). The event may be experienced directly or may be witnessed or learned about, as when someone learns about the murder of a loved one.

Table 1.1 lists the current diagnostic criteria for PTSD (American Psychiatric Association, 1994). There are six required elements, also known as Criteria A through F. Criterion A is exposure to a traumatic event, along with a reaction of fear, helplessness, or horror to the event. There are three sets of symptom criteria: B, reexperiencing symptoms, such as intrusive thoughts or flashbacks; C, avoidance and numbing symptoms, such as avoiding reminders of the trauma or having a restricted range of affect; and D, hyperarousal, such as insomnia or exaggerated startle. To receive a diagnosis of PTSD, a person must have at least one of the five reexperiencing symptoms, three of the seven avoidance and numbing symptoms, and two of the five hyperarousal symptoms. Criterion E specifies that the necessary B, C, and D symptoms must be present for at least one month, and Criterion F specifies that the symptoms cause extreme distress or functional impairment.

In the United States, 8% to 14% of traumatized men and 20% to 31% of traumatized women develop PTSD, which translates to a population prevalence of 5% to 6% in men and 10% to 12% in women (Breslau et al., 1991; Kessler et al., 1995; Resnick, Kilpatrick, Dansky, Saunders, & Best, 1993). Comparable epidemiological information from other countries is not available. However, in countries with a high number of war-exposed civilians, prevalence is considerably higher. For example, in a study in four postconflict situations involving low-income populations, lifetime PTSD prevalence ranged from 16% in Ethiopia to 37% in Algeria (de Jong et al., 2001). Thus, even though PTSD occurs only in a subset of those who are

TABLE 1.1
Diagnostic Criteria for Posttraumatic Stress Disorder
(American Psychiatric Association, 1994)

Criterion	Elements
A. Traumatic exposure (both 1 and 2 required)	1. experiencing, witnessing, or being confronted with an event that involved death, life threat, serious injury, or a threat to the physical integrity of self or others 2. a response of fear, helplessness, or horror
B. Reexperiencing symptoms (need at least 1 item)	1. intrusive recollections 2. distressing dreams 3. flashbacks 4. intense distress following exposure to traumatic reminders 5. physiological reactivity to traumatic reminders
C. Avoidance/numbing symptoms (need at least 3 items)	1. avoidance of thoughts, feelings, or conversations about the trauma 2. avoidance of activities, places, or people that arouse traumatic memories 3. inability to recall an important aspect of the trauma 4. diminished interest or participation in activities 5. detachment or estrangement from others 6. restricted range of affect 7. sense of foreshortened future
D. Hyperarousal symptoms (need at least 2 items)	1. insomnia 2. irritability or outbursts of anger 3. difficulty concentrating 4. hypervigilance 5. exaggerated startle
E. Duration	B, C, D, symptoms must last at least one month
F. Severity	Symptoms must cause either clinically significant distress or functional impairment.

exposed to traumatic events, it affects large numbers of people around the world.

Numerous studies have shown that trauma exposure and PTSD have substantial and diverse effects on many aspects of well-being, such as an increased likelihood of depression, substance abuse, and most other psychiatric disorders; personality disorder; and severe social and occupational impairment (e.g., Kessler et al., 1995; Kulka et al., 1990). This book focuses on a topic that has received relatively less attention in research on trauma and PTSD: physical health. Individuals who have been exposed to traumatic stressors have adverse physical health outcomes, including poor self-reported health status, a greater number of self-reported medical problems, increased morbidity and mortality, and greater service utilization (Friedman &

Schnurr, 1995; Schnurr & Jankowski, 1999; see chaps. 2 and 3, this volume). Next we briefly describe the conceptual framework that underlies the book's content and then present an overview of the chapters that follow.

CONCEPTUAL FRAMEWORK

Physical health is a multidimensional construct that is expressed across a variety of objective and subjective domains. Wilson and Cleary (1995, p. 60) present a useful model in which health domains exist "on a continuum of increasing biological, social, and psychological complexity" that is affected by objective and subjective factors. At the most basic level are biological and physiological variables. At the next level are the symptoms experienced by the individual. Next comes functional status—how the individual is affected by symptoms—and then health perceptions. The most complex level is health-related quality of life. Characteristics of both people and environments influence all levels of this continuum from symptoms through quality of life. For example, functional status is affected by symptoms, and also by a person's motivation and socioeconomic supports.

Accepting Wilson and Cleary's (1995) or any other model that posits objective and subjective influences on health also requires acceptance of self-reports as valid measures of health. There is abundant evidence that self-reports of physical health are affected by psychological and emotional factors such as negative affectivity (Watson & Pennebaker, 1989). We do not dispute these findings but disagree with those who would use them to completely dismiss self-reports as invalid. Instead, we encourage readers to view self-reports as a component, along with medical exams and laboratory tests, necessary for thoroughly capturing the multidimensional complexity of physical health.

Research on the physical health effects of stress has evolved in three distinct tracks. The largest has focused on serious, but generally non-life-threatening, stressors; we refer to these stressors as *life events*. A much smaller literature has focused on the physical health effects associated with exposure to extreme stressors, particularly sexual and other criminal victimization, and natural and human-made disasters. An even smaller literature has focused on the health effects of PTSD.

These tracks have emerged relatively independently, with little overlap or cross-referencing. Most research into the physical health effects of life events has not included traumatic stressors. For example, a review of the literature on stress and infectious disease in humans suggested that the "impact of severe events would provide the fairest test of a stress-disease relationship" (Cohen & Williamson, 1991, p. 18) but then suggested divorce, bereavement, and job loss as examples of severe events. Furthermore, studies of trauma in primary and specialty care populations (e.g., Walker et al., 1999) have only recently begun to examine PTSD, and most PTSD studies have been conducted with military veterans. Finally, traumatic stress researchers have tended to avoid discussing their findings in terms of knowledge about everyday stress and health.

An important question in understanding all of these literatures is *how* stressors affect physical health. Cohen and Williamson (1991) discussed the distinction between stress (i.e., a stressor) and distress (the reaction to a stressor) in their review of findings on everyday stress and infectious disease. We believe that a similar event–reaction distinction is useful when considering the physical health consequences of exposure to a traumatic event and suggest that PTSD plays a crucial role in mediating the relationship between traumatic exposure and poor physical health. Posttraumatic stress disorder is not the only adverse outcome of traumatic exposure, however. Other serious distress reactions like depression may be important as well, and this is noted throughout the book when appropriate. We emphasize PTSD because it appears to be distinctive among these adverse posttraumatic outcomes for its potential impact on physical health. This impact seems to occur directly, through PTSD's associated biology and psychoneuroimmunology, as well as indirectly, through other cognitive and behavioral mechanisms such as coping and risky health behaviors, which are conceptually distinct from PTSD and other mental disorders, although probably overlap with them.

ABOUT THIS BOOK

This book provides a comprehensive summary of findings on trauma and physical health and aims to integrate these findings with research on the health effects of nontraumatic stress. It is based on a model, described fully in the final chapter, in which PTSD and other psychological reactions to traumatic exposure are the essential mechanism through which exposure affects physical health. The model, which extends prior work by Friedman and Schnurr (1995) and Schnurr and Jankowski (1999), includes biological, attentional, and behavioral components as additional mechanisms.

The book is divided into five parts. Part I summarizes the literature on trauma and PTSD in relation to physical health. Green and Kimerling (chap. 2) review findings on health status and disease, as indicated by self-reported health or symptoms, physician diagnosis, laboratory exam, and mortality. Their review indicates that PTSD, and to a lesser extent, other types of trauma-related psychological distress, are crucial for mediating the relationship between trauma and poor health. Their review also indicates that PTSD has effects independent of other comorbid disorders such as depression. In chapter 3, Walker, Newman, and Koss discuss what is known about how trauma survivors seek medical care and how this impacts costs to the health care system and society at large. The authors use a mental health services research perspective to present evidence that exposure to traumatic experiences is related to medical treatment seeking and service utilization.

The next three parts review evidence on possible mechanisms through which trauma and physical health could be related. Part II discusses psychological factors. Although a number of the psychological correlates of PTSD are associated with adverse physical health outcomes, this part focuses on depression and coping because of the relatively large amount of evidence linking these factors with poor health. In chapter 4, Ford examines the relationship between depression and cardiovascular disease as a model for addressing mental disorders and their impact on disease processes, covering such topics as mechanisms linking depression to cardiovascular disease and the impact of depression treatment on disease outcomes. Because PTSD and depression are so often comorbid, these findings are likely to have important implications for the study of PTSD and cardiovascular health. Aldwin and Yancura (chap. 5) review findings on coping. They provide a context for their review by describing theoretical and methodological approaches to conceptualizing coping and then examining similarities and differences between coping with nontraumatic stressors and coping with trauma. They conclude that coping affects health and that interventions designed to enhance coping can have beneficial effects on disease.

Part III discusses biological factors. In chapter 6, Dougall and Baum present findings on trauma and psychoneuroimmunology. They consider the evidence for immune system mediation of associations between trauma and infectious illness, cancer, HIV disease progression, and other aspects of physical health. Their review is supplemented by a basic discussion of relationships between severe stress and immune system regulation and by consideration of the ways in which immune system effects of traumatic stress could affect health or disease course. Friedman and McEwen (chap. 7) review findings on the neurobiology of PTSD and suggest that abnormalities in physiological reactivity and neuroendocrinology might constitute risk factors for medical illness among people with PTSD. They discuss the concept of allostatic load (McEwen & Stellar, 1993) to explain how subtle changes in PTSD-related biology could collectively lead to illness and propose a new construct, *allostatic support*, to explain how subtle positive biological changes could collectively buffer an individual against becoming ill following traumatic exposure.

Part IV includes information about attentional and behavioral factors, focusing on the problem of physical symptoms for which there is no obvious medical explanation. Engel (chap. 8) discusses this problem in terms of *multiple idiopathic physical symptoms*, or MIPS, rather than more traditional terms such as somatoform symptoms. He argues that MIPS is a useful construct because it embodies three important aspects of somatization: the lack of a clear medical explanation for physical symptoms, the physical (versus only emotional) nature of symptoms, and the existence of symptoms in a pattern that is associated with functional disability. His review indicates that trauma in both childhood and adulthood is associated with MIPS, at least in part through an association with PTSD. In chapter 9, Rheingold, Acierno, and Resnick discuss health behaviors such as smoking and substance abuse, and describe how these behaviors relate both to trauma and to PTSD. Trauma may increase the likelihood of poor health behaviors. Alternatively, health behaviors such as substance abuse may increase risk of retraumatization. The chapter outlines interactions among these factors and suggests both assessment and treatment strategies in health care service delivery.

The final part of the book, which features chapter 10 by Schnurr and Green, presents an integrative model that relates trauma to physical health through psychological, behavioral, attentional, and biological mechanisms that are triggered by PTSD and other significant distress reactions following a traumatic event. The chapter synthesizes the practice implications suggested by contributing authors and ends by discussing the clinical, training, and health policy implications of medical problems that result from traumatization. Both clinicians and researchers are encouraged to recognize that medical problems may be bona fide outcomes of traumatization.

We hope that the consolidation and integration of findings presented in this book will support future research on trauma and physical health by scholars from both the stress and traumatic stress fields, as well as those studying mental health in medical settings. We also hope that the emphasis on clinical relevance is useful to mental health clinicians whose patients may be struggling with medical illnesses, and to health care providers in both primary and specialty care settings, who often are confronted with the short and long-term consequences of trauma exposure in their patients. And last, we hope that this book leads to increasing recognition of the multiple ways that trauma affects individuals and society.

REFERENCES

American Psychiatric Association. (1980). *Diagnostic and statistical manual of mental disorders* (3rd ed.). Washington, DC: Author.

American Psychiatric Association. (1994). *Diagnostic and statistical manual of mental disorders* (4th ed.). Washington, DC: Author.

Babington, A. (1997). *Shell shock: A history of the changing attitudes to war neurosis.* London: Leo Cooper.

Breslau, N., Davis, G. C., Andreski, P., & Peterson, E. L. (1991). Traumatic events and posttraumatic stress disorder in an urban population of young adults. *Archives of General Psychiatry, 48,* 216–222.

Cohen, S., & Williamson, G. M. (1991). Stress and infectious disease in humans. *Psychological Bulletin, 109,* 5–24.

de Jong, J. T., Komproe, I. H., Van Ommeren, M., El Masri, M., Araya, M., Khaled, N., et al. (2001). Lifetime events and posttraumatic stress disorder in 4 postconflict settings. *Journal of the American Medical Association, 286,* 555–562.

Friedman, M. J., & Schnurr, P. P. (1995). The relationship between PTSD, trauma, and physical health. In M. J. Friedman, D. S. Charney, & A. Y. Deutch (Eds.), *Neurobiological and clinical consequences of stress: From normal adaptation to PTSD* (pp. 507–527). Philadelphia: Lippincott-Raven.

Kessler, D. C., Sonnega, A., Bromet, E., Hughes, M., & Nelson, C. B. (1995). Posttraumatic stress disorder in the National Comorbidity Survey. *Archives of General Psychiatry, 52,* 1048–1060.

Kulka, R. A., Schlenger, W. E., Fairbank, J. A., Hough, R. L., Jordan, B. K., Marmar, C. R., et al. (1990). *Trauma and the Vietnam War generation.* New York: Brunner/Mazel.

McEwen, B. S., & Stellar, E. (1993). Stress and the individual: Mechanisms leading to disease. *Archives of Internal Medicine, 153,* 2093–2101.

Norris, F. H. (1992). Epidemiology of trauma: Frequency and impact of different potentially traumatic events on different demographic groups. *Journal of Consulting and Clinical Psychology, 60,* 409–418.

Resnick, H. S., Kilpatrick, D. G., Dansky, B. S., Saunders, B. E., & Best, C. L. (1993). Prevalence of civilian trauma and posttraumatic stress disorder in a representative national sample of women. *Journal of Consulting and Clinical Psychology, 61,* 984–991.

Schnurr, P. P., & Jankowski, M. K. (1999). Physical health and posttraumatic stress disorder: Review and synthesis. *Seminars in Clinical Neuropsychiatry, 4,* 295–304.

Trimble, M. R. (1981). *Post-traumatic neurosis: From railway spine to the whiplash.* Chichester, England: Wiley.

Walker, E. A., Gelfand, A. N., Katon, W. J., Koss, M. P., Von Korff, M., Bernstein, D. E., et al. (1999). Adult health status of women with histories of childhood abuse and neglect. *American Journal of Medicine, 107,* 332–339.

Watson, D., & Pennebaker, J. W. (1989). Health complaints, stress, and distress: Exploring the central role of negative affectivity. *Psychological Review, 96,* 234–254.

Wilson, I. B., & Cleary, P. D. (1995). Linking clinical variables with health-related quality of life. *Journal of the American Medical Association, 273,* 59–65.

I

PHYSICAL HEALTH
OUTCOMES IN
TRAUMATIZED
POPULATIONS

2

TRAUMA, POSTTRAUMATIC STRESS DISORDER, AND HEALTH STATUS

BONNIE L. GREEN AND RACHEL KIMERLING

This chapter begins the process of building an integrated model of the mechanisms that may link trauma to health by reviewing the empirical literature on this topic. We examine the literature on empirically based links between trauma exposure and impaired health status, and then address associations between posttraumatic stress disorder (PTSD) and impaired health. We also examine the evidence for PTSD as a specific mediator of the relationship between exposure and health status. We refer the interested reader to several excellent articles for a more detailed literature review (Friedman & Schnurr, 1995; Koss & Heslet, 1992; Resnick, Acierno, & Kilpatrick, 1997; Schnurr & Jankowski, 1999). The present review focuses on key studies that illustrate relationships among trauma, PTSD, and health, including those recently added to this literature. Finally, we address issues of screening for trauma and PTSD in primary care as a prelude for a discussion of implications and recommendations for intervention in the final chapter of the book.

BACKGROUND AND CONCEPTUALIZATION

Health status is a multidimensional construct that refers to an individual's biological regulation, the presence or absence of organic pathology, symptom perception, and physical function (Wilson & Cleary, 1995). To understand the association between traumatic stress and health status, one needs to evaluate a wide range of studies targeting different facets of health status, including self-reported health, morbidity, and mortality measures, for consistency of results. The majority of studies examining trauma and health have focused on self-reported health, including physical symptom reports obtained from checklists, or on a global rating of self-perceived health, which has empirical support as a proxy for disease conditions, poor medical prognoses, and medical comorbidity (Hennessy, Moriarty, Zack, Scherr, & Brackbill, 1994), as well as for mortality risk (Idler & Angel, 1990; Idler & Kasl, 1991). It is important to determine the extent to which findings in these self-report studies are corroborated by those that include other health outcomes. More objective indicators of health status use physician diagnoses, morbidity, or laboratory tests to detect organic pathology and disease states. These data are usually obtained from medical charts or from study protocols that include physician exams. Limited mortality data are also available.

Several methodological issues must be addressed when interpreting these studies. Each type of measure reflects a different aspect of health status. Where we observe consistent relationships between trauma and health across domains, we can be more confident that a relationship exists. However, although inconsistent effects may reflect unreliability, they also may provide information about the specificity of a given relationship. For example, physical symptoms may be manifested in the absence of detectable organic pathology. This type of inconsistency can result from a number of factors, including imperfect medical knowledge or sociocultural factors. However, the negative affect associated with traumatic stress may cause biased reports of health status, if individuals interpret physical sensations as symptomatic of illness. Analysis of these consistencies and inconsistencies can help to distinguish whether traumatic stress affects only individual *perceptions* of health status, or actually impairs physical health.

Critical biological functions can also be severely disrupted (e.g., a compromised immune system, occluded arteries) without the subjective experience of physical symptoms. Therefore, laboratory tests and physician diagnoses provide unique information regarding health status. Only a small number of studies have included laboratory tests or physician exams; most have used diagnostic codes from hospital administrative databases, likely because tests and exams are difficult and expensive for larger sample sizes. These health status outcomes are free of potential method variance confounds such as those posed by a negative affect reporting bias. However, detection of morbidity via chart review or administrative databases requires the individual to (a) seek treatment, (b) receive a diagnosis, and (c) have that diagnosis documented in the medical chart. Even documented morbidity is subject to error and bias (e.g., methods of insurance reimbursement that influence charting procedures), and diagnoses often rely to a significant extent on patient report, with its attendant problems. One of the major strengths of laboratory studies is the ability to examine specificity: Trauma exposure may be associated with health impairment over certain organ systems or have a greater impact on the severity of certain disease states.

Most studies cited in this review are cross-sectional, and all data are nonexperimental. These studies provide information about the association between trauma and health, but cannot support causal inferences. Even in cases in which reported trauma precedes the physical health complaints or conditions, one must still be cautious, because memories of trauma may be influenced by current physical or mental health, and other factors may be related to both. Thus we comment on potential confounding factors controlled in statistical analyses while highlighting consistent associations among trauma exposure, PTSD, and health outcomes.

Although we have made important distinctions among different types and measures of health status, *trauma exposure* is not as easily classified. The trauma literature reveals myriad ways to define exposure to traumatic events. In most studies, only one type of exposure is assessed—for example, combat, sexual assault, physical abuse, and so forth. Indeed, this literature is often confounded regarding types of trauma studied, nature of the population, and the detail with which exposure is measured. For example, studies of childhood abuse experiences have largely used clinical populations consisting of women, and rarely have examined the presence of psychiatric disorders. Conversely, studies of combat exposure are conducted primarily with male participants from nonmedical populations, and include evaluations of the presence or absence of PTSD. In some studies, a single question serves as the indicator of exposure, whereas other studies have used more detailed assessments (e.g., Leserman, Li, Drossman, & Hu, 1998). Even detailed approaches vary with regard to how they obtain trauma information, with some addressing the experiences directly ("did you ever experience [event]?"), whereas others approach the assessment more subjectively or subtly (e.g., Walker et al., 1999).

The measurement of trauma history is a challenge in and of itself (Corcoran, Green, Goodman, & Krinsley, 2000), and few studies have attempted to assess the reliability and validity of trauma assessment measures. Furthermore, studies addressing one target event have rarely screened for the presence of other events in a participant's trauma history, making it impossible to link specific exposures with specific outcomes (Green et al.,

2000). Given this state of the art, we review a range of studies with trauma exposure defined and measured in various ways.

TRAUMA EXPOSURE AND HEALTH

In this section, we review studies that have addressed the relationship of trauma exposure to self-reported health, objective health indicators, and mortality.

Trauma Exposure and Self-Reported Health

As previous reviews (Friedman & Schnurr, 1995; Koss & Heslet, 1992; Resnick et al., 1997; Schnurr & Jankowski, 1999) have indicated, there is good evidence for self-reports of impaired physical health among individuals exposed to traumatic stressors. The strongest case for this association can be made from epidemiological data from the general adult population of the United States and from national samples of veteran populations. These data suggest that individuals who are exposed to one or more traumatic events over their lifetime report poorer self-rated health, more physical symptoms, and a greater number of chronic health conditions than do nonexposed individuals. One comprehensive study that relied on self-report health data was the Epidemiologic Catchment Area study (ECA), which included assessments of trauma history and self-reported health outcomes in representative United States samples. In the ECA, a lifetime history of trauma exposure was associated with reports of poor self-rated health and a greater number of chronic medical conditions, even with demographic characteristics, psychiatric history, and other stressful life events controlled (Ullman & Siegel, 1996). Sexual assault was associated with poor self-rated health and increased reports of medical symptoms over a number of organ systems (Golding, 1994), including reproductive health symptoms such as irregular menstruation, painful intercourse, and lack of sexual pleasure (Golding, 1996). A large study of a representative sample of New Zealanders found similar results (Flett, Kazantzis, Long, MacDonald, & Millar, 2002). Although levels of trauma exposure among the 1,500 residents surveyed were somewhat lower than exposure estimates from the United States, exposure to criminal victimization and accidents were each associated with higher levels of current physical symptoms and total chronic symptoms, as well as with chronic limitations in daily functioning.

The health correlates of lifetime trauma exposure among older adults appear similar. A study of 102 adult women over age 60 found that a history of exposure to interpersonal violence was associated with a greater number of self-reported physical symptoms and more current medication use when compared to nonexposed women (Higgins & Follette, 2002).

Trauma exposure has also been associated with a range of self-reported health symptoms among national samples of veterans. This consistency is important because veterans are screened for health problems before entering the military, and these samples may be typically healthier than representative community samples (Schnurr, 1996). The National Vietnam Veterans Readjustment Study (NVVRS) included face-to-face interviews with a nationally representative probability sample of 1,632 male and female Vietnam veterans, and found that degree of combat exposure was significantly associated with poorer reported health status (Kulka et al., 1990). Elder, Shanahan, and Clipp (1997) modeled the effect of combat exposure on self-reports of health status using a sample of World War II veterans from the Stanford-Terman data archives. In the 15 years following the war, individuals exposed to combat showed greater risk of physical decline than noncombat veterans, even when rank, theater, and post-war self-reported physical health were controlled. One of the most comprehensive analyses of combat exposure and health used data from the Veterans Affairs (VA) Normative Aging Study (Schnurr, Spiro, Aldwin, & Stukel, 1998). This 35-year prospective analysis of World War II and Korean Conflict veterans statistically modeled physical symptom trajectories among veterans who experienced no trauma, combat trauma only, noncombat (civilian) trauma only, or both. Men with both types reported 16% more symptoms across all ages.

A cross-sectional study of men and women on active duty in the Army found that noncombat trauma exposure was correlated with increased physical symptom reports (Martin, Rosen, Durand, Knudson, & Stretch, 2000). These results were corroborated by a study evaluating the levels of physical symptom reporting on the Brief Symptom Inventory (Derogatis & Melisaratos, 1983) in a sample of 358 Gulf War mortuary workers before and after their military exposure (McCarroll, Ursano, Fullerton, Liu, & Lundy, 2002). Veterans with the most exposure to the dead reported significantly more physical symptoms following their mortuary experiences when compared with baseline, even when volunteer status, age, gender, depression, fear, and prior exposure were statistically controlled.

However, some data suggest caution in interpreting the strength of the relationship between combat exposure and health status. In a study of more than 4,000 participants in the Vietnam era twin registry studies, a significant relationship was found between combat trauma and reports of hypertension, respiratory conditions, persistent skin conditions, gastrointestinal disorders, joint disorders, and hearing problems. However, when heredity and shared environmental experiences were accounted for, combat trauma explained a much smaller, although still significant, proportion of variance in health complaints (Eisen et al., 1998), suggesting that environmental variables, such as exposure to toxins or early environment, also play a role in the trauma–health relationship, probably by influencing both exposure and health.

In studies of current health status and childhood trauma, there may be a higher likelihood that the exposure preceded the health outcomes. The initial report of the Adverse Childhood Experiences (ACE) study (Felitti et al., 1998) described a mailed survey of 9,500 adult health mainte-nance organization (HMO) patients that investigated the correlation be-tween adverse childhood experiences and adult health risk behavior and disease. Adverse experiences included traumatic exposure and other adverse conditions: sexual, physical, or psychological abuse; exposure to interparental violence; or living in a household in which a member was a substance abuser, mentally ill, suicidal, or imprisoned. Individuals who reported four or more types of adverse childhood experiences were more likely to report chronic bronchitis or emphysema, stroke, cancer, and ischemic heart disease. They were also more likely to report a history of skeletal fractures and hepatitis, and to rate their health status as fair or poor. The authors argued that such adverse childhood experiences contribute to the development of risk behaviors, which may be considered part of the fundamental cause of the reported medical morbidity.

Trauma Exposure and Objective Health Indicators

Several major studies have corroborated self-reports of health status following trauma exposure with physician diagnoses or laboratory tests. One of the largest studies of this type was an investigation of 1,225 randomly selected women subscribers of a large HMO (Walker et al., 1999). Women who were classified as having experienced childhood maltreatment on the basis of a standardized psychometric instrument evidenced greater numbers of medically documented psychiatric and nonpsychiatric medical diagnoses including minor infectious disease, pain disorders, and other conditions (hypertension, diabetes, asthma, allergy, and abnormal uterine bleeding) in the past year, consistent with women's self-reports. In a study of 191 women seen at an outpatient obstetrics and gynecology clinic, those who reported sexual, physical, or emotional abuse during childhood were more likely than nonabused women to be diagnosed with a medical disorder, including excessive bleeding, vaginitis, cervical dysplasia, dysmenorrhea, and infertility (Letourneau, Holmes, & Chasedunn-Roark, 1999).

The Centers for Disease Control (CDC) conducted a large-scale inves-tigation of the health of Vietnam veterans, the Vietnam Experience Study. This study included a telephone survey of more than 7,000 male veterans, and detailed psychological, medical, and laboratory follow-ups on a subsample of

42% of these men. Those who served in Vietnam reported more current use of prescription drugs and a greater prevalence of diseases, somatic symptoms, and fertility problems than those who did not serve (CDC Vietnam Experience Study, 1988). Objective indicators showed more high-frequency hearing loss, occult blood in the stool, history of hepatitis B infections, lower sperm counts, and lower proportions of morphologically normal sperm in the veteran sample. In a comparison of former prisoners of war (POWs) to a demographically matched group of non-POW veterans, investigators examined medical diagnoses based on annual medical exams in the 14 years following military service (Nice, Garland, Hilton, Baggett, & Mitchell, 1996). The POW group had an increased risk for disorders of the peripheral nervous system, joint problems, back problems, and peptic ulcer than the non-POW group. The authors suggested that these illnesses were due in large part to physical effects of torture sustained during captivity.

Corroborating self-reported health with objective indictors of health status in population-based studies is both difficult and expensive. Thus, some investigations have explored the relationship between trauma exposure and medical morbidity by administering trauma history surveys to individuals with and without specific medical diagnoses, finding that those with the medical diagnoses tend to have more extensive trauma histories. For example, among a sample of women in advanced stages of HIV, the prevalence of trauma exposure was significantly higher than in a demographically matched comparison group from the same community who reported negative HIV serostatus (Kimerling, Armistead, & Forehand, 1999). Other researchers have hypothesized that exposure is associated with medically unexplained illness, but not objective disease states. A study of treatment-seeking men and women found higher reports of childhood emotional and physical abuse among individuals diagnosed with either chronic fatigue syndrome or fibromyalgia, compared to demographically similar individuals diagnosed with multiple sclerosis, rheumatoid arthritis, and healthy control groups (Van Houdenhove et al., 2001).

Additional research is still needed to fully understand the relationship between trauma exposure and specific disease states. Research on gastrointestinal disorders, for example, has shown that traumatic exposure may not be related to the presence of these disorders per se, but to a greater frequency of unexplained symptoms, a more severe course of illness, and an increased likelihood of being seen in specialty care (Drossman, 1995; Longstreth & Wolde-Tsadik, 1993). This latter association could result in an upwardly biased estimate of trauma exposure among individuals seen in these settings. More frequent contact with the medical system may also result in a greater likelihood of diagnoses appearing in medical charts. Course of disease may also differ based on trauma history. For example, among women in symptomatic stages of HIV, extent of prior victimization was associated with reports of physical symptoms, poorer functional status, and a faster rate of disease progression (Kimerling, Calhoun, et al., 1999).

Trauma Exposure and Mortality

Several studies have examined the association between trauma exposure and mortality. Sibai, Fletcher, and Armenian (2001) conducted a 10-year follow-up of a group of 1,567 men and women who were exposed to war-related stressors in Lebanon. Increased number of war-related stressors was associated with increased risk for both cardiovascular disease specific deaths and all-cause mortality. Women who experienced loss-related trauma, and men and women who were displaced by war-related events, showed the greatest mortality risks.

The Vietnam Experience Study (CDC Vietnam Experience Study, 1987) also found that the risk of early mortality was 17% higher among Vietnam veterans than among Vietnam-era veterans. This effect occurred primarily in the first 5 years following discharge and was largely attributed to accidental deaths. A study of mortality risk among 4,600 women Vietnam veterans and 5,300 women veterans who served elsewhere suggests that this issue is complex (Thomas, Kang, & Dalager, 1991). All-cause mortality rates did not differ between the two groups. Both groups were at less risk for all-cause mortality compared to U.S. women in general, primarily due to a lower likelihood of death from circulatory disease. However, although suicide rates were similar, there was a small effect for increased mortality from external causes among the Vietnam veterans, primarily due to an excess of motor vehicle accidents. The most pronounced effect was for cancers. Although rates were similar for all cancers combined, Vietnam veterans had twice the risk for mortality from cancers of the pancreas and uterine corpus, compared with non-Vietnam veterans, and to U.S. women in the general population.

Summary

Individuals exposed to trauma report poorer health status and more physical symptoms than do similar nonexposed individuals. Both self-report studies and studies of medical morbidity suggest that this may be due to a greater prevalence of illness for trauma-exposed groups. There is also evidence that trauma exposure is associated with greater functional impairment and a poorer course of disease among individuals with specific medical conditions. Additional research should clarify the conditions under which trauma exposure may impact medical morbidity, as well as how it moderates disease progression. Either increased morbidity or a poorer course of disease could lead to greater mortality risk for trauma-exposed individuals. Future investigations that disentangle the stress-related effects of exposure from associated environmental and behavioral factors that could also contribute to health status would help to clarify our knowledge of the exposure–health relationship.

PTSD AND HEALTH

In this section, we focus on PTSD and health outcomes, including self-reported health, objective health indicators, and mortality.

PTSD and Self-Reported Health

Schnurr and Jankowski (1999) provide an excellent overview of the research findings that have linked PTSD with reports of poor health outcomes. In this section we briefly review several major studies of this link, as well as recent additions to this literature as a prelude to a more in-depth analysis of the literature that has included other health outcomes. The NVVRS data indicated that men and women with PTSD reported a greater number of chronic physical health conditions, and perceived their health to be poorer, than men and women without PTSD (Kulka et al., 1990). Among participants in the VA Normative Aging Study, more severe PTSD was associated with poorer health status as measured by the physical health component score on the SF-36, even when behaviors such as smoking and alcohol consumption were taken into account (Schnurr & Spiro, 1999). In a sample of 363 male World War II veterans exposed to mustard gas, veterans with PTSD reported more chronic health conditions and poorer functional status when compared with veterans without PTSD (Schnurr, Ford, et al., 2000).

One of the largest and most comprehensive studies of PTSD and self-reported health is the CDC Vietnam Experience Study (Boscarino, 1997). A lifetime diagnosis of PTSD was associated with increased risk for reports of chronic disorders including circulatory, digestive, musculoskeletal, endocrine, respiratory, and non-sexually transmitted infectious disease. These analyses controlled for a number of factors thought to affect onset or reports of onset of illness, including intelligence, race, region of birth, enlistment status, army medical profile, hypochondriasis, age, smoking, substance abuse, education, and income. In a telephone survey of 3,682 veterans deployed during the Persian Gulf conflict, veterans who screened positive for current PTSD reported more physical symptoms, medical conditions, and poorer health-related functioning when compared with veterans without PTSD (Barrett et al., 2002). These results persisted even if deployment status, age, sex, ethnicity, rank, branch, military status, and smoking status were controlled.

A recent study of civilians demonstrated the link between self-reported health and PTSD as well. Zatzick, Jurkovich, Gentillelo, Wisner, and Rivara (2002) studied 101 randomly selected survivors of intentional and unintentional injuries who were interviewed, once while hospitalized at a Level 1 trauma center and again a year later. They found that patients who met criteria for PTSD at one year showed significantly worse outcomes (10–40 points lower) on 7 of 8 scales of the SF-36 than those who did not meet PTSD criteria.

PTSD and Objective Health Indicators

In a longitudinal analysis of a community sample of 605 older male veterans of the Korean Conflict and World War II, physical examination revealed that PTSD symptoms were associated with risk of onset for several categories of physician-diagnosed medical problems common to older males: arterial disorders, gastrointestinal disorders, dermatological problems, and musculoskeletal disorders (Schnurr, Spiro, & Paris, 2000). These investigators accounted for factors predictive of health status, such as age, smoking, body mass index (BMI), and alcohol use. A study of 327 male combat veterans seeking trauma-related mental health treatment assessed participants using standardized questionnaires and medical chart review (Beckham et al., 1998). Veterans with PTSD demonstrated more physician-diagnosed medical disorders than veterans without PTSD, even if health behaviors such as smoking were controlled.

Several studies have examined the association between PTSD and cardiovascular health using laboratory findings as outcome measures. In the CDC Vietnam study sample, chronic PTSD was associated with electrocardiogram (ECG) abnormalities, atrioventricular defects, and infarctions (Boscarino & Chang, 1999). The analyses accounted for other factors related to coronary heart disease, including age, ethnicity, education, location of service, medications, drug and alcohol use, body mass index, and cigarette smoking. In another study, Israeli veterans with combat-related PTSD demonstrated poorer performance on laboratory stress tests when compared with noncombat veterans, although no differences were observed in heart rate, blood pressure, or physical exam findings (Shalev, Bleich, & Ursano, 1990). This study controlled for behavioral risk factors for cardiovascular disease, including smoking and substance abuse. Beckham and colleagues (2002) used an anger recall task to study cardiovascular responses to in vivo anger states among 118 male Vietnam combat veterans. Veterans with PTSD demonstrated greater diastolic blood pressure (DBP) in response to anger states and in recovery from anger states when compared with veterans without PTSD. The interaction between PTSD status and a measure of covert hostility significantly predicted DBP during both anger states and recovery, as well as systolic blood pressure (SBP) during recovery from anger states. These analyses accounted for medication, ethnicity, and comorbid psychiatric disorders.

Although not much data exist to inform the link between PTSD and specific disease states, preliminary evidence suggests that, as with trauma exposure, PTSD may be associated with an increased likelihood of being seen in medical settings, with poorer functional outcomes, and with course of disease. A study of untreated PTSD in primary care found poor functional status among these individuals, comparable to chronic medical illness (Fifer et al., 1994). A study of 368 primary care patients also found higher rates of PTSD than in the general population and more health related functional impairment among those diagnosed with PTSD than in individuals without mental health diagnoses (Stein, McQuaid, Pedrelli, Lenox, & McCahill, 2000). In a sample of medical-treatment-seeking patients with irritable bowel syndrome, approximately 36% of patients met criteria for a PTSD diagnosis that preceded the onset of irritable bowel syndrome, suggesting that PTSD is overrepresented in patients with this diagnosis (Irwin et al., 1996). Another study found higher rates of PTSD among HIV-infected women than among a demographically matched comparison group at risk for HIV (Kimerling, Calhoun, et al., 1999). The HIV-infected women with PTSD also showed a more accelerated disease progression over a 1-year observation period.

PTSD and Mortality

One published study thus far has examined PTSD and mortality. In a study of 16,257 male Vietnam veterans from the Agent Orange Registry, investigators compared mortality rates between men with and without PTSD, and compared both groups with standardized mortality ratios for United States men (Bullman & Kang, 1994). Veterans with PTSD were almost four times as likely to die from suicide, and approximately three times more likely to die from accidental poisoning, when compared with veterans without PTSD. Results were similar when veterans with PTSD were compared with standard data of men in the United States of similar age and ethnicity, except that mortality risk for digestive diseases was also elevated.

Summary

The pattern of results for PTSD and health outcomes parallels that for trauma exposure and health. There is some evidence for increased rates of morbidity among individuals with PTSD, and findings attest to the role of PTSD in the course and impact of illness. It therefore follows that PTSD may mediate the relationship between trauma exposure and health outcomes.

PTSD AS A MEDIATOR BETWEEN TRAUMA EXPOSURE AND HEALTH

Friedman and Schnurr (1995) and Schnurr and Jankowski (1999) have proposed that PTSD may be a major pathway by which exposure affects physical health, and this premise is further developed in the remainder of the book. Increasing evidence addresses this mediation hypothesis. Most studies are based on self-report data, but a few studies including medical evaluations have also been conducted. In the remainder of this section, we review the studies that have tested PTSD as a mediator for the relationship between trauma and physical health outcomes. Finally, we review reports that have further tested whether PTSD has a specific impact on health over and above that of mental disorder or distress more generally.

Mediation effects can be demonstrated in several ways, but generally involve a change in the relationship between two variables when a third is introduced in multivariate analysis (Baron & Kenny, 1986). Many studies have linked trauma exposure and health. PTSD would be a mediator of this relationship to the extent that the trauma–health relationship was reduced, or no longer significant, once PTSD was taken into account. This could be assessed in several ways. Physical symptoms or functioning could be assessed for those with and without trauma exposure, and with and without PTSD. It would be demonstrated if only those with trauma *and* PTSD had high levels of physical symptoms or poor physical health (technically, a moderator relationship according to Baron and Kenny). Regression techniques test whether adding PTSD to a regression equation reduces the relationship between exposure and health, and path analysis can test models of the direct and indirect (through PTSD) influence of trauma on health. Studies that examined effects of PTSD in multivariate models controlling for exposure are also reported as consistent with mediation.

Mediation via PTSD

Wolfe, Schnurr, Brown, and Furey (1994) examined 109 female veterans of the Vietnam War via repeated mail surveys of trauma exposure, PTSD, and reported health problems. Although exposure was correlated with all of the health problems, these relationships were reduced when PTSD was controlled, suggesting that PTSD was an important link between the exposure and health. In a further examination of these same data, Friedman and Schnurr (1995) used path analysis to test the direct and indirect effects of exposure on health. For current health, most of the effect of war-zone trauma was indirectly mediated through PTSD (56%), although there was a direct effect as well. Only indirect effects were found for the number of problems reported. Kimerling, Clum, and Wolfe (2000) studied 52 female soldiers from the Vietnam War and found that exposure significantly predicted self-reported physical symptoms and health perceptions in the first step of the regression. Adding PTSD decreased the contribution of exposure to insignificant levels, supporting PTSD as a mediator of the relationship between trauma and health.

Taft, Stern, King, and King (1999) examined the relationships among exposure, PTSD, and health in 1,632 male and female veterans of the Vietnam War (NVVRS) using path analysis. For both genders, combat exposure was directly associated with physical health conditions, but was even more strongly associated through the effect of PTSD on the health conditions. There were no direct effects of combat on functional status. For men, physical health conditions and PTSD both predicted functional status. For women, only health conditions led to functional status. Schnurr and Spiro (1999) examined similar questions using path analysis in more than 900 male veterans as part of the Normative Aging Study. The path model indicated that 90% of the effect of combat on health, measured by the SF-36, was accounted for through PTSD scores. The direct effect of combat on health was not significant.

Wagner, Wolfe, Rotnitsky, Proctor, and Erickson (2000) examined 2,301 Gulf War veterans on their return from the Middle East and again 18–24 months later. Combat was a significant predictor of later health status, and it remained a significant predictor, but its relationship was reduced when PTSD was added to the regression equation. In the sample of World War II veterans exposed to mustard gas (Schnurr, Ford, et al., 2000), Ford and colleagues (2003) examined health conditions, functioning, and service utilization through veteran self-reports obtained in interview sessions. Number of exposures to mustard gas, which was correlated with health in bivariate analyses, had no direct relationship with health status on the SF-36 in the final path model. The health measures were predicted by PTSD symptoms, which were associated with exposure. Health problems and functional status, in turn, predicted self-reported outpatient utilization of services.

Several self-report studies in civilian samples show similar findings. In a sample of 534 Bosnian refugees living in Croatia, Mollica and colleagues (1999) found that disability, as measured by the MOS-20, was significantly related to the combination of PTSD and depression, whereas PTSD alone (an infrequent outcome) was not related. In their regression model, cumulative trauma continued to predict disability, but psychiatric status added significantly to the prediction. In a small sample of sexual assault victims, Clum, Calhoun, and Kimerling (2000) examined PTSD and depression outcomes and their association with exposure and health. Although exposure, especially the perceived severity of the incidents, predicted self-reported symptoms and health perceptions when they were initially entered into the regression equation, exposure no longer significantly predicted these outcomes if depression, and then PTSD, were entered.

In a study of 247 victims of trauma who presented in a regional trauma center following injury (Michaels et al., 2000), Injury Severity Scores were assigned by staff, and initial health and functional status were assessed, along with health-related work status and psychological symptoms. At 6 and 12 months, mailed surveys collected data on PTSD and repeated the initial measures. The investigators found that, controlling for injury severity, 12-month PTSD symptom scores significantly predicted health-related work status at 12 months. A similar study examined 101 injured patients admitted to a trauma center (Zatzick et al., 2002). At 1-year follow-up, PTSD was the strongest predictor of low scores on all subscales of the SF-36 except physical functioning after analyses were adjusted for age, sex, chronic medical conditions, injury severity, and alcohol use. After adjusting for PTSD, injury severity no longer predicted outcome. In a study of 342 Canadian bus drivers (Vedantham et al., 2001), including all those who had experienced a work-related accident, and a random sample of other drivers, the authors compared three groups on health complaints and use of health services: those who had not experienced any work-related trauma, those who were exposed but did not develop PTSD, and those with exposure and PTSD. Findings showed that only the group with exposure *and* PTSD had elevated complaints and service use, indicating that the PTSD, rather than the exposure per se, was driving the health complaints and service use.

A recent study in primary care showed similar findings with regard to PTSD specificity. A multisite study of 502 primary care patients assessed with the SCID DSM–IV (Weisberg et al., 2002) examined trauma, PTSD, and self-reported nonpsychiatric medical conditions in a sample of patients with one or more anxiety disorders. In this study, 46% of patients reported a trauma history, and 37% met full criteria for PTSD. Patients with PTSD reported a significantly greater number of current and lifetime medical conditions than did participants with other anxiety disorders but without PTSD. PTSD was a stronger predictor of reported medical problems than trauma history, physical injury, lifestyle factors, or comorbid depression.

Although self-report data provide an important source of information about health, questions can still be raised about the extent to which reporting biases could account for some of the findings. Thus, it is fortunate that investigators are now looking beyond self-report data to clarify these relationships. Two studies examined physician-diagnosed abnormalities or illness in models that allowed the assessment of mediation effects. In the Schnurr et al. (2000) study of World War II and Korean Conflict combat veterans, PTSD mediation was tested by hierarchical survival analysis for each disorder. Combat exposure predicted onset of arterial, pulmonary, and upper gastrointestinal disorders, as well as other heart disorders. When PTSD was added to the models, only the effect for pulmonary disorders retained significance, indicating a mediation effect for PTSD. The authors noted, however, that the absolute changes were small, and except for arterial disorders, failed to meet established criteria for mediation. They hypothesized that the low base rates of PTSD may have contributed to this finding. A study of 4,462 veterans who served during the Vietnam War evaluated the impact of PTSD on cardiac abnormalities (Boscarino & Chang, 1999). Controlling for demographic variables, service in Vietnam (i.e., exposure), and use of medications and substances, PTSD increased the odds of any ECG abnormality, of atrioventricular conduction defects, and of infarction.

Although PTSD has most often been the diagnosis used in examining the mediating role of mental disorders, a few studies have examined this question more generally (e.g., Holman, Silver, & Waitzkin, 2000). However, these studies examined other disorders without measuring or controlling for PTSD. For this reason, they are somewhat inconclusive and will not be presented here. Depression (in particular) may be an important mediator between traumatic exposure and physical health problems. But it also often co-occurs with PTSD, so that studies not assessing for PTSD are not able to eliminate it as an explanatory factor.

Specificity of PTSD as a Mediator

Fortunately, some studies have now evaluated the specific impact of PTSD on physical health by controlling for other mental disorders and evaluating its unique contribution. Most of these studies have not examined mediation per se, but have assessed whether, with other psychological symptoms or mental disorders controlled, PTSD explains unique variance in an equation predicting health outcomes. In civilian samples, Zoellner, Goodwin, and Foa (2000) found that, among rape victims with chronic PTSD, PTSD severity predicted self-reported physical symptoms even with anger and depression controlled. Clum and colleagues (2000) examined depression and PTSD simultaneously as mediators of physical health outcomes among rape victims. Each contributed unique additional variance to the outcomes of self-reported symptoms and global health perceptions if entered in a regression equation simultaneously. In the Bosnian refugee study of disability, Mollica and colleagues (1999) found that while depression was a significant bivariate predictor of disability, once PTSD and depression combined were accounted for, depression alone no longer predicted health outcomes, or mediated the relationship between trauma and physical health. Andreski, Chilcoat, and Breslau (1998) found that PTSD significantly increased the risk of somatization symptoms in 1,007 HMO participants over and above the total number of psychiatric disorders (anxiety and substance abuse on the Diagnostic Interview Schedule [DIS]), although the role of PTSD was substantially reduced in this model, suggesting that both PTSD *and* other disorders accounted for the relationship with somatic symptoms. The Zatzick and colleagues (2002) study of injured patients at a trauma center controlled for injury severity and concurrent problem drinking and still found that PTSD 1 year after the injury predicted all but 1 of 8 SF-36 scores. Finally, in a study of 326 men and women seeking treatment for anxiety disorders, individuals with PTSD demonstrated poorer scores on the bodily pain, general health, and physical functioning subscales of the SF-36 than did individuals with other anxiety disorders or major depression (Zayfert, Dums, Ferguson, & Hegel, 2002). PTSD continued to demonstrate a unique effect on physical health subscales when the effects of age, depression, and co-morbid anxiety disorders were controlled.

In military samples, Beckham and colleagues (1998) controlled for demographics, combat exposure, smoking, alcohol use, depression, and hypo-chondriasis, and still found that PTSD severity predicted several health outcomes in their sample of combat veterans. Hypochondriasis significantly predicted most of the health outcomes as well. In the anger response study (Beckham et al., 2002), the association of PTSD with cardiovascular re-sponses to anger in Vietnam veterans held even with comorbid psychiatric disorders controlled in the analysis. The Zatzick and colleagues (Zatzick, Marmar, et al., 1997; Zatzick, Weiss, et al., 1997) studies of the NVVRS data sets on male and female Vietnam veterans found significant odds of poorer health outcomes associated with PTSD, even with comorbid disorders taken into account. Currently not working and fair or poor health status continued to be significantly predicted by PTSD in both studies, and addi-tional health variables remained significant in one or the other. Odds ratios for PTSD tended to be reduced somewhat in these models that included comorbid disorders. Boscarino's (1997) analysis of the CDC Vietnam Experi-ence Survey controlled for substance abuse and found that PTSD was asso-ciated with more circulatory, digestive, musculoskeletal, nervous system, respiratory, and infectious diseases. In the cardiovascular study performed with this sample (Boscarino & Chang, 1999), controlling for the effects of other anxiety disorders and depression disorders rendered the nonspecific ECG findings no longer significantly predicted by PTSD. However, the effects for atrioventricular (AV) conduction defect remained the same, whereas those for infarction actually increased.

Taken together, these findings suggest both a general and a specific effect of PTSD on physical health. If other disorders are controlled, the effect of PTSD on health is typically reduced, suggesting that part of the PTSD effect is one associated with psychological distress or psychiatric disorder more generally. The most common other disorder is depression, and these studies suggest that it may play a unique role in health outcomes (see Ford, chap. 4, this volume). However, PTSD clearly plays a unique role as well, beyond what can be explained by distress or disorder more generally, and even depression specifically. This appears to be true for self-reported physical symptoms and distress or disorder, as well as laboratory findings. Although more studies including physical findings are warranted, strong evidence is accumulating that psychiatric disorders in general, and PTSD in particular, play an important role in the link between exposure to traumatic events and adverse health outcomes.

IMPLICATIONS FOR SCREENING

Most people with mental disorders do not seek mental health treatment (Kessler et al., 1994), including those with PTSD (Kessler, Sonnega, Bromet, Hughes, & Nelson, 1995). Furthermore, given the associations with health noted here, and the reluctance of many individuals to seek mental health care in specialty care settings, individuals with trauma and PTSD may be more likely to seek medical treatment for symptoms, and to seek help in primary care settings. Thus, it may make the most sense to screen for trauma and PTSD in these settings. This issue comprises the remainder of our discussion.

Detection of Depression in Primary Care

The literature on mental disorders in primary care has largely focused on depression. Researchers have examined alternative models for assessment of depression in primary care, and have tested these for clinical and cost-effectiveness. Much can be learned from these studies that may apply to PTSD. The Depression Treatment Guidelines, developed by the Agency for Health Care Policy and Research (now the Agency for Healthcare Research and Quality), incorporate some of this research into their treatment guidelines. They note, for example, that psychopharmacologic treatment of depression "transfers" well from specialty to primary care: that is, rates of improvement (50–60%) are similar between the two sites (Schulberg, Katon, Simon, & Rush, 1998). Other research has indicated that treatments in these settings must be enhanced in some way to be effective; that is, "treatment as usual" by primary care physicians is not as effective as treatments that include either specific training of primary care physicians to administer medications or the involvement of mental health professionals in the treatment. Both medication treatments by primary care physicians trained in manualized pharmacotherapy protocols, and interpersonal psychotherapy by trained psychologists and psychiatrists have been shown to be better than usual care for treatment of depression (Schulberg et al., 1996). Collaborative models also work well: either primary care physicians with psychiatrists (medication plus education), or psychiatrists with psychologists (medication plus psychotherapy; Katon et al., 1997). Although findings are mixed regarding whether these treatments, which consistently improve adherence, satisfaction with treatment, and depression outcomes, are cost-effective (Lave, Frank, Schulberg, & Kamlet, 1998; Von Korff et al., 1998; Zhang, Rost, & Fortney, 1999), all of the studies clarify that the involvement of mental health professionals is important for the effective treatment of depression in primary care.

The treatment of depression assumes that it has been initially detected, however, and studies indicate that detection of depression by primary care physicians is low (e.g., Perez-Stable, Miranda, Munoz, & Ying, 1990). Even with interventions to teach physicians how to detect depression, however, treatment has not automatically improved (Katon & Gonzales, 1994; Rost et al. 1998). One of the reasons for this, ironically, is that the presence of chronic medical problems may decrease the likelihood of detecting depression (Rost et al., 2000). A recent study estimated that annual screening for depression would not be cost-effective unless screenings were very inexpensive, there was a high prevalence of depression in the patient population, treatment was initiated in 80% of cases diagnosed, and 85% of patients treated achieved remission (Valenstein, Vijan, Zeber, Boehm, & Buttar, 2001). Periodic screening every 3 to 5 years is cost-effective under more plausible, but still optimistic, assumptions (Valenstein et al., 2001). These results do not contraindicate screening for depression in health care settings but suggest that universal screening alone may not provide benefits to patients commensurate with the effort required. In a review of the literature on screening for depression in primary care, Coyne, Thompson, Palmer, Kagee, and Maunsell (2000) indicated that many screening instruments yield high numbers of false positives due to the difficulties in discriminating depression from general distress. They concluded that routine screening should only be undertaken if (a) resources are available for interpreting the significance of positive screen scores (which do not always indicate a diagnosis), (b) appropriate and acceptable interventions are available, and (c) potential negative effects of screening can be avoided. In fact, a recent study indicated that when routine depression screening is administered in conjunction with treatment enhancement (training and resources for medication or psychotherapy treatments), the package is a cost-effective method (relative to usual care) to increase patient access to effective treatment, and to reduce depression and its associated quality of life and economic burdens (Schoenbaum et al., 2001).

Screening for Traumatic Experiences (Past and Present)

The findings that detection of depression alone is not sufficient to change depression outcomes should give us pause. Nearly all of the studies of the physical health effects of trauma and PTSD conclude with recommendations for routine screening in primary care settings. This proposal seems logical in that primary care is a likely setting for patients with trauma-related physical symptoms to present for treatment. The previously reviewed studies have shown that rates of trauma exposure are relatively high in these settings. For these reasons, the American Medical Association (AMA) has developed guidelines for medical settings and goals for one group of traumatized medical patients: women exposed to interpersonal violence (Council on Scientific Affairs, AMA, 1992). The AMA suggests the importance of training physicians, routine protocols for assessing current and past victimization, the development of response staff within the medical setting, if possible, and the development of referral resources in the community. They go so far as to recommend routine screening, emphasizing the importance of validating the woman's experience, adding such information to medical records, and rapid referral following disclosure. For recommendations of some brief screening strategies in medical settings, see Resnick, Acierno, Holmes, Dammeyer, and Kilpatrick (2000).

Although these recommendations ring true for mental health professionals, even physicians who agree with the logic of such recommendations, and have the time to inquire in the course of an otherwise typically short primary care visit, may be reluctant to do so. A number of studies have documented the low rates of inquiry about ongoing or current domestic violence. For example, Rodriguez, Bauer, McLoughlin, and Grumbach (1999) surveyed 900 family care practitioners and found that only 10% routinely screened new patients for family violence, although most *injured* patients were screened (79%). They cited barriers to screening that suggest physician discomfort with discussing violence, including expectations of patients' fear of retaliation from victimizers, expectation of nondisclosure, potential police involvement, and cultural differences between patient and provider. In a qualitative study of family practitioners, Sugg and Inui (1992) found that physicians were reluctant to screen for domestic violence because of lack of comfort, fear of offending patients by asking, personal or professional powerlessness, loss of control, and time constraints. Although such reluctance is understandable from the standpoint of time and uncertainty about responding, including potential reporting requirements, it also seems to apply to past abuse. McNutt, Carlson, Gagen, and Winterbauer (1999) surveyed 80 women from urban family practice settings about screening for domestic violence. About one quarter of the abused women reported that a physician had previously asked them about violence, whereas only 8% of the nonabused women had been asked. Most women agreed that health care providers should screen women patients for abuse, but some also admitted that they would be inhibited from discussing abuse with physicians. Qualitative studies suggest that women patients often report feeling hesitant to disclose violence if physicians do not address the issue in an open and direct manner as part of their health care (Bauer, Rodriguez, Quiroga, & Flores-Ortiz, 2000; Gerbert, Abercrombie, Caspers, Love, & Bronstone, 1999; McNutt et al., 1999). Patients cite helpful responses as those that validate the experience in a nonblaming manner (Gerbert et al., 1999). In a survey of 164 patients and 27 physicians at public and private primary care sites (Friedman, Samet, Roberts, Hudlin, & Hans, 1992), more than three quarters of the patients (78%) favored routine inquiry about prior physical abuse, and more than two thirds (68%) supported their physicians asking them about past sexual abuse. Nearly all believed that physicians could help with these problems. Yet only 6–7% reported ever being asked about these experiences by their physicians. One third of the physicians reported that they believed these questions should be asked, but only 11% inquired about sexual abuse initially and 15% at a follow-up visit. Physical abuse questions were more common: 33% at initial visit and 40% at follow-up visits. These figures suggest a disconnect between the wishes of abuse survivors, who may or may not link their physical symptoms to prior abuse experiences, and physician behavior.

Interventions that educate providers about intimate partner violence and effective screening methods appear to increase the detection of abuse, to increase referrals to community services (Parker, McFarlane, Soeken, Silva, & Reel, 1999; Wiist & McFarlane, 1999), and to enhance health care providers' comfort in discussing violence with their patients (Thompson et al., 1998). Policies that integrate screening protocols with standard clinic procedures increase detection of and referrals for violence as well (Parker et al., 1999; Waalen, Goodwin, Spitz, Petersen, & Saltzman, 2000; Wiist & McFarlane, 1999). Unfortunately, these positive outcomes are not always linked to improvements in patient well-being. Even with increased screening and detection, physician referrals to community services are not always associated with increased use of these resources (McFarlane, Soeken, Reel, Parker, & Silva, 1997), or with fewer medical visits for abuse-related injuries (Muelleman & Feighny, 1999). Perhaps, in a way similar to depression, greater emphasis on linking enhancement of treatment beyond usual care with these screening practices would result in more effective treatment for violence in health care settings.

Screening for PTSD

We know even less about screening for PTSD in primary care settings. Stein and colleagues (2000) used the Posttraumatic Stress Disorder Checklist—Civilian Version (PCL–C) to screen for PTSD among patients attending a primary care clinic. The investigators screened 368 patients and found that 9% screened positive for PTSD. Those individuals were scheduled for a diagnostic evaluation, and 58% followed through. The remaining 42% either refused or could not be contacted. Diagnoses of PTSD were made using a paper-and-pencil version of the Comprehensive International Diagnostic Interview (CIDI; Kessler et al., 1994). Fewer than half of those who screened positive and took the CIDI met full criteria for PTSD. Sixty-one percent of the patients had comorbid major depression. Thus, of the original 368 patients screened, 8, or about 2%, screened positive and ultimately were diagnosed with PTSD. And it is difficult to know how many of these might have followed through with treatment, if it was offered.

A study at Georgetown University (Krupnick, 2002) provides data on screening, diagnosis, and treatment initiation for a study evaluating the effects of interpersonal group treatment of PTSD for interpersonal trauma. Low-income women are recruited in three county health departments and screened with a 5-item questionnaire about exposure to interpersonal trauma. The 8-item screen developed by Breslau and colleagues (Breslau, Peterson, Kessler, & Schultz, 1999) is used to assess probable PTSD. Very few women (fewer than 5%) have refused screening. Women who screen positive and are not otherwise ineligible are screened a second time and then complete a face-to-face diagnostic interview, including the Stressful Life Events Screening Questionnaire for trauma history (Goodman, Corcoran, Turner, Yuan, & Green, 1998) and the CAPS (Weathers, 1996) for PTSD. Women with PTSD are provided free, on-site treatment or are placed in a wait-list control group. About 8% of the women screen positive for current PTSD, and about two thirds of those have comorbid major depression. The 8% figure is congruent with Stein and colleagues (2000), as well as other studies of PTSD in the general population, in which rates based on diagnostic interview are about 4–5% for current PTSD in women.

Of the 161 women who screened positive and were assigned to the study, 30% decided not to continue on with screening or treatment for various reasons. Of those who initially screened positive, 11% of those who received a second screening about 1 week later no longer screened positive. Of those who did rescreen positive, all but one met full criteria for PTSD at clinical interview, indicating good validity for the screener and suggesting that sequential screening was an excellent way to identify those with bona fide PTSD. Forty-five women began treatment or were assigned to a wait list, approximately 28% of the initial screen positive sample, whereas 20% indicated lack of interest following administration of the CIDI. Only five patients dropped out of treatment once they had started.

These figures suggest that it is labor intensive to screen relative to the number of women who ultimately follow through with treatment (or are willing to, in the case of the control groups). This may in part be due to multiple stages of screening. For some women, it was related to their schedules; many were working shifts or more than one job, or were caring for young children or relatives, and they may not have been able to make a commitment to a course of treatment. However, of all of the women initially screened, only about 2–3% had PTSD *and* made it into treatment (or to the wait list). Although having 28% of those with PTSD carry through with randomization represents a good participation rate, it took multiple calls and conversations with the women to get each of the interviews scheduled. The women who started treatment tended to continue it, and to improve, but the cost was high. It seems important then, to develop multiple approaches to helping patients with trauma exposure and PTSD.

Going forward, it seems important to do more than call for screening in primary care. We need to be clear about the purpose of screening for trauma and for PTSD. In cases of current abuse, it may be for intervention in the violence, reporting to authorities, getting patients to a safe setting, and so forth. In other cases, it may be to help the physician or other care providers understand better whether or not the patient's current health picture is related to his or her trauma experiences, so they might have more information for diagnostic purposes, or to help the patient understand their current problems. In still other cases, it may be to determine if the patient needs mental health treatment, either medication or therapy, administered either by the primary care physician or a mental health specialist, and if so, whether the patient is psychologically ready to accept the diagnosis and the need for treatment. In future studies, it will be important to assess how patients get to treatment and whether it improves their mental and physical health. There is much to learn.

CONCLUSIONS AND FUTURE DIRECTIONS

In summary, individuals exposed to trauma report poorer health status and more physical symptoms than do similar nonexposed individuals; and objective indicators of physical health, such as medical diagnosis and laboratory findings, support this relationship as well. Trauma exposure is also associated with greater functional impairment and a poorer course of disease among individuals with specific medical conditions. The pattern of results for PTSD and health outcomes appears to parallel that for trauma exposure and health, with self-reports, objective indicators, and course of illness being associated with PTSD. PTSD consistently mediates the relationship between trauma exposure and health outcomes, with several studies indicating that this mediation holds, although the absolute effect may be reduced, even if other psychiatric disorders are taken into account. These latter studies support both general and specific effects of PTSD on physical health. Although more studies including physical findings are needed, it seems clear that PTSD plays an important role in the link between exposure to traumatic events and adverse health outcomes. Although PTSD screening studies in primary care are just beginning, and useful guidelines for such screening are still to be developed, the role of PTSD in medical outcomes clearly suggests that it needs to be more carefully attended to in primary care settings.

REFERENCES

Andreski, P., Chilcoat, H. D., & Breslau, N. (1998). Post-traumatic stress disorder and somatization symptoms: A prospective study. *Psychiatry Research, 79,* 131–138.

Baron, R. M., & Kenny, D. A. (1986). The moderator-mediator variable distinction in social psychological research: Conceptual, strategic, and statistical considerations. *Journal of Personality and Social Psychology, 51,* 1173–1182.

Barrett, D. H., Doebbeling, C. C., Schwartz, D. A., Voelker, M. D., Falter, K. H., Woolson, R. F., et al. (2002). Posttraumatic stress disorder and self-reported physical health status among U. S. military personnel serving during the Gulf War period: Population-based study. *Psychosomatics, 43,* 195–205.

Bauer, H. M., Rodriguez, M. A., Quiroga, S. S., & Flores-Ortiz, Y. G. (2000). Barriers to health care for abused Latina and Asian immigrant women. *Journal of Health Care for the Poor and Underserved, 11,* 33–44.

Beckham, J. C., Moore, S. D., Feldman, M. E., Hertzberg, M. A., Kirby, A. C., & Fairbank, J. A. (1998). Health status, somatization, and severity of posttraumatic stress disorder in Vietnam combat veterans with posttraumatic stress disorder. *American Journal of Psychiatry, 155,* 1565–1569.

Beckham, J. C., Vrana, S. R., Barefoot, J. C., Feldman, M. E., Fairbank, J. A., & Moore, S. D. (2002). Magnitude and duration of cardiovascular responses to anger in Vietnam veterans with and without posttraumatic stress disorder. *Journal of Consulting and Clinical Psychology, 70,* 228–234.

Boscarino, J. A. (1997). Diseases among men 20 years after exposure to severe stress: Implications for clinical research and medical care. *Psychosomatic Medicine, 59,* 605–614.

Boscarino, J. A., & Chang, J. (1999). Electrocardiogram abnormalities among men with stress-related psychiatric disorders: Implications for coronary heart disease and clinical research. *Annals of Behavioral Medicine, 21*, 227–234.

Breslau, N., Peterson, E. L., Kessler, R. C., & Schultz, L. R. (1999). Short screening scale for DSM-IV posttraumatic stress disorder. *American Journal of Psychiatry, 156*, 908–911.

Bullman, T. A., & Kang, H. K. (1994). Posttraumatic stress disorder and the risk of traumatic deaths among Vietnam veterans. *Journal of Nervous and Mental Disease, 182*, 604–610.

Centers for Disease Control Vietnam Experience Study. (1987). Postservice mortality among Vietnam veterans. *Journal of the American Medical Association, 257*, 790–795.

Centers for Disease Control Vietnam Experience Study. (1988). Health status of Vietnam veterans. II. Physical health. The Centers for Disease Control Vietnam Experience Study. *Journal of the American Medical Association, 259*, 2708–2714.

Clum, G. A., Calhoun, K. S., & Kimerling, R. (2000). Associations among symptoms of depression and posttraumatic stress disorder and self-reported health in sexually assaulted women. *Journal of Nervous and Mental Disease, 188*, 671–678.

Corcoran, C. B., Green, B. L., Goodman, L., & Krinsley, K. (2000). Conceptual and methodological issues in trauma history assessment. In A. Shalev, R. Yehuda, & A. McFarlane (Eds.), *International handbook of human response to trauma* (pp. 223–232). New York: Kluwer Academic/Plenum Publishers.

Council on Scientific Affairs, American Medical Association. (1992). Violence against women: Relevance for medical practitioners. *Journal of the American Medical Association, 267*, 3184–3189.

Coyne, J. C., Thompson, R., Palmer, S. C., Kagee, A., & Maunsell, E. (2000). Should we screen for depression? Caveats and potential pitfalls. *Applied and Preventive Psychology, 9*, 101–121.

Derogatis, L. R., & Melisaratos, N. (1983). The Brief Symptom Inventory: An introductory report. *Psychological Medicine, 13*, 595–605.

Drossman, D. A. (1995). Sexual and physical abuse and gastrointestinal illness. *Scandinavian Journal of Gastroenterology (Supplement), 208*, 90–96.

Eisen, S. A., Neuman, R., Goldberg, J., True, W. R., Rice, J., Scherrer, J. F., et al. (1998). Contribution of emotionally traumatic events and inheritance to the report of current physical health problems in 4,042 Vietnam era veteran twin pairs. *Psychosomatic Medicine, 60*, 533–539.

Elder, G. H., Jr., Shanahan, M. J., & Clipp, E. C. (1997). Linking combat and physical health: The legacy of World War II in men's lives. *American Journal of Psychiatry, 154*, 330–336.

Felitti, V. J., Anda, R. F., Nordenberg, D., Williamson, D. F., Spitz, A. M., Edwards, V., et al. (1998). Relationship of childhood abuse and household dysfunction to many of the leading causes of death in adults: The Adverse Childhood

Experiences (ACE) study. *American Journal of Preventive Medicine, 14,* 245–258.

Fifer, S. K., Mathias, S. D., Patrick, D. L., Mazonson, P. D., Lubeck, D. P., & Buesching, D. P. (1994). Untreated anxiety among adult primary care patients in a health maintenance organization. *Archives of General Psychiatry, 51,* 740–750.

Flett, R. A., Kazantzis, N., Long, N. R., MacDonald, C., & Millar, M. (2002). Traumatic events and physical health in a New Zealand community sample. *Journal of Traumatic Stress, 15,* 303–312.

Ford, J. D., Schnurr, P. P., Friedman, M. J., Green, B. L., Adams, G., & Jex, S. (2003). *Posttraumatic stress disorder symptoms, physical health outcomes, and health care utilization fifty years after exposure to a toxic gas.* Manuscript submitted for publication.

Friedman, L. S., Samet, J. H., Roberts, M. S., Hudlin, M., & Hans, P. (1992). Inquiry about victimization experiences: A survey of patient preferences and physician practices. *Archives of Internal Medicine, 152,* 1186–1190.

Friedman, M. J., & Schnurr, P. P. (1995). The relationship between trauma, post-traumatic stress disorder, and physical health. In M. J. Friedman, D. S. Charney, & A. Y. Deutch (Eds.), *Neurobiological and clinical consequences of stress: From normal adaptation to post-traumatic stress disorder* (pp. 507–524). Philadelphia: Raven.

Gerbert, B., Abercrombie, P., Caspers, N., Love, C., & Bronstone, A. (1999). How health care providers help battered women: The survivor's perspective. *Women and Health, 29,* 115–135.

Golding, J. M. (1994). Sexual assault history and physical health in randomly selected Los Angeles women. *Health Psychology, 13,* 130–138.

Golding, J. M. (1996). Sexual assault history and women's reproductive and sexual health. *Psychology of Women Quarterly, 20,* 101–121.

Goodman, L. A., Corcoran, C., Turner, K., Yuan, N., & Green, B. L. (1998). Assessing traumatic event exposure: General issues and preliminary findings for the Stressful Life Events Screening Questionnaire. *Journal of Traumatic Stress, 11,* 521–542.

Green, B. L., Goodman L. A., Krupnick, J. L., Corcoran, C. B., Petty, R. M., Stockton, P., et al. (2000). Outcomes of single versus multiple trauma exposure in a screening sample. *Journal of Traumatic Stress, 13,* 271–286.

Hennessy, C. H., Moriarty, D. G., Zack, M. M., Scherr, P. A., & Brackbill, R. (1994). Measuring health-related quality of life for public health surveillance. *Public Health Reports, 109,* 665–672.

Higgins, A. B., & Follette, V. M. (2002). Frequency and impact of interpersonal trauma in older women. *Journal of Clinical Geropsychology, 8,* 215–226.

Holman, E. A., Silver, R. C., & Waitzkin, H. (2000). Traumatic life events in primary care patients. *Archives of Family Medicine, 9,* 802–810.

Idler, E. L., & Angel, R. J. (1990). Self-rated health and mortality in the NHANES-I Epidemiologic Follow-up Study. *American Journal of Public Health, 80*, 446–452.

Idler, E. L., & Kasl, S. (1991). Health perceptions and survival: Do global evaluations of health status really predict mortality? *Journal of Gerontology, 46*, S55–S65.

Irwin, C., Falsetti, S. A., Lydiard, R. B., Ballenger, J. C., Brock, C. D., & Brener, W. (1996). Comorbidity of posttraumatic stress disorder and irritable bowel syndrome. *Journal of Clinical Psychiatry, 57*, 576–578.

Katon, W. J., & Gonzales, J. (1994). A review of randomized trials of psychiatric consultation-liaison studies in primary care. *Psychosomatics, 35*, 268–278.

Katon, W. J., Von Korff, M., Lin, E., Simon, G., Walker, E. A., & Ludman, E. (1997). Collaborative management to achieve depression treatment guidelines. *Journal of Clinical Psychiatry, 58*(Suppl. 1), 20–23.

Kessler, R. C., McGonagle, K. A., Zhao, S., Nelson, C. B., Hughes, M., Eshleman, S., et al. (1994). Lifetime and 12-month prevalence of DSM-III-R psychiatric disorders in the United States. *Archives of General Psychiatry, 51*, 8–19.

Kessler, R. C., Sonnega, A., Bromet, E., Hughes, M., & Nelson, C. B. (1995). Posttraumatic stress disorder in the National Comorbidity Survey. *Archives of General Psychiatry, 52*, 1048–1060.

Kimerling, R., Armistead, L., & Forehand, R. (1999). Victimization experiences and HIV infection in women: Associations with serostatus, psychological symptoms, and health status. *Journal of Traumatic Stress, 12*, 41–58.

Kimerling, R., Calhoun, K. S., Forehand, R., Armistead, L., Morse, E., Morse, P., et al. (1999). Traumatic stress in HIV-infected women. *AIDS Education and Prevention, 11*, 321–330.

Kimerling, R., Clum, G. A., & Wolfe, J. (2000). Relationships among trauma exposure, chronic posttraumatic stress disorder symptoms, and self-reported health in women: Replication and extension. *Journal of Traumatic Stress, 13*, 115–128.

Koss, M. P., & Heslet, L. (1992). Somatic consequences of violence against women. *Archives of Family Medicine, 1*, 53–59.

Krupnick, J. L. (2002, November). Interpersonal psychotherapy groups with low-income women with PTSD. In N. Talbot (Chair), *Emerging findings on psychotherapies for PTSD in community settings.* Symposium conducted at the meeting of the International Society for Traumatic Stress Studies, Baltimore, MD.

Kulka, R. A., Schlenger, W. E., Fairbank, J. A., Hough, R. L., Jordan, B. K., Marmar, C. R., et al. (1990). *Trauma and the Vietnam war generation: Report of findings from the National Vietnam Veterans Readjustment Study.* New York: Brunner/Mazel.

Lave, J. R., Frank, R. G., Schulberg, H. C., & Kamlet, M. S. (1998). Cost-effectiveness of treatments for major depression in primary care practice. *Archives of General Psychiatry, 55*, 645–651.

Leserman, J., Li, Z., Drossman, D. A., & Hu, Y. J. B. (1998). Selected symptoms associated with sexual and physical abuse history among female patients with gastrointestinal disorders: The impact on subsequent health care visits. *Psychological Medicine, 28,* 417–425.

Letourneau, E. J., Holmes, M. M., & Chasedunn-Roark, J. (1999). Gynecologic health consequences to victims of interpersonal violence. *Women's Health Issues, 9,* 115–120.

Longstreth, G. F., & Wolde-Tsadik, G. (1993). Irritable bowel-type symptoms in HMO examinees: Prevalence, demographics, and clinical correlates. *Digestive Diseases and Sciences, 38,* 1581–1589.

Martin, L., Rosen, L. N., Durand, D. B., Knudson, K. H., & Stretch, R. H. (2000). Psychological and physical health effects of sexual assaults and nonsexual traumas among male and female United States Army soldiers. *Behavioral Medicine, 26,* 23–33.

McCarroll, J. E., Ursano, R. J., Fullerton, C. S., Liu, X., & Lundy, A. (2002). Somatic symptoms in Gulf War mortuary workers. *Psychosomatic Medicine, 64,* 29–33.

McFarlane, J., Soeken, K., Reel, S., Parker, B., & Silva, C. (1997). Resource use by abused women following an intervention program: Associated severity of abuse and reports of abuse ending. *Public Health Nursing, 14,* 244–250.

McNutt, L. A., Carlson, B. E., Gagen, D., & Winterbauer, N. (1999). Reproductive violence screening in primary care: Perspectives and experiences of patients and battered women. *Journal of the American Medical Women's Association, 54,* 85–90.

Michaels, A. J., Michaels, C. E., Smith, J. S., Moon, C. H., Peterson, C., & Long, W. B. (2000). Outcome from injury: General health, work status, and satisfaction 12 months after trauma. *Journal of Trauma: Injury, Infection, and Critical Care, 48,* 841–850.

Mollica, R. F., McInnes, K., Sarajlic, N., Lavelle, J., Sarajlic, I., & Massagli, M. P. (1999). Disability associated with psychiatric comorbidity and health status in Bosnian refugees living in Croatia. *Journal of the American Medical Association, 282,* 433–439.

Muelleman, R. L., & Feighny, K. M. (1999). Effects of an emergency department-based advocacy program for battered women on community resource utilization. *Annals of Emergency Medicine, 33,* 62–66.

Nice, D. S., Garland, C. F., Hilton, S. M., Baggett, J. C., & Mitchell, R. E. (1996). Long-term health outcomes and medical effects of torture among U.S. Navy prisoners of war in Vietnam. *Journal of the American Medical Association, 276,* 375–381.

Parker, B., McFarlane, J., Soeken, K., Silva, C., & Reel, S. (1999). Testing an intervention to prevent further abuse to pregnant women. *Research in Nursing and Health, 22,* 59–66.

Perez-Stable, E. J., Miranda, J., Munoz, R. F., & Ying, Y. W. (1990). Depression in medical outpatients: Underrecognition and misdiagnosis. *Archives of Internal Medicine, 150,* 1083–1088.

Resnick, H. S., Acierno, R., Holmes, M., Dammeyer, M., & Kilpatrick, D. (2000). Emergency evaluation and intervention with female victims of rape and other violence. *Journal of Clinical Psychology, 56,* 1317–1333.

Resnick, H. S., Acierno, R., & Kilpatrick, D. G. (1997). Medical and mental health outcomes: Part 2. Health impact of interpersonal violence. *Behavioral Medicine, 23,* 65–78.

Rodriguez, M. A., Bauer, H. M., McLoughlin, E., & Grumbach, K. (1999). Screening and intervention for intimate partner abuse: Practices and attitudes of primary care physicians. *Journal of the American Medical Association, 282,* 468–474.

Rost, K. M., Nutting, P., Smith, J., Coyne, J., Cooper-Patrick, L., & Rubenstein, L. (2000). The role of competing demands in the primary care of patients with major depression. *Archives of Family Medicine, 9,* 150–154.

Rost, K. M., Zhang, M., Fortney, J., Smith, J., Coyne, J., & Smith, G. R., Jr. (1998). Persistently poor outcomes of undetected major depression in primary care. *General Hospital Psychiatry, 20,* 12–20.

Schnurr, P. P. (1996). Trauma, PTSD, and physical health. *PTSD Research Quarterly, 7*(3), 1–6.

Schnurr, P. P., Ford, J. D., Friedman, M. J., Green, B. L., Dain, B. J., & Sengupta, A. (2000). Predictors and outcomes of posttraumatic stress disorder in World War II veterans exposed to mustard gas. *Journal of Consulting and Clinical Psychology, 68,* 258–268.

Schnurr, P. P., & Jankowski, M. K. (1999). Physical health and post-traumatic stress disorder: Review and synthesis. *Seminars in Clinical Neuropsychiatry, 4,* 295–304.

Schnurr, P. P., & Spiro, A., III. (1999). Combat exposure, posttraumatic stress disorder symptoms, and health behaviors as predictors of self-reported physical health in older veterans. *Journal of Nervous and Mental Disease, 187,* 353–359.

Schnurr, P. P., Spiro, A., III, Aldwin, C. M., & Stukel, T. A. (1998). Physical symptom trajectories following trauma exposure: Longitudinal findings from the Normative Aging Study. *Journal of Nervous and Mental Disease, 186,* 522–528.

Schnurr, P. P., Spiro, A., III, & Paris, A. H. (2000). Physician-diagnosed medical disorders in relation to PTSD symptoms in older male military veterans. *Health Psychology, 19,* 91–97.

Schoenbaum, M., Unutzer, J., Sherbourne, C., Duan, N., Rubenstein, L., Miranda, J., et al. (2001). Cost-effectiveness of practice-initiated quality improvement for depression: Results of a randomized controlled trial. *Journal of the American Medical Association, 286,* 1325–1330.

Schulberg, H. C., Block, M. R., Madonia, M. J., Scott, C. P., Rodriguez, E., Imber, S. D., et al. (1996). Treating major depression in primary care practice: Eight-month clinical outcomes. *Archives of General Psychiatry, 53,* 913–919.

Schulberg, H. C., Katon, W., Simon, G. E., & Rush, A. J. (1998). Treating major care depression in primary care practice: An update of the Agency for Health Care Policy and Research Practice Guidelines. *Archives of General Psychiatry, 55,* 1121–1127.

Shalev, A., Bleich, A., & Ursano, R. J. (1990). Posttraumatic stress disorder: Somatic comorbidity and effort tolerance. *Psychosomatics, 31,* 197–203.

Sibai, A. M., Fletcher, A., & Armenian, H. K. (2001). Variations in the impact of long-term wartime stressors on mortality among the middle-aged and older population in Beirut, Lebanon, 1983–1993. *American Journal of Epidemiology, 154,* 128–137.

Stein, M. B., McQuaid, J. R., Pedrelli, P., Lenox, R., & McCahill, M. E. (2000). Posttraumatic stress disorder in the primary care medical setting. *General Hospital Psychiatry, 22,* 261–269.

Sugg, N. K., & Inui, T. (1992). Primary care physicians' response to domestic violence: Opening Pandora's box. *Journal of the American Medical Association, 267,* 3157–3160.

Taft, C. T., Stern, A. S., King, L. A., & King, D. W. (1999). Modeling physical health and functional health status: The role of combat exposure, posttraumatic stress disorder, and personal resource attributes. *Journal of Traumatic Stress, 12,* 3–23.

Thomas, T. L., Kang, H. K., & Dalager, N. A. (1991). Mortality among women Vietnam veterans, 1973–1987. *American Journal of Epidemiology, 134,* 973–980.

Thompson, R. S., Meyer, B. A., Smith-DiJulio, K., Caplow, M. P., Maiuro, R. D., Thompson, D., et al. (1998). A training program to improve domestic violence identification and management in primary care: Preliminary results. *Violence and Victims, 13,* 395–410.

Ullman, S. E., & Siegel, J. M. (1996). Traumatic events and physical health in a community sample. *Journal of Traumatic Stress, 9,* 703–720.

Valenstein, M., Vijan, S., Zeber, J. E., Boehm, K., & Buttar, A. (2001). The cost-utility of screening for depression in primary care. *Annals of Internal Medicine, 134,* 345–360.

Van Houdenhove, B., Neerinckx, E., Lysens, R., Vertommen, H., Van Houdenhove, L., Onghena, P., et al. (2001). Victimization in chronic fatigue syndrome and fibromyalgia in tertiary care: A controlled study on prevalence and characteristics. *Psychosomatics, 42,* 21–28.

Vedantham, K., Brunet, A., Boyer, R., Weiss, D. S., Metzler, T. J., & Marmar, C. R. (2001). Posttraumatic stress disorder, trauma exposure, and the current health of Canadian bus drivers. *Canadian Journal of Psychiatry, 46,* 149–155.

Von Korff, M., Katon, W., Bush, T., Lin, E., Simon, G., Saunders, K., et al. (1998). Treatment costs, cost offset, and cost-effectiveness of collaborative management of depression. *Psychosomatic Medicine, 60,* 143–149.

Waalen, J., Goodwin, M. M., Spitz, A. M., Petersen, R., & Saltzman, L. E. (2000). Screening for intimate partner violence by health care providers: Barriers and interventions. *American Journal of Preventive Medicine, 19,* 230–237.

Wagner, A. W., Wolfe, J., Rotnitsky, A., Proctor, S. P., & Erickson, D. J. (2000). An investigation of the impact of posttraumatic stress disorder on physical health. *Journal of Traumatic Stress, 13,* 41–55.

Walker, E. A., Gelfand, A. N., Katon, W. J., Koss, M. P., Von Korff, M., Bernstein, D. E., et al. (1999). Adult health status of women with histories of childhood abuse and neglect. *American Journal of Medicine, 107,* 332–339.

Weathers, F. W. (1996). Psychometric review of the Clinician Administered PTSD Scale (CAPS). In B. H. Stamm (Ed.), *Measurement of stress, trauma, and adaptation* (pp. 106–107). Lutherville, MD: Sidran Press.

Weisberg, R. B., Bruce, S. E., Machan, J. T., Kessler, R. C., Culpepper, L., & Keller, M. B. (2002). Nonpsychiatric illness among primary care patients with trauma histories and posttraumatic stress disorder. *Psychiatric Services, 53,* 848–854.

Wiist, W. H., & McFarlane, J. (1999). The effectiveness of an abuse assessment protocol in public health prenatal clinics. *American Journal of Public Health, 89,* 1217–1221.

Wilson, I. B., & Cleary, P. D. (1995). Linking clinical variables with health-related quality of life. *Journal of the American Medical Association, 273,* 59–65.

Wolfe, J., Schnurr, P. P., Brown, P. J., & Furey, J. (1994). Posttraumatic stress disorder and war-zone exposure as correlates of perceived health in female Vietnam War veterans. *Journal of Consulting and Clinical Psychology, 62,* 1235–1240.

Zatzick, D., Jurkovich, G. J., Gentillelo, L., Wisner, D., & Rivara, F. P. (2002). Posttraumatic stress, problem drinking, and functional outcomes after injury. *Archives of Surgery, 137,* 200–205.

Zatzick, D., Marmar, C. R., Weiss, D. S., Browner, W. S., Metzler, T. J., Golding, J. M., et al. (1997). Posttraumatic stress disorder and functioning and quality of life outcomes in a nationally representative sample of male Vietnam veterans. *American Journal of Psychiatry, 154,* 1690–1695.

Zatzick, D., Weiss, D. S., Marmar, C. R., Metzler, T. J., Wells, K., Golding, J. M., et al. (1997). Post-traumatic stress disorder and functioning and quality of life outcomes in female Vietnam veterans. *Military Medicine, 162,* 661–665.

Zayfert, C., Dums, A. R., Ferguson, R. J., & Hegel, M. T. (2002). Health functioning impairments associated with posttraumatic stress disorder, anxiety disorders, and depression. *Journal of Nervous and Mental Disease, 190,* 233–240.

Zhang, M., Rost, K. M., & Fortney, J. (1999). Earnings changes for depressed individuals treated by mental health specialists. *American Journal of Psychiatry, 156,* 108–114.

Zoellner, L. A., Goodwin, M. L., & Foa, E. B. (2000). PTSD severity and health perceptions in female victims of sexual assault. *Journal of Traumatic Stress, 13,* 635–649.

3

COSTS AND HEALTH CARE UTILIZATION ASSOCIATED WITH TRAUMATIC EXPERIENCES

EDWARD A. WALKER, ELANA NEWMAN, AND MARY P. KOSS

Although the past decade of research has documented the use of health care facilities by trauma survivors and has provided evidence about the need to address traumatic symptoms in non-mental health facilities, there is now a need to use more advanced approaches that have greater potential to affect public health care policy. To shape mental and physical health care policy to meet the needs of trauma-exposed people, researchers need to integrate economic analytic approaches in their work.

This chapter is an overview of the issues facing the next generation of research in trauma treatment. It summarizes the economic consequences of the detection and nondetection of trauma status in health care settings, associated costs and impacts on utilization, and how research and policy barriers might be overcome by targeted health services research designs. We are just beginning to see the first well-designed studies of the actual cost to medical care plans of the trauma response itself as well as its treatment.

We appreciate the editorial comments of Caroline Pyevich, University of Tulsa.

Because of the small number of studies, we spend the majority of this chapter outlining some design challenges that face health services researchers, as investigators might benefit from recognizing the complexities of measuring and analyzing these data. By understanding these issues, trauma specialists interested in creating, testing, and evaluating treatments can be better equipped to influence policy changes in future service delivery.

We review core concepts of service utilization, cost analysis, and the potential impact of disclosure of trauma histories on eligibility for insurance. We also examine statistical issues regarding the proper interpretation of cost data with particular focus on analytic methods and study design that are appropriate to account for the large variability in service utilization and medical system design.

Exposure to traumatic life events has long been associated with the development of a wide range of immediate and later-appearing psychological outcomes, particularly depression and anxiety (Neumann, Houskamp, Pollock, & Briere, 1996; Saunders, Kilpatrick, Hanson, Resnick, & Walker, 1999; Widom, 1999). During the past decade we have become aware of an additional connection between traumatic life events and adverse medical symptoms (Allers, Benjack, White, & Rousey, 1993; Dickinson, deGruy, Dickinson, & Candib, 1999; Golding, 1996, 1999; Schnurr & Jankowski, 1999; Spak, Spak, & Allebeck, 1998; Widom & Kuhns, 1996; see also Green & Kimerling, chap. 2, this volume).

As the authors of these publications have shown, a remarkable amount of data have recently been collected in medical settings on the prevalence of individuals who have had traumatic experiences, as well as on their medical symptoms. Nevertheless, these findings are only a first step in translating these epidemiological data into meaningful changes in health care policy. A second generation of research is now investigating how trauma-related responses impact medical care utilization, costs, access to care, and eligibility for insurance. This literature ultimately may change the way treatment is provided for trauma survivors, as health care policy planners quantitatively assess how to spend diagnostic and treatment dollars.

HOW DO PEOPLE DECIDE TO USE HEALTH CARE?

The use of medical services is a complex behavior. Individuals exhibit great variability as to whether and how they present for care. Imagine for a moment that we could create an unpleasant physical symptom in a large group of individuals. The decision about what to do about that symptom will be a function of a number of constitutional, personal, economic, and cultural factors (Andersen, 1995). Personality characteristics such as stoicism or hypochondriasis, cultural beliefs about illness, past experiences of sickness (both personal and family), sense of control and mastery, and individual genetic predispositions to physical disease will ultimately converge into a decision about whether to pursue medical care.

Furthermore, availability of insurance, access to a health care provider, socioeconomic status, availability of appointments that do not cause one to lose time at work, and availability of child care also contribute to use of services. For example, proximity to a Veterans Affairs (VA) Medical Center outpatient clinic and receipt of VA compensation were positively associated with timeliness, as well as access and intensity of service use among veterans with mental disorders (Druss & Rosenheck, 1997). Finally, cultural factors, including attitudes toward health professionals and religiosity, can influence health care utilization. These factors (most of which are not measured in studies of trauma-related health effects) confound our ability to understand the link between trauma and health care utilization (Andersen, 1995).

DEFINING AND MEASURING UTILIZATION

More and more trauma experts are examining service or health care utilization (e.g., Golding, Stein, Siegel, Burnam, & Sorenson, 1988; Schnurr, Friedman, Sengupta, Jankowski, & Holmes, 2000). Utilization includes primary care services, specialist visits, use of pharmacy services, ancillary services (e.g., laboratory), emergency room visits, and inpatient hospitalization. Studying utilization data yields intuitively helpful information and is consistent with local practitioners and administrators' approaches to provide services, the process of counting visits. Utilization data are often helpful in comparing systems when charges and collection rates vary in different insurance markets.

Nevertheless, this approach may have significant shortcomings because the data may not generalize across differing heath care systems. For example, health care systems can vary in the way patients access providers, with some allowing patients to seek treatment in expensive emergency room or specialty care settings, whereas others encourage a more cost-effective primary care gatekeeping strategy. Equal numbers of visits in these settings do not generate comparable costs, and studies that rely on utilization data must carefully stratify by type of service. Furthermore, utilization data may not describe ease of access. Systems that do not provide primary care entry points tend to force initial contacts into specialty or emergency room services in which volume or appointment delays may discourage utilization. This is particularly true in managed mental health systems in which patients ultimately may not make or keep appointments due to the number of barriers (e.g., preauthorization by insurance carrier, difficulty getting to the mental health clinic) placed in their way. It is likely that ultimate health care policy will be determined with respect to cost, not usage. Hence, utilization data per se do not necessarily help policymakers in their overall approach to managing a health care system.

ARE THERE DIFFERENCES BETWEEN OBJECTIVE AND SELF-REPORTED UTILIZATION?

Although automated utilization data captured in health plans is most desirable, self-report utilization sometimes is an appropriate substitute. In fact, most published studies examining trauma survivors' health care use have relied solely on self-report (e.g., Amaya-Jackson et al., 1999; Boscarino, 1997; Golding et al., 1988; Rosenheck & Fontana, 1994; Rosenheck & Massari, 1993; Schnurr, Friedman, et al., 2000; Shariat, Mallonee, Kruger, Farmer, & North, 1999; Switzer et al., 1999). Unfortunately, like most self-report data, there is high variability within these data if correlated with actual utilization, and there can be substantial distortion in the reported utilization (Bellon, Lardelli, Luna, & Delgado, 2000; Roberts, Bergstralh, Schmidt, & Jacobsen, 1996). This effect becomes more pronounced as the number of visits increases over longer units of time. A patient who makes one visit per year for a defined purpose (e.g., pelvic exam) is likely to accurately recall this visit due to its unusual salience. However, patients who make multiple visits per month to a variety of clinical settings, both primary and specialty, are less likely to give accurate estimates of their visit frequency. In general, patients will recall visits in the past few months, but may have more difficulty recalling utilization earlier in the year. More important, self-reported visit data does not capture visit length or complexity, which are major factors in estimating impact on the health care system.

These limitations may be mitigated somewhat by taking a subsample of the self-report data and auditing clinical records. Yet, even this additional validation may not account for utilization that occurs at health care settings outside the particular clinical site being studied. In general, nonvalidated self-report utilization data should be used with caution. Although it may be useful to show direction of utilization (either higher or lower with respect to a particular condition), the effect size cannot be reliably determined by these data alone. There is a real need for trauma researchers to increase the complexity of their approaches by focusing on cost rather than utilization.

DEFINING AND MEASURING COSTS IN HEALTH CARE

The increasingly competitive health care market of the past 20 years has had major impacts on the way in which medical care is planned and delivered. Since 1980, the health care industry has seen remarkable growth: It currently constitutes approximately 14% of the gross domestic product, or approximately $1.2 trillion (Braden et al., 1998). As medical care costs rose substantially faster than inflation during that period, health plan managers have noticed increasingly narrow profit margins despite substantial improvements in efficiency and cuts in unnecessary costs.

These economic factors have forced health plan providers to scale back the number and degree of covered services, resulting in diminished payment for some treatments (i.e., a high copayment) and the complete exclusion of other services (e.g., mental health benefits) known as "carve-outs." Insured patients often find themselves carefully comparing plans during open enrollment periods to weigh the type and extent of coverage provided given their known or anticipated risk for illness. Meanwhile the uninsured population frequently obtains care in settings that are not cost-effective (e.g., emergency rooms and specialty care clinics) in which little coordination and long-term planning of care is possible (Kasper, Giovannini, & Hoffman, 2000). Ultimately, costs become one of the most important issues in planning services, and medical care systems that cannot adequately control costs will eventually fail.

Many mental health professionals are uncomfortable with the concept of evaluating services according to cost. Nonetheless, given the reality that services do cost money, it is important to identify the most efficient use of resources. The amount of money and resources devoted to health care is fixed, and small relative to the demand. Health care finance planners thus face difficult decisions about how to allocate these resources and frequently use costs as one way of comparing the impact of different medical conditions on individuals or society.

What Constitutes a Cost?

As can be seen in Table 3.1, costs can be direct or indirect. In health care, direct costs are the monetary value of all the goods and resources used to provide a medical treatment. Direct health care costs include the costs of tests, drugs, supplies, salaries of health care providers, and tangible expenses of operating treatment facilities. These costs are the most visible and easily measured. Indirect costs are sometimes not immediately obvious. From the perspective of the health care system, these costs include infrastructure overhead (telephone, transcription services, utilities, billing services, and so forth) and the fixed costs of production that occur regardless of whether health care is administered (the bank will want the clinic's mortgage paid whether it is making money or not). From the perspective of the patient, indirect costs might include lost work time, transportation costs, and need for extra child care. Indirect costs are a substantial fraction of the

TABLE 3.1
Illustrative Examples of Types of Cost According to the
Contextual Perspective

Perspective	Direct	Indirect
Health care system	Tests Medication Supplies Salaries of providers Expenses of operating facility	Infrastructure overhead Telephone service Transcription service Utilities Fixed costs of production Mortgage
Patient	Payment for appointment Payment for medication or test	Lost work time Transportation costs Extra child care
Society	Publicly funded health insurance Emergency care for uninsured patients	Days off work Decreased productivity Loss of employment by patient Loss of employment by family Family burdens

total costs of health care and are often overlooked in the assessment of treatment costs.

Some costs are very difficult to measure and are often overlooked in analyses. Societal costs such as days off work, decreased productivity, loss of employment by the patient, loss of employment by family members who must care for the patient, and other family burden issues are important indirect costs associated with medical disorders.

Costs are more easily measured in some health systems than in others. Most health maintenance organizations (HMOs) are well suited to conduct research on costs. They often contain automated tracking systems that are able to monitor each service used and diagnosis provided that are paid by the health plan. They can also capture the actual cost of production by amortizing the total costs (both direct and indirect) to each unit of service. Most, if not all, utilization occurs within the plan, although even the out-of-plan use can be captured. HMOs and highly integrated care systems such as the VA medical system, therefore, have a distinct advantage in the development of cost-effective care due to their ability to track the true costs of care and to make informed choices about competing treatment priorities. Although not all health care systems track the true costs of care, most health care systems do use some type of accounting system to make health policy decisions. In many systems, case billing documents are reviewed to estimate charges, and these documents become the next-best option for researchers.

What Are Charges, and How Do They Relate to Costs?

Charges are the fees that care providers bill to patients and insurance payers for their services. Charges vary by diagnosis and visit complexity, and they are usually substantially higher than costs due to an added profit margin. Nevertheless, providers are not usually reimbursed for full charges. In fact, the majority of insurers only pay a fraction of billed charges through the use of adjustments.

A series of reductions occur as charges move through the payment system. First, the clinic may expect the patient to make a "co-pay," which reduces the overall share of the charge borne by the insurance payer. Next, previously agreed upon contractual adjustment may further lower the amount of charge allowed. Furthermore, for certain services the payer may elect to reimburse only a fraction of the allowable charge (e.g., mental health treatment may be reimbursed at only 50% of the allowable charge). Thus, a clinic visit charge of $100 may actually be reduced by a $10 co-pay, adjusted to a maximum allowable charge (by contract) of $70, and then reimbursed at 50% of that maximum for a total reimbursement from the payer of $35. This renders charge and billing data more difficult to interpret, and these data may not accurately estimate costs due to the wide variability in these factors across insurance plans. This is sometimes dealt with by adjusting the data using charge-to-cost ratios. However, even if average charge to cost ratios can be determined for a large practice, there is no guarantee that these ratios accurately reflect the performance of subsectors of the clinic population. For example, survivors of childhood trauma may be disproportionately represented in state-sponsored public insurance programs (e.g., Medicaid), possibly rendering average charge-to-cost ratios inaccurate for that group.

Despite these limitations, it is sometimes possible to convert charge data to standardized Medicare costs using a formula that is adjusted for regional differences in costs of living and costs of providing medical care to compare health services research from different institutions.

What About Claims Data?

Health care providers may request payment for a given medical service or item by filing a claim with the insurance carrier. There are significant limitations to using claims data as a proxy for costs. In addition to being subject to the limitations of charge data just mentioned, claims data overestimate costs because they exclude several classes of consumers: (a) nonusers, (b) patients whose utilization level is below the plan deductible, (c) those who use services above the upper limit on covered services, (d) those who do not file claims, and (e) those that use uncovered services. The failure to correct for these limitations may also result in substantial distortions in estimations of the cost of care.

What Is Opportunity Cost?

If resources are used to provide medical care for one patient or condition, they then become unavailable for other patients and other societal uses. Health care policy decisions are strongly determined by political and financial factors that create value conflicts as limited resources are apportioned. For example, should a plan pay for prenatal care for many people or organ transplant services for a few? Trauma survivors must compete with other patients for an appropriate share of these limited resources, yet the type and extent of their need is poorly recognized by most health care organizations.

What Is Cost-Effectiveness?

Cost-effectiveness is the cost per unit of improved health status (e.g., number of dollars spent per successfully treated patient). Cost-effectiveness is analogous to "bang for the buck" and is considered a measure of the financial efficiency with which care is being delivered. This measure has been used as one way to decide which treatments for which disorders will be covered in health plans. Once the health planners agree to cover a treatment, the most cost-effective approach is desirable. Marginal or incremental cost-effectiveness is the preferred metric because it compares an existing treatment (usual care) with a newer treatment and computes the ratio of the differences in costs to the differences in effect sizes.

One of the frequently unrealized dreams of health planners is to have a treatment recoup its cost by the prevention of more serious disease, a concept known as a *cost-offset*. The idea is that a well-timed intervention that prevents the appearance of a disease or delays the worsening of a chronic condition may save the plan money at a later date by decreasing the amount of future care required. For example, smoking prevention and cessation programs may be viewed as decreasing the later appearance of expensive chronic lung and heart disease. Cost-offset sometimes leads to interesting paradoxes, however. It may be actually less expensive for a health plan to allow individuals to continue to smoke uninterrupted because cancer and heart disease mortality often remove individuals from the insured pool long before the appearance of chronic expensive disease. This irony underscores the complexity of health plan coverage decisions, and shows the intersection of societal and ethical values with cost-effectiveness.

Over the past 20 years, health services researchers have attempted to determine whether the provision of mental health treatment provides a compensatory offset of medical care costs. The argument is that the cost of treating the psychiatric disorder is compensated by deferring medical care costs that inefficiently are misdirected at the mental health problem, such as repeated visits for somatization. Despite years of well-designed research in a variety of health care settings, it has been very difficult to demonstrate a consistent cost-offset for the treatment of any mental disorder.

Despite the difficulty in demonstrating actual cost-offsets, several recent studies have shown that collaborative interventions between behavioral clinicians and primary care or medical specialty providers can increase the efficiency of care by making available cost-effective approaches to the treatment of disorders such as major depression (Von Korff et al., 1998). Thus, cost-effectiveness is a consideration once the health plan has decided to treat a disorder and attempts to make the cost per treated case as low as possible using various efficiencies of service.

The Cost to Whom?

The determination of actual costs (both direct and indirect) is the best method to ascertain the impact of trauma on medical care services. Costs can allow health planners to make value judgments on the merits of treating different conditions. However, even in systems in which these cost data are available, there may still be differences in how the costs are calculated. One problem is defining the perspective from which the costs are being viewed. Costs can be seen from the vantage point of the patient, family members, the health care provider, the clinic, the health plan, or society (Drummond, Richardson, O'Brien, Levine, & Heyland, 1997). Failure to understand these multiple perspectives can result in paradoxes in which potentially cost-effective interventions are misperceived as ineffective depending on the context within which they are understood.

For example, suppose a primary care clinic in an HMO decides to start actively screening for trauma victims to provide a hypothetical, cost-effective, evidence-based antidepressant treatment for posttraumatic stress disorder (PTSD). The cost-effectiveness of this treatment is based on data that show a net reduced cost in providing medical care to trauma survivors due to a decrease in the number of unnecessary clinic visits for medically unexplained physical symptoms. Although not a cost-offset, this program is judged to be cost-effective because it reduces psychological morbidity and increases overall quality of life to a degree that the doctors within the clinic agree that it represents good, efficient care.

Although the quality of care for trauma survivors will increase in this clinic without a significant increase in the clinic's budget (the prescription writing time is a negligible increase in the length of a visit), a major increase in the budget of the HMO pharmacy results due to the large number of new antidepressant prescriptions. Let us assume that the most robust clinical results occur using the newer, more expensive antidepressant medications such as selective serotonin reuptake inhibitors. To the pharmacy administrator, there is a substantial increase in costs associated with the program, resulting in a 15% increase in the pharmacy budget. This increase triggers several requests for cost-reduction measures from upper level pharmacy administrators or may even lead to layoffs in pharmacy personnel. Thus, the same program that is perceived as cost-effective by the clinic medical staff is not desirable to the pharmacy administrators because they have a fixed budget. The opportunity cost of supporting this treatment means that they must cut other pharmacy services or provide less coverage for other conditions. This may result in a decision at an even higher organizational level in the HMO central office not to pursue the effective antidepressant treatment program due to an unfavorable financial cost to the HMO, from the perspective of the overall health plan.

However, as the denominator of the calculation (the part that contains the stakeholders) widens, it again changes the possible outcome. The small increase in the pharmacy budget may be substantially offset in the workplace by reduced numbers of sick days, with a resultant increase in productivity considerably greater than the cost of the treatment to the pharmacy. If this HMO were linked to a self-insured corporation, then senior corporate managers might overrule the health plan pharmacy managers by pointing to the greater good of the business and possibly even shifting additional money into the pharmacy budget. This productivity increase will also likely be mirrored by increased quality of life as viewed by the patient's family and community.

Now let us imagine the same program occurring not at a self-insured corporation, but at an HMO not tied to the workplace. From the widest possible perspective, this program may still be producing substantial quality of life and economic gains at the level of the workplace, society, the family, and the patient's quality of life, yet it produces localized, unfavorable financial outcomes at a critical decision level of the HMO (which does not have an obligation to maximizing society's well-being), possibly dooming the program. This example shows the importance of carefully defining the perspective from which the costs were determined. The same program can simultaneously be viewed as cost-effective or not cost-effective depending on whose costs are being considered.

Over What Time Period?

In addition to addressing stakeholder issues, time is also an important consideration. Most contemporary health services research uses the perspective of the health plan for a defined time, such as 1 year, to allow for seasonal variations in the use of health care. Longer time periods may be necessary for some disorders that occur infrequently (e.g., closed head injury), whereas shorter time periods may be appropriate for disorders that involve frequent, regular follow-up (e.g., diabetes). The time frame for evaluation is critical if examining programs that might not be cost-effective in a shorter time period but which become more favorable if viewed from a longer time perspective. Conversely, in systems in which a sizable fraction of the covered population moves to another health plan each year, cost-effective interventions that are favorable in the short run lose their value over time as treated patients leave the system and newer, untreated members become eligible for treatment.

DESIGN ISSUES FOR COST AND UTILIZATION RESEARCH

Although it is relatively straightforward to investigate the epidemiology of individuals exposed to traumatic experiences in health care settings, it is far more difficult to design studies to measure and interpret cost and utilization data attributable to these exposures. It is tempting to simply identify individuals who have experienced a trauma and compare them with individuals who have not with respect to how their health care utilization and costs differ after adjusting for confounding variables. Nevertheless, this kind of research is more complicated than first envisioned.

This baseline of health utilization unrelated to the response to trauma exposure is always occurring in the background, and care must be taken in attributing trauma-related causes to differences between the groups with respect to cost variables. Even well-designed studies of utilization using complex models containing dozens of potentially relevant variables rarely explain more than 10% to 20% of the variance in visits or costs (Russo, Katon, Sullivan, Clark, & Buchwald, 1994). This sobering starting point should be kept in mind when interpreting relationships between trauma and subsequent utilization, no matter how clear the connection intuitively appears at first.

More precision may be gained, however, by considering specific health outcomes and costs. Certain health outcomes have been shown to have a more robust correlation with trauma, and studies that focus on these outcomes are more likely to produce useful utilization and cost data. Trauma interacts with health-related outcomes in at least three ways (see Schnurr & Green, chap. 10, this volume, for a model of these relationships). First it has been shown to cause direct health effects. For example, exposure to traumatic life events can result in wounds, blood loss, head injuries, malnutrition, toxin poisoning, and hypoxic or anoxic episodes that require immediate medical attention. Specific long-term health risks have been associated with certain types of trauma exposure. Among male Vietnam veterans, skin disease and decreased sperm count have been noted (Centers for Disease Control, 1988). Increased incidence of breast disease, bladder infections, two or more yeast infections a year, and pregnancy complications were found among sexually abused women as compared with non-sexually abused women (Springs & Friedrich, 1992). Four to thirty percent of all rape victims contract sexually transmitted diseases (Murphy, Munday, & Jeffries, 1990) and approximately 5% of all rapes result in pregnancy (Beebe, 1991; Koss, Koss, & Woodruff, 1991).

A second category involves health risk behaviors. These behaviors are lifestyle choices that can adversely affect health status, resulting in important, but indirect, contributions to medical morbidity and costs. For example, survivors of childhood maltreatment have an increased risk of becoming obese (Felitti et al., 1998; Walker, Gelfand, et al., 1999). Obesity has multiple causes and occurs in individuals without traumatic experiences, yet it may be an intermediate variable in the causal chain between trauma exposure and increased costs or utilization. It can lead to serious physical diseases such as hypertension, heart disease, and diabetes. Similarly, high-risk health behaviors such as smoking and failure to use a seat belt are also associated with histories of childhood sexual abuse (Springs & Friedrich, 1992). Hence, injuries or diseases associated with smoking or lack of seat belt use may occur and bring the person to medical attention.

The third category is somatization. One of the most robust effects of trauma exposure seems to be the strong association with development and maintenance of medically unexplained physical symptoms, in both veterans and civilians (Eisen, Goldberg, True, & Henderson, 1991). These unexplained physical symptoms (both those related to trauma and those that are not related) have been shown to account for as much as 80% of health-care utilization in primary care clinics, representing a costly and inefficient use of clinic resources (Kroenke & Mangelsdorff, 1989).

Paradoxically, subgroups of trauma survivors may have either higher or lower rates of utilization depending on personal, historical, and socioeconomic factors. For some individuals help seeking may be a therapeutic part of the resolution of their trauma-related difficulties and cooperating with medical care providers may provide a desirable focus for their healing. This might result in higher than expected utilization by these individuals. For others, whose trauma exposure involved early childhood neglect and abuse, there may be an ongoing distrust of caregivers, with a resultant disincentive to consult medical providers. This might result in lower than expected utilization or delay in seeking care for a potentially serious problem such as a breast lump. Although overutilizers have been documented in the literature on traumatic stress, very few studies have adequately depicted the costs and consequences of underutilization, particularly if underutilization ultimately increases medical morbidity and associated costs at a later time due to delay. Clearly, failing to separate out the effects of these differing groups of under- and overutilizers can result in analyses that show no effects of trauma on mean visits and costs, whereas, in reality, there may be opposing, self-canceling effects of considerable magnitude.

This bimodal utilization pattern has been seen in people with dental phobia, who have long periods of lower use of routine prophylactic dental services but then require substantially more expensive treatments due to advanced dental disease brought on by lack of preventive care (Gordon, Dionne, & Snyder, 1998; Walker, Milgrom, Weinstein, Getz, & Richardson, 1996). For many patients, nonparticipation in preventive care ultimately results in increased morbidity over time, suggesting that the overall effect of trauma on utilization and costs ultimately increases medical care costs, even in cases in which there is decreased utilization for a short period.

Designs that do not assess health care costs across a wide range of settings may miss observations in which health care is merely diverted to another unmeasured setting. In a highly regulated primary care system such as an HMO, costs are most clearly seen in the primary care sector, and there is little spillover into emergency and specialty services. However, in fee-for-service systems that do not have highly developed primary care linkages, specialty and emergency room settings are frequently the forum in which care utilization takes place. Measuring health care costs in only one location may underestimate the total costs.

Investigators planning cost and utilization studies should consult with a health economist in the design stages to gain a greater appreciation for the difficulties involved in conducting such research. One of the most unpleasant initial surprises can be the realization of how large the sample must be to reach any meaningful conclusions about costs. Power calculations will normally reveal that sample sizes of 500–1,000 patients are needed to deal with the large variances found in health care cost and utilization data (Diehr, Yanez, Ash, Hornbrook, & Lin, 1992; Gold, Siegel, Russell, & Weinstein, 1996).

DATA ANALYSIS ISSUES

Even the most competent biomedical or behavioral researchers need to be cautious when examining health care data, as there are many important issues to consider. This section offers the reader some direction in understanding the complexity of the problem, interpreting the literature, and recognizing when consultation is needed in conducting such studies. First, health care data often violate assumptions of traditional statistical approaches. For example, participants often have more than one visit or hospitalization, and these health care uses are frequently correlated (violating the independence assumption). Furthermore, almost all health care utilization data are distributed in a nonnormal manner. A significantly large number of insured patients use no services over a defined time, whereas a small number use services an extraordinarily large number of times. This results in right-skewed distributions with a mode of zero (having a shape resembling the right half of a normal distribution) that makes parametric analyses difficult to interpret. Typical transformations can be difficult because a sizable fraction of the sample will have zero costs or utilization, and certain transformation procedures (e.g., log transformations) of zero are undefined. One customary solution is to add one dollar or half a visit to each subject to allow an acceptable transformation of the data. This minor distortion does not significantly alter the distribution after transformation. However, transformed data are often difficult to interpret in many designs. The transformed units have now become "log dollars" or "log visits," which are difficult to interpret as meaningful health care data. Simple back-transformation (e.g., performing parametric analyses such as ANOVA on the log data and then taking the anti-log of the results) distorts the variance estimates severely enough to cause concern about validity of the findings. Several techniques such as "smearing" have been used to retransform the data back to more usable form. This technique adjusts the transformed data back to dollars or visits but compensates for the errors in variance created by the transformation (Diehr et al., 1992).

Alternatively, two-part analytic plans have been implemented (Diehr et al., 1992). In this case, the probability of any utilization first is computed for all patients. Next the level of use of those who have had any health care is computed, removing those with zero utilization. The predicted level of use for any patient is then the product of the two. On the other hand, nonparametric techniques such as median regression or multichotomous logistic regression often can be used with such complicated data. Regardless of which method is chosen, investigators should be aware of the distortions that may be introduced by the manner in which costs and utilization data are collected. Because multiple observations are taken over a time period (e.g., 1 year), one needs to be concerned about autocorrelations within subjects (i.e., individuals with high costs at one point are likely to have high costs at another). Consultation with a biostatistician or a health economist may be helpful in the planning stages of the study and especially prior to data analysis.

One of the most confusing design issues in cost and utilization research is the classification of intermediate variables as either confounders or effect modifiers. Confounders are variables that have an association with both the cause and the effect. Removing the effects of these variables gives a more accurate picture of costs. Effect modifiers, on the other hand, serve as indirect pathways for the effect. A good example of this problem in childhood trauma research is what to do with marital status and education. Traditionally, these variables have been treated as confounders (i.e., marital status and education cause medical outcomes independent of the trauma and therefore these effects should be removed from the analysis).

On the other hand, childhood trauma survivors may have reduced opportunities for education and marriage (Walker, Gelfand, et al., 1999), making these variables effect-modifying mediators. It is inappropriate to remove the effects of mediating variables. This concern can be addressed by a sensitivity or scenario analysis that estimates costs both ways (using the variables first as confounders, then as mediators) and presents a range of values into which the costs are contained. In a sensitivity and scenario analysis, the worst and best cases for each variable are ascertained and then combined to construct a worst and best case model. More sophisticated approaches such as Monte Carlo simulations are also possible in which repeated sampling is taken from the probability distributions of the uncertain variables. Regardless of the method chosen, the models illustrate the possible range of reasonably expected outcomes. Studies on health utilization among veterans with PTSD that include marital status as a variable (e.g., Williams, Weiss, Edens, Johnson, & Thornby, 1998) could be improved by use of this strategy.

Another important issue in the analysis of cost and utilization data is that they must be adjusted for the presence of chronic medical illness. Are observed differences in costs between trauma and nontrauma groups attributable to differences in the prevalence of chronic medical conditions unrelated to trauma? Measures such as the *chronic disease score* (Clark, Von Korff, Saunders, Baluch, & Simon, 1995) can perform this adjustment, and these measures highly correlate with physician ratings of physical disease severity, predicted mortality, and hospital use.

The mean annual costs per patient are only meaningful if they are placed in the context of how these costs will impact the entire health plan. An interesting application of the results to the real world can be affected by using the concept *of population attributable risk*. Population attributable risk allows one to extrapolate how specific risks (costs, utilization) found in one's results might apply to a larger appropriate reference group. This analysis involves multiplying the costs per patient by the number of affected patients in the system. For highly prevalent conditions such as childhood trauma exposure, even small annual costs are magnified over the entire insured population. In a study of 1,225 women in a Seattle HMO, we found that 42.8% of the women in the HMO had maltreatment experiences and that mean additional cost per maltreated woman per year for medical care related to maltreatment was approximately $116. This finding does not seem impressive until one estimates the total attributable cost associated with maltreatment in this HMO, which turns out to be $8,175,816 per year (42.8% × total population of 163,844 women × cost difference per patient; Walker, Unutzer, et al., 1999).

HEALTH-RELATED COSTS AND UTILIZATION ASSOCIATED WITH TRAUMA EXPOSURE

With this background we can now turn to the existing literature to address the issue of how traumatic experiences contribute to medical health care costs. A literature review of the effects of trauma on costs and utilization of health care is surprisingly difficult to do given a variety of classification and methodological problems that must first be sorted through before studies can be meaningfully compared. Very few published studies address costs or utilization in survivors of trauma, and these existing studies vary widely in methodological sophistication. Before one can consider the impact of trauma on health care costs and utilization, it is important to address three main areas of concern: case identification, measurement, and analytic strategy (see Table 3.2).

TABLE 3.2
Issues to Consider When Evaluating Cost and Utilization Studies

Issue	Question
Case identification	How were cases recruited?
	Type of trauma?
	How long ago was event relative to medical outcome assessment?
	Valid and reliable measures of exposure and psychological impact?
	Were underutilizers identified?
Cost or utilization measurement	Is it self-report? If so, was a subset audited with verified information?
	Were all costs determined (patient, system, society)?
	Was a range of heath care services and costs evaluated?
	Were out-of-hospital or -network costs examined?
	Was the time frame reasonable?
Analytic strategy	Were appropriate statistical procedures for nonparametric health care data used if needed?
	Were intermediate variables properly classified as confounders or effect mediators?
	Were chronic medial illnesses adjusted for?
	Were outcomes expressed in meaningful units (e.g., not log dollars)?
	Are results meaningful to policy analysts, clinicians, and researchers?

Case Identification

What kinds of trauma have been studied (e.g., rape, war experiences, domestic violence, accident trauma)? It should not be assumed that each type of trauma will lead to similar changes in utilization and cost. Is there an attempt to combine dissimilar trauma categories in the same study? When did the traumatic event occur relative to the measured medical outcomes (e.g., rape in the past year vs. sexual abuse 25 years ago)? What is the validity and reliability of the trauma measurement (e.g., how certain are we that this experience produced a trauma response such as PTSD)?

Cost or Utilization Measurement

How are the visits or costs measured (e.g., self-report, chart review, charges, automated data)? To what degree does the assessment method cover all possible costs (e.g., does the individual obtain care in any setting that is not measured)? Is the specified time period long enough to capture the variability inherent in utilization? What kinds of costs are captured? What is the perspective of the study (the costs to whom)? Does the sample size create enough power to detect a meaningful difference?

Analytic Strategy

Has the study used appropriate statistical procedures that account for nonparametric characteristics of health care data? Have appropriate confounders and mediators been measured so that predictive models can be built to explain the proportionate role of trauma in the production of health care visits and costs? Are the outcomes expressed in meaningful units (e.g., not log dollars)? Are the results meaningful to policy analysts, clinicians, and researchers?

A number of early studies have documented increased health utilization associated with trauma exposure in various samples, although the case identification, measurement, and analytic strategies used were limited. Nonetheless, a pattern has emerged from all these studies. Across a range of studies, sexual assault survivors appear to use medical services at elevated rates compared with individuals who have not experienced assault in the years following the assault (Felitti, 1991; Golding et al., 1988; Moeller, Bachmann, & Moeller, 1993; Walker et al., 1992). Similarly, several studies have suggested greater health care utilization among women who experienced child sexual abuse (Finestone et al., 2000). Battered women have been shown to use emergency room services for physical injuries obtained during violence from a partner (Stark & Flitcraft, 1988). Veterans with PTSD also have reported greater health care utilization (e.g., Schnurr, Ford, et al., 2000).

The majority of these studies have not examined confounder and effect variables, autocorrelations, or chronic medical illnesses unrelated to trauma. Instead, they have relied on self-report utilization and used parametric analyses without examining distributions of data. Although consistent, these data need to be reexamined with more sophisticated techniques and validated records of utilization to assure the pattern is an accurate one, especially given the possibility that trauma survivors who are not using health care may affect these findings.

Early studies in the field used innovative approaches to examine how health and cost might be related. For example, Golding and colleagues (1988) used self-report data to find an interaction between sexual assault status and insurance status for sexual assault survivors. There was a larger increase of medical service use among those without private health insurance than among those with private health insurance. However, assault was associated with increased utilization among those without Medicaid but was unrelated to utilization among those with Medicaid. Although important early in the field, the self-report data and other confounds in this approach may make it difficult to interpret.

Given the state of the art at this time and the history of this research in the field, we reviewed the available literature using the following stringent minimum criteria:

1. Studies were required to have a validated assessment measure for case identification. These included standardized assessments for PTSD, childhood maltreatment, domestic violence, or other traumatic conditions.

2. Objective cost and utilization data were obtained either from automated data systems (e.g., HMO or claims data) or systematic record review with validation using multiple sources (e.g., cross-referenced with claims and billing data). Self-report utilization was included if an effort was made to validate the self-report with clinical records.

3. Only studies that had sufficient power and used appropriate statistical analyses were included.

There are currently very few studies that meet this level of methodological rigor. Although several studies have attempted to measure self-reported utilization as one of several health variables, most have not cross-validated these findings with chart reviews or actual utilization data. Five studies have obtained these data in a more methodologically accurate manner.

Koss and colleagues (1991) studied 390 adult women (74 nonvictims and 316 victims of crime). The severely victimized women, compared with nonvictims, reported more distress and less well-being, made physician visits twice as frequently in the index year, and had outpatient costs that were 2.5 times greater. Criminal victimization severity was the most powerful predictor of physician visits and outpatient costs. Utilization data across 5 years preceding and following the crime were obtained from 15 rape victims, 26 physical assault victims, and 27 noncontact crime victims and were compared with five continuous years of utilization among 26 nonvictims. Victims' physician visits increased 15% to 24% during the year of the crime compared with less than 2% change among nonvictims.

Scholle, Rost, and Golding (1998) retrospectively assessed domestic violence health services use over 1 year in a cohort of 303 depressed women from a random community sample from Arkansas. Measures included the Conflict Tactics Scale and a structured medical records review protocol. After controlling for sociodemographic and severity-of-illness factors, recently abused, depressed women were much less likely to receive outpatient care for mental health problems as compared to other depressed women (odds ratio [OR] = 0.3; p = .013), although they were more likely to receive health care for physical problems (OR = 5.7, p = .021).

Walker, Unutzer, and colleagues (1999) examined differences in annual health care use and costs in a random sample of 1,225 women HMO members with and without validated histories of childhood sexual, emotional, or physical abuse or neglect. Health care costs and use data were obtained from the automated cost-accounting system of the HMO, including total costs, outpatient and primary care costs, and emergency department visits. Women who reported any abuse or neglect had median annual health care costs that were $97 (95% confidence interval = $0.47 – $188.26) greater than women who did not report maltreatment. Women who reported sexual abuse had median annual health care costs that were $245 (95% confidence interval = $132.32 – $381.93) greater than costs among women who did not report abuse. Women with sexual abuse histories had significantly higher primary care and outpatient costs and more frequent emergency department visits than women without these histories. Maltreatment was also significantly associated with an increased number of physician-coded ICD–9 diagnoses (excluding health maintenance codes such as routine gynecologic exams) for the 18-month period prior to the study. This increase was not only due to mental health diagnoses and medically unexplained pain complaints, but also to physical diseases.

Using the same sample and the aforementioned automated cost-accounting system of the HMO, Walker and colleagues (2003) examined total and component health care cost by PTSD status. PTSD status was measured using the PTSD Checklist (Weathers, Litz, Herman, Huska, & Keane, 1993), which had been validated in a subset of 268 participants. The total unadjusted mean annual health care costs were $3,060 ± $6,381 (median $1,283) for the high group, $1,779 ± $3,008 (median $829) for the moderate group, and $1,646 ± $5,156 (median $609) for the low group. Even if controlling for depression, chronic medical illness, and psychological distress, women with high PTSD Check List (PCL) scores had significantly greater odds of having non-zero health care costs compared to women with low PCL scores (OR = 13.14, CI = 1.70 – 101.19). Compared with women in the low PCL score group, those in the moderate group had on average a 38% increase in adjusted total annual median costs, and those in the high group had a 104% increase.

Arnow and colleagues (1999) examined the relationships among reported history of childhood sexual abuse (CSA), psychological distress, and medical utilization for 206 women in an HMO waiting room setting. Participants were classified, using screening questionnaires and the revised Symptom Checklist 90, as (a) CSA-distressed, (b) distressed only, (c) CSA only, or (d) control participants. Medical utilization rates were generated from the computerized database of the HMO for (a) nonpsychiatric outpatient, (b) psychiatric outpatient, (c) emergency room (ER), and (d) inpatient admissions. CSA-distressed and distressed-only groups both used significantly more nonpsychiatric outpatient visits than CSA only and control participants, but were not different from one another. CSA-only and control participants did not differ on nonpsychiatric outpatient utilization. CSA-distressed participants used significantly more ER visits and were more likely to visit the ER for pain-related complaints than other participants. Among CSA-distressed participants, those who met criteria for physical abuse had significantly more ER visits than those who did not. There were no differences among the four groups in inpatient utilization rates. Thus, psychological distress was associated with higher outpatient medical utilization, independent of CSA history. History of CSA with concomitant psychological distress was associated with significantly higher ER visits, particularly for those with a history of physical abuse. History of CSA without distress was not associated with elevated rates of medical utilization.

All five studies show clear increases in health care costs and utilization for trauma survivors. Nevertheless, each of the studies is limited in the scope of problems it examined and the generalizability of the findings. Even the larger studies by Walker and colleagues (1999, 2003) provide data appropriate only for health planners considering HMO-based interventions for women with childhood maltreatment. It is clear that large, systematic investigations of the full range of traumatic experiences are needed in systems that can provide long-term observations using automated data and, if possible, use the family as the unit of analysis rather than just the individual patient. This systems view is particularly important given the fact that traumatic experiences frequently involve the entire support system of the victim, shifting increased costs and utilization across several individuals.

IMPLICATIONS FOR ACCESS TO HEALTH INSURANCE

Researchers who investigate the connections between trauma exposure and health are forced to ponder a dilemma. Although we now know more about how traumatic events produce adverse health outcomes and how to provide effective treatment for survivors, the same studies can potentially be used against patients with trauma histories to deny or decrease their eligibility for medical insurance.

On the positive side, identification of victimization status presents an opportunity for a health plan to proactively offer specialty services designed to help that individual cope with the effects of trauma. Early identification of trauma survivors upon enrollment in a health plan could allow care providers to focus on meeting special needs (for example, those with mood or anxiety disorders, particularly major depression and PTSD, who might benefit from treatment). A special case management approach utilizing a combination of group and individual therapy might be combined with a specific track through the primary care clinics that allows prompt recognition of anxiety and depression that might otherwise present as medically unexplained physical symptoms. Much of the epidemiological data already collected on trauma survivors could be used to design such programs. Like many other "chronic disease management" programs for disorders such as diabetes, initial high costs for stabilization of trauma-related disorders would gradually yield to lower maintenance costs. Certainly such economic analyses can help promote prevention and community outreach programs designed for trauma survivors.

Nevertheless, as promising as this initially sounds, in our current multi-payer medical system, disenrollment rates would tend to quickly dilute the value of such a program. In certain for-profit HMOs it is common for as much as 50% of the enrolled population to become ineligible or to move out of the plan any given year. Cumulatively this attrition tends to decrease the cost-effectiveness of such interventions because the members at the final stages of maintenance treatment leave the plan and are replaced by those requiring initial stabilization and costly intervention. In the United States VA health care delivery system this is less likely to be the case due to widespread implementation across clinics. Yet not all veterans use the services, and even among those that do, a proportion receives services outside the system. If the United States implemented a national health insurance plan, an early identification, prevention, and disease management system would not be problematic to implement. However, such ambitious case management in our current system would tend to penalize health systems that chose to implement such programs by exposing them to a disproportionate share of the cost of diagnosis and stabilization.

A more ominous possibility is that insurers might use the information from these studies to deny people insurance or to delay the start of benefits based on preexisting conditions. Many of these health care policy issues are currently being worked out with diseases such as HIV (Daniels, 1990). It is one thing to change health insurance rates for individuals who voluntarily choose to continue a health risk behavior such as smoking, and quite another to refuse insurance or diminish coverage for victims of criminal behavior who have no choice. As researchers and clinicians, we have an obligation to be vigilant that the data we collect are not used in ways that could jeopardize the ability of survivors of trauma to obtain health care.

CONCLUSIONS AND FUTURE DIRECTIONS

As we have suggested, a paradigm shift in the field of health research and traumatic stress is necessary for the field to reach its true potential. The next generation of trauma research must take into account costs and utilization if we are to make lasting changes in health care policy. Although there is value in continuing to increase our understanding about the epidemiology of trauma in medical settings, our main focus should be studying the impact of trauma patients on health care delivery systems as well as the impact of health care delivery systems on trauma patients. This priority involves understanding how quality improvements in health care can be made for trauma survivors using traditional health services models.

One of the most commonly used theoretical models of health care quality improvement is the classic work of Donabedian (1980). In this framework, positive health care outcomes for a condition result from attention to three characteristics of the health care delivery process: the patient, the provider, and the health care system. Our research to date has been too narrowly focused on the patient. Although we have a good understanding of how trauma can precipitate symptoms, disease, and clinic visits, we do not have a comparable depth of knowledge in how well health care providers recognize these connections, or how able they are to intervene once they do recognize them.

Nor do we understand how health care systems can interact with these individuals. Although we have good evidence of how to treat trauma survivors in highly structured experimental settings (e.g., Foa, Keane, & Friedman, 2000), these efficacy studies contribute little to the "real world" of medical care. Effectiveness studies are essential in translating these evidence-based therapies into the clinic. Furthermore, even if these effectiveness studies are commissioned, we still need to show that this care can be accomplished in a cost-effective manner compared with other health care priorities. Nonetheless, if clinical researchers integrate measures of cost into efficacy and effectiveness studies of mental health and physical health interventions, we will be able to provide data to help improve services for trauma survivors.

Cost and utilization research will be a central part of the process that translates these findings into policy. As we envision and design these future studies, we must be careful to hold our research to the absolutely highest methodological standards possible to get meaningful planning data. Future studies should attempt to illuminate the full range of costs, including societal costs related to loss of productivity and impact on the family.

REFERENCES

Allers, C. T., Benjack, K. J., White, J., & Rousey, J. T. (1993). HIV vulnerability and the adult survivor of childhood sexual abuse. *Child Abuse and Neglect, 17,* 291–298.

Amaya-Jackson, L., Davidson, J. R., Hughes, D. C., Swartz, M., Reynolds, V., George, L. K., et al. (1999). Functional impairment and utilization of services associated with posttraumatic stress in the community. *Journal of Traumatic Stress, 12,* 709–724.

Andersen, R. M. (1995). Revisiting the behavioral model and access to medical care: Does it matter? *Journal of Health and Social Behavior, 36,* 1–10.

Arnow, B. A., Hart, S., Scott, C., Dea, R., O'Connell, L., & Taylor, C. B. (1999). Childhood sexual abuse, psychological distress, and medical use among women. *Psychosomatic Medicine, 61,* 762–770.

Beebe, D. K. (1991). Emergency management of the adult female rape victim. *American Family Physician, 43,* 2041–2046.

Bellon, J. A., Lardelli, P., Luna, J. D., & Delgado, A. (2000). Validity of self reported utilization of primary health care services in an urban population in Spain. *Journal of Epidemiology in Community Health, 54,* 544–551.

Boscarino, J. A. (1997). Diseases among men 20 years after exposure to severe stress: Implications for clinical research and medical care. *Psychosomatic Medicine, 59,* 605–614.

Braden, B. R., Cowan, C. A., Lazenby, H. C., Martin, A. B., McDonnell, P. A., Sensenig, A. L., et al. (1998). National health expenditures, 1997. *Health Care Financial Review, 20,* 83–126.

Centers for Disease Control. (1988). Health status of Vietnam veterans: II. Physical health. *Journal of American Medical Association, 259,* 2708–2714.

Clark, D. O., Von Korff, M., Saunders, K., Baluch, W. M., & Simon, G. E. (1995). A chronic disease score with empirically derived weights. *Medical Care, 33,* 783–795.

Daniels, N. (1990). Insurability and the HIV epidemic: Ethical issues in underwriting. *Milbank Quarterly, 68,* 497–525.

Dickinson, L. M., deGruy, F. V. III, Dickinson, W. P., & Candib, L. M. (1999). Health-related quality of life and symptom profiles of female survivors of sexual abuse in primary care. *Archives of Family Medicine, 8,* 35–43.

Diehr, P., Yanez, D., Ash, A., Hornbrook, M., & Lin, D. Y. (1992). Methods for analyzing health care utilization and costs. *Annual Review of Public Health, 20,* 125–144.

Donabedian, A. (1980). *Explorations in quality assessment and monitoring (Vol. 1): The definition of quality and approaches to its assessment.* Ann Arbor, MI: Health Administration Press.

Drummond, M. F., Richardson, W. S., O'Brien, B. J., Levine, M., & Heyland, D. (1997). User's guide to the medical literature. How to use an article on economic analysis of clinical practice: Are the results of the study valid? *Journal of the American Medical Association, 19,* 1552–1557.

Druss, B. G., & Rosenheck, R. (1997). Use of medical services by veterans with mental disorders. *Psychosomatics, 38,* 451–458.

Eisen, S. A., Goldberg, J., True, W. R., & Henderson, W. G. (1991). A co-twin control study of the effects of the Vietnam war on the self-reported physical health of veterans. *American Journal of Epidemiology, 134,* 49–58.

Felitti, V. J. (1991). Long–term medical consequences of incest, rape, and molestation. *Southern Medical Journal, 84,* 328–331.

Felitti, V. J., Anda, R. F., Nordenberg, D., Williamson, D. F., Spitz, A. M., Edwards, V., et al. (1998). Relationship of childhood abuse and household dysfunction to many of the leading causes of death in adults: The Adverse Childhood Experiences (ACE) Study. *American Journal of Preventative Medicine, 14,* 245–258.

Finestone, H. M., Stenn, P., Davies, F., Stalker, C., Fry, R., & Koumanis, J. (2000). Chronic pain and health care utilization in women with a history of childhood sexual abuse. *Child Abuse and Neglect, 24,* 547–556.

Foa, E. B., Keane, T. M., & Friedman, M. J. (2000). *Effective treatments for PTSD.* New York: Guilford.

Gold, M. R., Siegel, J. E., Russell, L. B., & Weinstein, M. C. (1996). *Cost-effectiveness in health and medicine.* New York: Oxford University Press.

Golding, J. M. (1996). Sexual assault history and limitations in physical functioning in two general population samples. *Research in Nursing and Health, 19,* 33–44.

Golding, J. M. (1999). Sexual assault history and long-term physical health problems: Evidence from clinical and population epidemiology. *Current Directions in Psychological Science, 8,* 191–194.

Golding, J. M., Stein, J. A., Siegel, J. M, Burnam, M. A., & Sorenson, S. B. (1988). Sexual assault history and use of health and mental health services. *American Journal of Community Psychology, 16*, 625–644.

Gordon, S. M., Dionne, R. A., & Snyder, J. (1998). Dental fear and anxiety as a barrier to accessing oral health care among patients with special health care needs. *Special Care Dentist, 18*, 88–92.

Kasper, J. D., Giovannini, T. A., & Hoffman, C. (2000). Gaining and losing health insurance: Strengthening the evidence for effects on access to care and health outcomes. *Medical Care Research Review, 57*, 298–318.

Koss, M. P., Koss, P. G., & Woodruff, W. J. (1991). Deleterious effects of criminal victimization on women's health and medical utilization. *Archives of Internal Medicine, 151*, 342–347.

Kroenke, K., & Mangelsdorff, A. D. (1989). Common symptoms on primary care: Incidence, evaluation, therapy and outcome. *American Journal of Medicine, 86*, 262–266.

Moeller, T. P., Bachmann, G. A., & Moeller, J. R. (1993). The combined effects of physical, sexual, and emotional abuse during childhood: Long-term health consequences for women. *Child Abuse and Neglect, 17*, 623–640.

Murphy, S., Munday, P.E., & Jeffries, D. J. (1990). Rape and subsequent seroconversion to HIV. *British Medical Journal, 300*, 118.

Neumann, D. A., Houskamp, B. M., Pollock, V. E., & Briere, J. (1996). The long-term sequelae of childhood sexual abuse in women: A meta-analytic review. *Child Maltreatment, 1*, 6–16.

Roberts, R. O., Bergstralh, E. J., Schmidt, L., & Jacobsen, S. J. (1996). Comparison of self-reported and medical record health care utilization measures. *Journal of Clinical Epidemiology, 49*, 989–995.

Rosenheck, R., & Fontana, A. (1994). Utilization of mental health services by minority veterans of the Vietnam Era. *Journal of Nervous and Mental Disease, 182*, 685–691.

Rosenheck, R., & Massari, L. (1993). Wartime military service and utilization of VA health care services. *Military Medicine, 158*, 223–228.

Russo, J., Katon, W. J., Sullivan, M., Clark, M., & Buchwald, D. (1994). Severity of somatization and its relationship to psychiatric disorders and personality. *Psychosomatics, 35*, 546–556.

Saunders, B. E., Kilpatrick, D. G., Hanson, R. F., Resnick, H. S., & Walker, M. E. (1999). Prevalence, case characteristics, and long-term psychological correlates of child rape among women: A national survey. *Child Maltreatment, 4*, 187–200.

Schnurr, P. P., Ford, J. D., Friedman, M. J., Green, B. L., Dain, B. J., & Sengupta, A. (2000). Predictors and outcomes of posttraumatic stress disorder in World War II veterans exposed to mustard gas. *Journal of Consulting and Clinical Psychology, 68*, 258–268.

Schnurr, P. P., Friedman, M. J., Sengupta, A., Jankowski, M. K., & Holmes, T. (2000). PTSD and utilization of medical treatment services among male Vietnam veterans. *Journal of Nervous and Mental Disease, 188,* 496–504.

Schnurr, P. P., & Jankowski, M. K. (1999). Physical health and post-traumatic stress disorder: Review and synthesis. *Seminars in Clinical Neuropsychiatry, 4,* 295–304.

Scholle, S. H., Rost, K. M., & Golding, J. M. (1998). Physical abuse among depressed women. *Journal of General Internal Medicine, 13,* 607–613.

Shariat, S., Mallonee, S., Kruger, E., Farmer, K., & North, C. S. (1999). A prospective study of long-term health outcomes among Oklahoma City bombing survivors. *Journal of the Oklahoma State Medical Association, 92,* 178–186.

Spak, L., Spak, F., & Allebeck, P. (1998). Sexual abuse and alcoholism in a female population. *Addiction, 93,* 1365–1373.

Springs, F. E., & Friedrich, W. N. (1992). Health risk behaviors and medical sequelae of childhood sexual abuse. *Mayo Clinic Proceedings, 67,* 527–532.

Stark, E., & Flitcraft, A. H. (1988). Personal power and institutional victimization: Treating the dual trauma of woman battering. In F. M. Ochberg (Ed.), *Posttraumatic therapy and victims of violence* (pp. 115–151). New York: Brunner/Mazel.

Switzer, G. E., Dew, M. A., Thompson, K., Goycoolea, J. M., Derricott, T., & Mullins, S. D. (1999). Posttraumatic stress disorder and service utilization among urban mental health center clients. *Journal of Traumatic Stress, 12,* 25–39.

Von Korff, M., Katon, W., Bush, T., Lin, E. H., Simon, G. E., Saunders, K., et al. (1998). Treatment costs, cost offset, and cost-effectiveness of collaborative management of depression. *Psychosomatic Medicine, 60,* 143–149.

Walker, E. A., Gelfand, A., Katon, W., Koss, M., Von Korff, M., Bernstein, D., et al. (1999). Adult health status of women HMO members with histories of childhood abuse and neglect. *American Journal of Medicine, 107,* 332–339.

Walker, E. A., Katon, W. J., Hansom, J., Harrop-Griffiths, J., Holm, L., Jones, M. L., et al. (1992). Medical and psychiatric symptoms in women with childhood sexual abuse. *Psychosomatic Medicine, 54,* 658–664.

Walker, E. A., Katon, W., Russo, J., Ciechanowski, P., Newman, E., & Wagner, A. (2003). Health care costs associated with posttraumatic stress disorder symptoms in women. *Archives of General Psychiatry, 60,* 369–374.

Walker, E. A., Milgrom, P. M., Weinstein, P., Getz, T., & Richardson, R. (1996). Assessing abuse and neglect and dental fear in women. *Journal of the American Dental Association, 127,* 485–490.

Walker, E. A., Unutzer, J., Rutter, C., Gelfand, A., Saunders, K., Von Korff, M., et al. (1999). Costs of health care use by women HMO members with a history of childhood abuse and neglect. *Archives of General Psychiatry, 56,* 609–613.

Weathers, F. W., Litz, B. T., Herman, D. S., Huska, J. A., & Keane, T. M. (1993, October). *PTSD Checklist: Description, use, and psychometric properties.* Paper presented at the annual meeting of the International Society for Traumatic Stress Studies, San Antonio, TX.

Widom, C. S. (1999). Posttraumatic stress disorder in abused and neglected children grown up. *American Journal of Psychiatry, 156,* 1223–1229.

Widom, C. S., & Kuhns, J. B. (1996). Childhood victimization and subsequent risk for promiscuity, prostitution, and teenage pregnancy: A prospective study. *American Journal of Public Health, 86,* 1607–1612.

Williams, W., Weiss, T. W., Edens, A., Johnson, M., & Thornby, J. I. (1998). Hospital utilization and personality characteristics of veterans with psychiatric problems. *Psychiatric Services, 49,* 370–375.

II

PSYCHOLOGICAL MECHANISMS LINKING TRAUMA AND HEALTH

4

DEPRESSION, TRAUMA, AND CARDIOVASCULAR HEALTH

DANIEL E. FORD

Numerous studies in the past 10 years have highlighted the potential risk that mental disorders pose for subsequent health conditions categorized under the broad category of physical illnesses. The majority of these studies have focused on depression. Depression has been consistently associated with elevated risk for a broad array of conditions within the category of cardiovascular disease. In this chapter, I review the extensive literature on mental disorders (primarily depression) and cardiovascular disease and consider the extent to which this research may be applicable to the association between posttraumatic stress disorder (PTSD) and physical disorders. The relationship between depression and coronary heart disease thus provides an excellent empirically based model that can inform questions about PTSD and health.

Depression is of particular relevance to understanding how PTSD relates to health because depression is frequently comorbid with PTSD. The National Comorbidity Survey estimated that the lifetime prevalence of major depression was 48% in men and 49% in women with PTSD, versus 12% and 19%, respectively, in men and women without PTSD (Kessler, Sonnega, Bromet, Hughes, & Nelson, 1995). In the majority of cases, PTSD is primary (Breslau, Davis, Peterson, & Schultz, 2000; Kessler et al., 1995), but even when it is not, the high comorbidity has significant implications for understanding research on the health effects of depression. Many individuals in depression studies are likely to have PTSD. For example, a recent study of women recruited for a depression treatment trial found that 52% of these women had current comorbid PTSD in addition to current major depression (Miranda et al., 2003). The influence of undetected PTSD on the depression studies reviewed in this chapter is impossible to estimate, but it is likely to enhance the generalizability of results to PTSD.

EPIDEMIOLOGY OF CARDIOVASCULAR DISEASE

Economically developed countries have experienced a true epidemic of coronary heart disease in the past century, with a peak incidence in the 1960s and 1970s. Through careful epidemiologic investigations, community interventions, and development of new methods to treat coronary heart disease, age-adjusted death rates have decreased by 50% (American Heart Association, 2001).

Atherosclerosis, or narrowing of the arteries due to plaque formation, is the underlying process leading to several manifestations of cardiovascular disease. In the heart, narrowing of the coronary artery vessels can lead to angina, a type of chest pain due to a decreased supply of blood to the heart muscle. With angina, it is generally believed that no permanent damage occurs to the heart. If the decreased supply of blood lasts too long, however, a myocardial infarction occurs, with permanent death of cardiac muscle. Both of these conditions comprise the general category of coronary artery disease (CAD). Other terms for CAD include coronary heart disease (CHD) and ischemic heart disease. Atherosclerosis in the cerebral vessels providing blood to the brain can lead to transient ischemic attacks (TIA) or stroke. Atherosclerosis in the aorta and arteries providing blood to the legs is called peripheral vascular disease. Peripheral vascular disease leads to intermittent claudication, or a deep pain in the legs with walking, that resolves in minutes if the individual stops walking. The most consistent risk factors for atherosclerosis, in addition to older age and male gender, are elevated blood pressure, elevated levels of low-density lipid (LDL) cholesterol, diabetes, and tobacco smoking. The search for new risk factors continues, as all of these risk factors just listed may predict as little as 50% of the variance in cases of myocardial infarction. Potential new risk factors of current interest include markers of inflammation and thrombosis.

DEPRESSION AND CORONARY ARTERY DISEASE

In the 1960s and 1970s, Type A personality was considered to be the most important behavioral syndrome elevating the risk of coronary artery disease. This syndrome consisted of competitive achievement striving, a sense of time urgency, aggressiveness, and easily aroused hostility, although all studies did not define it in exactly the same way (Booth-Kewley & Friedman, 1987). Over time, evidence pointed to hostility–anger and depression as the key components of Type A personality for predicting CAD (Booth-Kewley & Friedman, 1987). Three relatively separate lines of research have converged to increase our confidence in the conclusion that depression is a risk factor for the development and progression of coronary artery disease. First are observational studies following patients hospitalized for depression to assess their subsequent health outcomes. Second are studies reporting decreased survival for patients with major depression who have experienced a clinical event, usually a myocardial infarction. Third is a rapidly increasing body of literature indicating that individuals with depression have increased risk for the development of new or incident cardiovascular disease. I briefly review each of these lines of research.

CAD in Patients Hospitalized With Depression

Between 1960 and 1985, a common study design was to determine the mortality experience of a sample of patients hospitalized for depression. Some of these studies included a standardized diagnostic assessment, but others relied on usual clinician assessments. One prime example of these studies is the Iowa record-linkage study. This study was initiated to examine death rates in individuals hospitalized for psychiatric disorders. Diagnostic classification was based on routine clinical assessments. Death certificates for 5,412 individuals hospitalized between 1972 and 1981 were identified and their death rates were compared to the general population after adjustment for age and gender. As expected, suicide rates were elevated. In addition, death from heart disease, especially in women, was modestly, but significantly, elevated (Black, 1998; Black, Winokur, & Nasrallah, 1987). A study from Israel using a similar design found elevated rates of mortality compared with the general population from a variety of diseases in addition to suicide (Zilber, Schufman, & Lerner, 1989). A meta-analysis examining the effect of depression on mortality reviewed these articles, as well as reports of mortality based on psychiatric assessments of community samples. A total of 57 studies were identified, with 21 receiving a rank above 8 on a 12-point index assessing quality of methods. However, few of the studies had controlled for important confounders such as severity of physical illness, smoking, or alcohol use. For example, only nine of the studies had controlled for smoking. The authors did not feel the available studies allowed a formal quantitative meta-analysis, but they concluded that depression seems to increase the risk for death by cardiovascular disease, particularly in men. However, they did not find that depression increased the risk of death from cancer (Wulsin, Vaillant, & Wells, 1999).

Impact of Depression on Survival After a Myocardial Infarction

Survivors of myocardial infarction who have depression are more likely to die or experience another cardiovascular event compared with survivors without depression (Glassman & Shapiro, 1998). Frasure-Smith and colleagues completed a careful follow-up of about 1,000 patients who had a myocardial infarction and found higher mortality for those with elevated Beck Depression Inventory scores, even after controlling for smoking and standard measures of cardiac function (Frasure-Smith, Lesperance, & Talajic, 1995). Increased mortality in the study was largely from higher rates of cardiac sudden death, and it was limited to those with a greater number of premature ventricular contractions at baseline. The increased risk applied to both women and men, and depressive symptoms were a stronger predictor of mortality than anxiety, anger, or lack of social support (Frasure-Smith, Lesperance, Juneau, Talajic, & Bourassa, 1999). Depression has also been found to predict increased mortality for individuals who have not experienced a recent myocardial infarction but had coronary artery disease documented by cardiac catheterization (Barefoot et al., 1996). Increased risk of mortality due to depressive symptoms was independent of the severity of coronary artery disease and left ventricular function (Barefoot et al., 2000).

Depression as a Risk Factor for Cardiovascular Disease in Community Samples

A growing body of literature is documenting that individuals with depression who have no known clinical heart disease are at an increased risk for subsequent or incident cardiovascular disease (Musselman, Evans, & Nemeroff, 1998). Although a few older studies found no relationship between depression and incident coronary artery disease, more recent studies have consistently reported a positive association (Goldberg, Comstock, & Hornstra, 1979; Vogt, Pope, Mullooly, & Hollis, 1994). The association is modest in strength: Individuals with depression have about twice the risk as those who never experienced depression. Study designs have been mostly prospective and observational. The association has been reported for populations in the United States, Great Britain, Canada, Finland, and the Netherlands (Everson et al., 1996; Hippisley-Cox, Fielding, & Pringle, 1998;

Murphy, Neff, Sobol, Rick, & Olivier, 1985; Penninx et al., 2001; Pratt et al., 1996). In addition to the cohort studies, a case-control study from Great Britain found a positive association between depression and coronary artery disease using a general practice case registry (Hippisley-Cox et al., 1998). In this study, a recorded diagnosis of depression was three times more common in men with a myocardial infarction than in controls of the same age who had not experienced a myocardial infarction.

The optimal datasets to assess the relationship between depression and coronary artery disease would have in-depth data on both psychiatric symptomatology and cardiovascular risk factors and outcomes. However, researchers usually have had to choose datasets that only measure one of the variables in depth. The Baltimore Epidemiology Catchment Area study is one of the best datasets measuring psychopathology in a community sample. However, data on cardiovascular disease and associated risk factors are limited. As part of this study, 3,481 individuals were selected from a 1981 household survey to have an assessment of their psychiatric and medical status. Trained lay interviewers completed the interviews with the Diagnostic Interview Survey (DIS). Affective disorders and some anxiety disorders (phobias, panic disorder, obsessive–compulsive) were measured, but not posttraumatic stress disorder or generalized anxiety disorder. Thirteen years later survivors were located and interviewed (Pratt et al., 1996). Sixty-four individuals reported that they had survived a myocardial infarction. Using these data, Pratt and colleagues reported that the adjusted relative risk for developing a myocardial infarction was 4.1 times higher in individuals who met criteria for an episode of major depression sometime in their lifetime. An intermediate risk was found for those only reporting dysphoria of 2 weeks duration or more. Interestingly, the anxiety disorders measured were not associated with an elevated risk for myocardial infarction. Results were adjusted for age, self-reported hypertension, diabetes, and smoking. There was no measurement of lipids, blood pressure, or exercise at baseline. In addition, the results were based on self-reported myocardial infarctions for survivors. At this time, additional analyses based on medical records and death certificates are under way. These results are important because they originate from a community sample followed for a relatively long period, and the effect of depressive disorders and anxiety disorders could be directly evaluated.

The Johns Hopkins Precursors Study provides a complementary perspective because excellent measures of cardiovascular risk factors were available, although the measure of depression was not standard. All of the participants are physicians, and they were asked for several decades if they had ever had an episode of clinical depression. Follow-up was more than 35 years in duration (Ford et al., 1998). Adjusting for the established cardiovascular risk factors did not substantially alter the risk estimate for clinical depression on subsequent coronary artery disease. As in other studies, those with depression had about a doubling of risk for subsequent myocardial infarction. An analysis of data from a randomized clinical trial of blood pressure treatment with excellent measures of potential cardiovascular risk factor confounders also indicated that increasing levels of depression predicted incident myocardial infarctions and stroke (Wassertheil-Smoller et al., 1996).

SPECIFICITY OF MEASUREMENT OF DEPRESSION AND RISK OF CHD

Depression is probably a heterogeneous condition that can be measured in multiple ways. One might question if the risk of coronary artery disease is present across a broad range of measurement techniques. In studies as of this writing, depression has most often been measured with self-report questionnaires like the Center for Epidemiologic Studies Depression questionnaire (CES-D; Simonsick, Wallace, Blazer, & Berkman, 1995; Wassertheil-Smoller et al., 1996) Two studies using the Minnesota Multiphasic Personality Inventory (MMPI) did not find an association (Brozek, Keyes, & Blackburn, 1966; Ostfeld, Lebovits, Shekelle, & Paul, 1964), but one did (Gillum, Leon, Kamp, & Becerra-Aldama, 2000). Major depression as assessed by the DIS had a stronger relationship than dysphoria to myocardial infarction in one study (Pratt et al., 1996). A recent study has found a clear stepwise relationship between the severity of depression and subsequent heart disease (Penninx et al., 2001). In this study, a sample of 2,847 men and women between 55 and 85 years of age living in the Netherlands completed the CES-D at baseline and were followed for 4 years. Endpoints included self-reported coronary artery disease, physician reports, and death certificates. Compared with those with CES-D scores less than 3, those with CES-D scores between 3 and 15 had a relative risk of 1.5, and those with a CES-D score above 24 had a relative risk of 3.2 for coronary artery disease. Overall, the evidence suggests that there is no clear threshold beyond which depression is associated with an elevated risk of coronary artery disease.

Some investigators have focused on depression-related symptoms or demoralization. Hopelessness and high scores on the depression subscale of the General Well-Being Scale predict coronary artery disease (Anda et al., 1993). A study of Finnish men (Kupio Ischemic Heart Disease Study) found that hopelessness predicted myocardial infarction even after controlling for depressive symptoms as measured with the MMPI Depression Scale (Everson et al., 1996). Excess fatigue or vital exhaustion has also been reported as a risk factor for myocardial infarction (Appels & Mulder, 1988). The evidence therefore supports the conclusion that depression, measured in multiple ways, is associated with coronary artery disease.

POPULATION SUBGROUPS AND RELATIONSHIP BETWEEN DEPRESSION AND CAD

Within several of the studies investigating depression and coronary artery disease, some subgroups were found to have a stronger association between depression and coronary heart disease. However, the subgroup with the highest risk has not been consistent. In the New Haven Established Populations for Epidemiologic Studies of the Elderly (EPESE) sample of adults age 65 and older, there was no relationship between depression and coronary heart disease in men; the association only held for women (Mendes de Leon et al., 1998). The SHEP study also found slightly stronger associations for older women than for men (Wassertheil-Smoller et al., 1996). Other studies have found the association between depression and coronary heart disease to be stronger in men than in women (Hippisley-Cox et al., 1998). The Precursors Study was almost exclusively male, yet found a significant association (Ford et al., 1998). However equivalent results were seen for the small number of women in the study. Neither the reports from the Baltimore Epidemiologic Catchment Area (ECA) nor the National Health and Nutrition Examination Survey (NHANES) sample described any differences by gender (Anda et al., 1993; Ferketich, Schwartzbaum, Frid, & Moeschberger, 2000; Hippisley-Cox et al., 1998; Prochazka et al., 1998; Turner-Cobb, Sephton, Koopman, Blake-Mortimer, & Spiegel, 2000). In general, there appear to be slightly stronger associations between depression and coronary heart disease for middle-age adults as compared with older adults. This would be similar to what is found with many cardiovascular risk factors. Older adults may include a subset of individuals who are not vulnerable to known cardiac risk factors present in young to middle age. The risk for coronary heart disease associated with depression appears to be stronger or more easily detected in older adults with minimal physical impairments as compared with those older adults with impairments (Mendes de Leon et al., 1998).

The data from all of the studies clearly indicate that the association between coronary heart disease and depression is not due to confusion about the temporal order of which condition came first. The risk of a cardiovascular event after an episode of depression does not appear to decrease over time. For example, in the Precursors Study, the median time between first report of depression and first cardiovascular event was 15 years (Ford et al., 1998). In the EPESE report, the association between depression and coronary heart disease mortality was much higher for coronary heart disease outcomes occurring after 3 years than for those outcomes occurring in the first 3 years of follow-up (Mendes de Leon et al., 1998). Most alarming is that the risk associated with depression has not been demonstrated to decrease with time. Risk for myocardial infarction was still elevated more than 10 years after report of first depression in the Precursor's sample (Ford et al., 1998). The Baltimore ECA data indicate that the elevated risk for myocardial infarction is the same in the later years of the 13-year follow-up as at the beginning when lifetime depression was assessed (Pratt et al., 1996). Even after more than 10 years of follow-up in the sample with known coronary artery disease, depression continued to predict poorer survival (Barefoot et al., 1996). Although the current evidence is not ideal because it does not include measures of resolution of depressive symptoms, the best interpretation of the data at this time is that once an individual has had a depressive episode, risk for cardiovascular disease remains elevated indefinitely. If this is the case, primary prevention of depression as well as investigation of the mechanisms for increased risk need to become research priorities. However, future research needs to more carefully assess the course of the depression, and, because it is a recurrent and chronic disorder, consider if multiple episodes are associated with higher risk than a single episode.

DEPRESSION AND STROKE

Although the vast majority of research has focused on coronary artery disease as the disease outcome, several recent studies have evaluated whether depression is a risk factor for incident stroke, another important clinical manifestation of vascular disease. There are now five naturalistic studies of community-based populations that have found depression to be associated with an elevated risk for stroke. These studies were conducted in several different countries. Each controlled for hypertension, the major known risk factor for stroke. A report based on the Alameda county sample found that individuals reporting five or more symptoms of depression were 50% more likely to die from a stroke-related cause during a 29-year follow-up period (Everson, Roberts, Goldberg, & Kaplan, 1998). Nonfatal strokes were not included in these analyses. The results were adjusted for educational level, smoking, alcohol consumption, body mass index, hypertension, and diabetes. A general observation is that adjustment for established cardiovascular risk factors does not substantially change the estimates for the risks associated with depression. An Australian study found that older adults in the highest tertile of depression symptoms as measured by the CES-D had a 41% higher risk for ischemic stroke than those in the lowest tertile (Simons, McCallum, Friedlander, & Simons, 1998).

Japanese populations have a different pattern of cardiovascular disease characterized by low levels of cholesterol, higher levels of blood pressure, and a relative predominance of strokes as compared to myocardial infarctions. Ohira reported on a sample of men and women living in a rural Japanese community who completed the Zung Self-Rating Depression Scale at baseline along with a complete assessment of cardiovascular risk factors (Ohira et al., 2001). The sample was followed for 10 years. Those in the highest tertile for depressive symptoms at baseline had a twofold increased risk for stroke compared with the lowest tertile, even after controlling for level of systolic blood pressure, alcohol intake, and cigarette smoking. Ninety percent of the strokes were confirmed by CT scans, which allowed the investigators to explore the possible mechanism for how depression might increase risk for stroke. Although power to detect an association between depressive symptoms and hemorrhagic stroke was limited, depressive symptoms were clearly related to ischemic, and not hemorrhagic, strokes. Such a pattern suggests that depression may cause stroke by promoting atherosclerosis.

Two reports have been based on samples in the United States. Jonas and collaborators (Jonas, Franks, & Ingram, 1997) found that depressive symptoms were associated with higher risk for incident stroke in the NHANES I sample after 22 years of follow-up. This study had excellent measures of blood pressure and clinical endpoints but a limited measurement of depression. The second report is based on the Baltimore Epidemiologic Catchment Area Study. Individuals with a lifetime history of major depression were 2.6 times more likely to have had a stroke even after the investigators adjusted for age, ethnicity, socioeconomic status, tobacco smoking, and a self-reported history of hypertension, diabetes, or heart disease. In this study, 11% of the strokes could be attributed to depression (Larson, Owens, Ford, & Eaton, 2001).

TREATMENT OF DEPRESSION AND RISK FOR CARDIOVASCULAR DISEASE

One reason for the interest in depression as a potential risk factor for cardiovascular disease is that effective treatment regimens for depression are available. Although the existing data do not provide confidence that treatment of depression reduces the risk for subsequent cardiac disease, methodically sound studies addressing the question have not been completed. In the Johns Hopkins Precursors Study, men who reported receiving treatment with antidepressants or psychotherapy with or without sedatives had slightly higher, although nonsignificant, risks for cardiovascular disease than those who reported no treatment for depression yet reported having a clinical depression (Ford et al., 1998). In the Baltimore ECA sample, lifetime use of psychotropic medication was associated with a slightly increased risk for myocardial infarction (relative risk = 1.36) as compared with not having used psychotropic medication, even after adjusting for depressive symptomatology. Use of tricyclic antidepressants, and a higher compared to a lower mean dose of tricyclic antidepressant, were associated with incident ischemic heart disease in the British case register sample (Hippisley-Cox et al., 1998, 2001). Several recent studies have also examined the effect of antidepressant medications on subsequent myocardial infarction without considering level of depressive symptoms (Cohen, Gibson, & Alderman, 2000; Sauer, Berlin, & Kimmel, 2001). The main conclusion is that the selective serotinergic reuptake inhibitors (SSRI) class of antidepressants seem to pose a lower risk for myocardial infarction than do the tricyclic antidepressants. These data certainly are not definitive because it is difficult to separate out severity of depression and use of medications in any naturalistic or observational study. However, it points out the need to understand the potential impact of treatment, a question of intense interest to health care providers and individuals with depression.

Results of interventions to improve survival for patients with depression and poor social support after a myocardial infarction have generally not been promising. However the interventions have not been focused specifically on depression and may not have been sufficiently powerful to reduce risks for subsequent cardiovascular disease. The Sertraline Anti-Depressant Heart Attack Trial (SADHAT), a randomized clinical trial evaluating the use of sertraline in patients with depression after a myocardial infarction, found sertraline to be safe, more effective than placebo in reducing depression, and associated with a trend toward reducing cardiovascular events (Glassman et al., 2002). Final results of the ENRICHD trial testing primarily a counseling approach for individuals with depression and myocardial infarction have not been published (The ENRICHD Investigators, 2000; Shapiro et al., 1999).

PROPOSED MECHANISMS FOR DEPRESSION INCREASING RISK FOR CARDIAC DISEASE

Several mechanisms have been proposed to explain the relationship between depression and coronary heart disease. As indicated in Figure 4.1, the simplest question is whether the health behaviors of patients with depression account for the elevated risk for cardiovascular disease. These health behaviors include tobacco smoking, alcohol use, dietary factors, physical activity, and adherence to treatment for cardiovascular risk factors like elevated blood pressure and hyperlipidemia. A second proposed pathway relates primarily to the underlying biology of depression (Musselman, Evans,

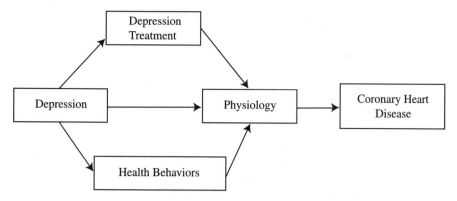

Figure 4.1. Potential mechanisms for depression causing coronary artery disease. Health behaviors include tobacco, alcohol, coffee, diet, physical activity, and adherence to treatment of cardiovascular risk factors. Physiology includes lipids, blood pressure, glucose, obesity, heart rate variability, inflammation, and platelet function (hypothalamic–pituitary–adrenocortical axis and sympathoadrenal axis as potential mediators).

& Nemeroff, 1998). The medications used to treat depression should also be considered. It is safe to assume that these pathways interact with each other in complex ways yet to be understood. Of interest is the extent to which changes in the hypothalamic–pituitary–adrenocortical (HPA) axis and sympathoadrenal axis are mediators for the other biological systems. Patients with depression consistently demonstrate changes in their HPA axis and sympathoadrenal system (see Friedman & McEwen, chap. 7, this volume). Patients with major depression have elevated levels of corticotropin releasing factor (CRF) along with other changes in their HPA axis (Banki, Karmasci, Bissette, & Nemeroff, 1992; Nemeroff et al., 1984). The dexa-methasone suppression test has been found to have lower specificity than one would like in a diagnostic test, but cortisol levels are consistently higher in patients with major depression, particularly those with the more severe form of the disorder. In addition, an abnormal dexamethasone suppression test may predict who has a higher risk of being resistant to treatment and relapsing in the future (Carroll, 1986; Ritchie, Belkin, Krishnan, Nemeroff, & Carroll, 1990). Administered corticosteroids adversely affect several well-established coronary heart disease risk factors such as impaired glucose metabolism and blood pressure.

In terms of the sympathoadrenal system, higher levels of catecholamines have also been associated with major depression. Not only do depressed patients have higher basal plasma concentrations of norepinephrine, but those with melancholia exhibit even greater elevations in plasma norepi-nephrine if orthostatically challenged as compared with individuals without depression or depressed patients without melancholia (Roy, Guthrie, Pickar,

& Linnoila, 1987). Catecholamines have multiple effects on the body that might be related to the development of cardiovascular disease, such as impacting on the function of the heart, blood vessels, and platelets.

At this time, there are two areas in which the direct effects of disturbances in the HPA and sympathoadrenal systems on cardiovascular disease have been demonstrated: platelet activation and heart rate variability. Platelets play a central role in hemostasis, thrombosis, development of atherosclerosis, and acute coronary syndromes through interactions both with subendothelial components of damaged vessel walls and plasma coagulation factors like thrombin. Platelets may affect both atherogenesis and acute thrombus formation on top of existing atherosclerotic plaques. Human platelets contain adrenergic, serotonergic, and dopaminergic receptors, which suggests a mechanism for how depression might impact on platelet function. Small studies of patients with depression have demonstrated that platelet function is altered in such a way that clotting would be more likely, and might be reversible, with use of the antidepressant paroxetine (Musselman et al., 1996, 2000). Overall, further research into platelet function of individuals with depression appears to be a promising area for future investigation.

Abnormalities of the sympathoadrenal system in patients with depression may also lead to changes in heart rate variability. Heart rate variability reflects the balance between sympathetic and parasympathetic tone on the cardiac pacemaker (Berntson et al., 1997). Several studies have reported that decreased heart rate variability is associated with increased mortality after a myocardial infarction (Kleiger, Miller, Bigger, & Moss, 1987; Odemuyiwa et al., 1991), and there is now evidence that decreased heart rate variability may predict cardiovascular mortality (Liao et al., 1997; Tsuji et al., 1994). Most, but not all studies, have found that depressed patients have lower heart rate variability (Beardsley, Gardocki, Larson, & Hidalgo, 1988; Carney et al., 1995; Miyawaki & Salzman, 1991; Rechlin, Weis, & Claus, 1994) perhaps reflecting decreased parasympathetic tone. There is considerably less information regarding whether treatment of depression increases heart rate variability. One nonblinded study found that heart rate variability returned to normal after effective treatment (Balogh, Fitzpatrick, Hendricks, & Paige, 1993). Another study found that some aspects of heart rate variability returned toward normal after treatment with cognitive–behavioral therapy in patients with known CHD and major depression (Carney et al., 2000). The early evidence is intriguing that heart rate variability might provide new insights into the biology of depression and the link between depression and coronary heart disease.

Green and Kimerling (chap. 2, this volume) cite several studies reporting that PTSD is associated with increased risk of cardiovascular disorder. Schnurr and Jankowski (1999) suggested that similar biological mechanisms might mediate the effects of PTSD on cardiovascular disorder: sympathoadrenal hyperactivity, diminished heart rate variability, and platelet aggregation. To date there is only limited evidence of diminished heart rate variability (Cohen, Benjamin, et al., 2000) in PTSD, and no information about platelet aggregation, but Friedman and McEwen (chap. 7, this volume) document substantial evidence of excessive sympathoadrenal activity in PTSD. Friedman and McEwen also present conflicting findings on the HPA axis in PTSD, but clear evidence of dysregulation. Thus, there is a reasonable probability that PTSD, like depression, is associated with coronary heart disease.

RELATIONSHIP BETWEEN DEPRESSION AND TRADITIONAL CARDIOVASCULAR RISK FACTORS

Even though we are learning more about the biological consequences of depression and how depression might increase risk for coronary artery disease, it is important to determine the extent to which the pathway includes changes in traditional cardiovascular risk factors. For example, if all of the cardiovascular risk related to depression was mediated by elevated lipid levels, the best approach to reducing risk would probably be to target lipid abnormalities. If the elevated risk is not mediated by known cardiovascular risk factors, a more creative strategy will be needed to reduce overall risk. A brief review of the relationship between depression and known cardiovascular risk factors follows.

There are several reports suggesting that depression is a risk factor for the development of hypertension. Probably the most rigorous study of this topic has been by Jonas, Franks, and Ingram (1997). They reported on the 14,407 individuals between the ages of 25 and 74 in the NHANES-I Epidemiologic Follow-up Study who were initially free of hypertension by standardized blood pressure measurement. Anxiety and depression were measured with two 4-item scales from the General Well-Being Schedule. The sample was followed for 16 years. Even after controlling for baseline age, gender, education, systolic blood pressure, body mass index, alcohol use, and history of diabetes, stroke, and coronary artery disease, high levels of anxiety and depression were associated with about twice the risk for developing hypertension. Depression and anxiety were so highly correlated they could not assess the independent contribution of each. It is important to note that for this study, alcohol use was measured in a rather crude fashion. Because alcohol consumption above two or three alcohol drinks per day strongly predicts the onset of hypertension, this deficiency may be important. They also could not adjust for the increased use of health care services associated with anxiety and depression that might have led to a biased determination of elevated blood pressure. Other studies have not found a clear relationship between depression or anxiety and the development of hypertension (Goldberg, Comstock, & Graves, 1980; Kahn, Medalie, Neufeld, Riss, & Goldbourt, 1972). If depression and anxiety are related to elevated blood pressure, the effect appears to be relatively small and probably would not account for the relationship between depression and coronary artery disease. Including blood pressure in multivariate models has not substantially changed the risk for coronary artery disease associated with depression.

The relationship between depression and lipid metabolism is somewhat more complicated. In general there does not appear to be a positive association between depression and elevated levels of total cholesterol. Patients with depression generally have similar mean levels of total cholesterol to those without depression. However, some evidence indicates that individuals with markedly low levels of total cholesterol are slightly more likely to develop depression. Observational studies have suggested that those who commit suicide are more likely to have a very low serum cholesterol level (Ellison & Morrison, 2001; Steegmans, Hoes, Bak, van der Does, & Grobbee, 2000). However, randomized clinical trials to lower cholesterol either through medication or dietary approaches have not found higher levels of depression in those who successfully lower their cholesterol (Stewart et al., 2000; Wardle et al., 2000). Long-term assessment of psychological well-being in a large randomized placebo controlled trial of cholesterol reduction with pravastatin did not find any increase in depression with lowering of lipids (Stewart et al., 2000). One possible explanation might be that a common genetic predisposition is associated with low total cholesterol and depression, but that one does not impact on the other. The possible inverse relationship between depression and total cholesterol makes it very unlikely that cholesterol is an important mediator for the effect of depression on coronary artery disease.

The one established cardiovascular risk factor most strongly associated with depression is tobacco smoking. Patients with depression are more likely to smoke cigarettes and are also less likely to be able to quit (Covey, Glassman, & Stetner, 1998; Glassman et al., 1990). These associations are primarily based on cross-sectional data, and risk is probably limited to regular smokers, particularly those who are nicotine dependent (Breslau, Kilbey, & Andreski, 1991). These relationships hold throughout the life course. Several studies have found that antidepressant medications like bupropion and nortriptyline can increase the probability that smoking cessation attempts are successful even in smokers who do not meet criteria for current depression (Hurt et al., 1997; Jorenby et al., 1999; Prochazka et al., 1998). It is possible that the observed association between depression and coronary artery disease could be at least partially be explained by a bias in reporting of tobacco use. For example, if smokers with depression systematically underreport the extent of their smoking compared with smokers without depression, this reporting discrepancy might account or partially account for the association between depression and coronary artery disease found in the observational studies. The risk attributed to depression might actually be due to greater exposure to tobacco than inferred from the measured data. In addition, several studies have found that tobacco smokers with depression are particularly prone to increased coronary artery disease as compared with nonsmokers with depression (Anda et al., 1993; Ford et al., 1998).

Individuals with depression may be more likely to have other unhealthy behaviors that would contribute to increased risk of coronary artery disease. Substantial research indicates that individuals with depression are more likely to drink alcohol. However, the relationship between alcohol consumption and coronary artery disease is complex. Abstainers from alcohol appear to have a higher risk for coronary artery disease than those consuming 1–2 drinks per day. Only if consumption goes above 3 alcoholic drinks per day does the risk for cardiovascular disease substantially increase.

Although most observational studies have found a negative association between depression and levels of physical activity, there have been exceptions (Byrne & Byrne, 1993; Farmer et al., 1988). However, many of these studies have not isolated the effect of exercise independent of the social interaction that frequently accompanies physical activity. One randomized clinical trial found that individuals with major depression randomized to an exercise regimen did as well as those randomized to sertraline (Blumenthal et al., 1999). The interaction between depressed mood and exercise is probably a complex phenomenon related to motivational levels and coping strategies. Current studies assessing the risk of depression and CAD have not consistently accounted for levels of physical activity. The few studies that have did not find that physical activity mediated the relationship.

DEPRESSION AND ADHERENCE TO MEDICAL TREATMENT

With the advent of multiple proven interventions to reduce risk of cardiac disease, nonadherence to recommended preventive interventions such as taking aspirin, antihypertensives, and lipid-lowering medications may now be considered a risk factor for development of CHD. Most health professionals believe that patients with depression are less adherent to medical care recommendations; however, empirical findings do not completely support this belief. Patients with depression have more ambulatory care visits to both general medical and specialty mental health providers than those without depression, and number of visits to providers is one of the best predictors of adherence to recommended treatments. One community-based study found that individuals with major depression who reported having a chronic medical condition were just as likely to be receiving regular medical care as those without major depression. Those individuals with chronic medical problems who were not in care were more likely to have other mental disorders like alcohol abuse and phobias (Cooper-Patrick, Crum, Pratt, Eaton, & Ford, 1999). The sense of pessimism and hopelessness associated with depression may influence health perceptions about their chronic medical conditions. For example, patients with depression may be more likely to feel susceptible to future disease or less likely to believe they can change their level of risk. These beliefs are components of the Health Belief Model, a moderate predictor of adherence to medical treatments. Surprisingly, even within the randomized clinical trials in which excellent markers of adherence should be available, investigators have not commented on the extent to which adherence might mediate the association between depression and coronary heart disease. Depression in individuals surviving myocardial infarctions has been associated with lowered adherence to aspirin intake, low-fat diets, regular exercise, and stress reduction (Carney et al., 1998). A meta-analysis found that there was a substantial relationship between depression and noncompliance with medical treatment, although the number and rigor of the studies was not high (DiMatteo, Lepper, & Croghan, 2000). The need to learn more about the causal mechanism for these relationships was the primary conclusion of this meta-analysis.

HOSTILITY AND HEART DISEASE

Hostility or anger is a common symptom in PTSD and increasingly is being found to be a risk factor for coronary artery disease. In cardiovascular research, hostility is usually measured with the Cook-Medley scale. This 50-item questionnaire was derived from the Minnesota Multiphasic Personality Inventory and measures the construct of cynical hostility (Barefoot, Dodge, Peterson, Dahlstrom, & Williams, 1989). Although not all studies have found an association between hostility and coronary artery disease (Helmer, Ragland, & Syme, 1991), hostility has been reported to be a risk factor for angiographically documented coronary artery disease (Barefoot et al., 1994), myocardial infarction (Dembroski, MacDougall, Costa, & Grandits, 1989; Everson, Kauhanen, & Kaplan, 1997), and total mortality (Hearn, Murray, & Luepker, 1989). A study of adults between 18 and 30 years old found that higher hostility scores were related to higher levels of calcification in the coronary arteries (Iribarren et al., 2000). Calcification of the coronary arteries is a measure of subclinical (the earliest form of) atherosclerosis and is not dependent on clinical diagnosis. These results were adjusted for demographic, lifestyle, and physiological risk factors. The results were not adjusted for depression or measures of social isolation, which is true for most of the studies of hostility and CHD. In addition, some data indicate that the risk for CAD is only present at the highest level of hostility (Chang, Ford, Meoni, Wang, & Klag, 2002) and that the contribution of hostility to overall CAD incidence is marginal (Myrteck, 2001). Hostility has been linked to increased cardiovascular reactivity, prolonged increased levels of catecholamines, and platelet activation. Although hostility may affect the long-term process of atherosclerosis, it has been linked in some studies as a trigger of immediate cardiac events (Mittleman et al., 1996). Future studies linking traumatic events and subsequent cardiovascular disease need to carefully measure both hostility and depression because both are common in individuals with PTSD.

CONCLUSIONS AND FUTURE DIRECTIONS

The large body of research related to depression and coronary artery disease provides one of the best examples for understanding the relationship between mental disorders and physical health outcomes. The field has moved forward by first concentrating on well-designed observational studies of individuals with preexisting coronary artery disease, followed by community studies of individuals without any known heart disease. A similar progression of research is needed to better understand the effects of PTSD on CAD. As in depression, the search to understand the mechanisms by which PTSD might increase risk for coronary artery disease needs to carefully account for the impact of both PTSD and depression on biological factors and the interaction with treatment regimens targeting both disorders and cardiovascular risk factors. Social factors cannot be ignored either. For example, the growing literature that low socioeconomic status and social isolation may act as risk factors for coronary artery disease has not been carefully considered in the studies linking depression with coronary artery disease.

However, there remain several important deficits in our understanding of how mental disorders might be causally related to physical illnesses. Existing research has not adequately addressed diagnostic issues regarding mental disorders. Although psychiatric comorbidity is common in the real world, many of the current studies do not consider psychiatric comorbidity in their interpretation of the findings. For example, community-based surveys indicate that the majority of individuals with PTSD meet criteria for an additional mental disorder. Many individuals with PTSD have three or more other mental disorders (Kessler et al., 1995). The overlap with depression, anxiety disorders, and substance abuse is considerable, and there may be differences, as well as similarities, among these disorders in both mechanisms for and risk of different physical disorders. Although clinically oriented researchers tend to focus on mental disorders, there has also been considerable research that psychological symptoms such as anger or insomnia may also act as risk factors for cardiovascular disease (Hemingway & Marmot, 1999; Schwartz et al., 1999). Future studies should evaluate whether the increased risk for coronary artery disease, and all medical diseases, can be linked to certain mental disorders, or symptom clusters within mental disorders.

Prospective observational studies will most likely remain the foundation for making inferences on whether depression, PTSD, or other mental disorders are independent risk factors for incident cardiovascular disease. Therefore skeptics will always suggest that potential confounders, like tobacco use, have not been accounted for with sufficient precision. Future studies clearly need to take these concerns to heart. For example, tobacco smoking measured only as "current," "past," or "never" is unlikely to be sufficient, as even small changes in tobacco exposure might be equivalent to the independent effect of the mental disorder. Smoking only 1–9 cigarettes per day has been associated with a statistically significant hazard ratio of 1.3 for total deaths even after adjusting for age, body mass index, serum cholesterol, systolic blood pressure, and the presence of clinical cardiovascular disease (Jacobs et al., 1999). Just as important is assessing tobacco smoking at more than one point in time. Around 50% of tobacco smokers in America quit smoking during their lifetime and the risk for cardiovascular disease approaches that of nonsmokers within 2–5 years. Multiple measurements of tobacco smoking, and probably other substances such as marijuana, should remain a priority for future studies.

Linking mental disorders to higher risk for subsequent physical illnesses is often difficult information to present to patients who have been diagnosed with these conditions. They are often already concerned about their physical health and facing many challenges in the recovery process. Clarifying the relationships between mental disorders and physical disorders may have a role in the effort to gain parity in insurance coverage for mental disorders. However, patients really want to know how they might reduce their increased risk for future disease. As expected, the most valuable knowledge related to whether treatment of mental disorders decreases risk for coronary artery disease is the most difficult to ascertain. Ongoing randomized clinical trials of interventions to reduce depression after a myocardial infarction will provide important first steps in our understanding of whether treatment will reduce subsequent risk for additional cardiovascular events or mortality. However, the long lag time between episodes of depression and first cardiovascular events makes it unlikely that randomized clinical trials assessing the impact of treatment of depression will be acceptable or ethical. Therefore, future research needs to also concentrate on understanding the biological mechanisms by which depression, PTSD, and other mental disorders may increase risk. Once these biological mechanisms are identified, we can begin to evaluate how different treatments for mental disorder affect subsequent risk for cardiac disease.

REFERENCES

American Heart Association. (2001). *Other cardiovascular diseases*. Retrieved July 26, 2001, from http://americanheart.org/statistics/othercvd.html

Anda, R., Williamson, D., Jones, D., Macera, C., Eaker, E., Glassman, A., et al. (1993). Depressed affect, hopelessness, and the risk of ischemic heart disease in a cohort of U.S. adults. *Epidemiology, 4*, 285–294.

Appels, A., & Mulder, P. (1988). Excess fatigue as a precursor of myocardial infarction. *European Heart Journal, 9*, 758–764.

Balogh, S., Fitzpatrick, D. F., Hendricks, S. E., & Paige, S. R. (1993). Increases in heart rate variability with successful treatment in patients with major depressive disorder. *Psychopharmacological Bulletin, 29*, 201–206.

Banki, C. M., Karmasci, L. I., Bissette, G., & Nemeroff, C. B. (1992). CSF corticotropin-releasing and somatostatin in major depression: Response to antidepressant treatment and relapse. *European Neuropsychopharmacology, 2*, 107–111.

Barefoot, J. C., Brummett, B. H., Clapp-Channing, N. E., Siegler, I. C., Vitaliano, P. P., Williams, R. B., et al. (2000). Moderators of the effect of social support on depressive symptoms in cardiac patients. *American Journal of Cardiology, 86*, 438–442.

Barefoot, J. C., Dodge, K. A., Peterson, B. L., Dahlstrom, W. G., & Williams, R. B., Jr. (1989). The Cook-Medley Hostility Scale: Item content and ability to predict survival. *Psychosomatic Medicine, 51*, 46–57.

Barefoot, J. C., Helms, M. J., Mark, D. B., Blumenthal, J. A., Califf, R. M., Haney, T. L., et al. (1996). Depression and long-term mortality risk in patients with coronary artery disease. *American Journal of Cardiology, 78*, 613–617.

Barefoot, J. C., Patterson, J. C., Haney, T. L., Cayton, T. G., Hickman, J. R., Jr., & Williams, R. B. (1994). Hostility in asymptomatic men and angiographically confirmed coronary artery disease. *American Journal of Cardiology, 74*, 439–442.

Beardsley, R. S., Gardocki, G. J., Larson, D. B., & Hidalgo, J. (1988). Prescribing of psychotropic medication by primary care physicians and psychiatrists. *Archives of General Psychiatry, 45*, 1117–1119.

Berntson, G. G., Bigger, J. T., Jr., Eckberg, D. L., Grossman, P., Kaufmann, P. G., Malik, M., et al. (1997). Heart rate variability: Origins, methods, and interpretive caveat. *Psychophysiology, 34*, 623–648.

Black, D. W. (1998). Iowa record-linkage study: Death rates in psychiatric patients. *Journal of Affective Disorders, 50*, 277–282.

Black, D. W., Winokur, G., & Nasrallah, A. (1987). Is death from natural causes still excessive in psychiatric patients? A follow-up of 1,593 patients with major affective disorder. *Journal of Nervous and Mental Disease, 175,* 674–680.

Blumenthal, J. A., Babyak, M. A., Moore, K. A., Craighead, W. E., Herman, S., Khatri, P., et al. (1999). Effects of exercise training on older patients with major depression. *Archives of Internal Medicine, 159,* 2349–2356.

Booth-Kewley, S., & Friedman, H. S. (1987). Psychological predictors of heart disease: A quantitative review. *Psychological Bulletin, 101,* 343–362.

Breslau, N., Davis, G. C., Peterson, E. L., & Schultz, L. R. (2000). A second look at comorbidity in victims of trauma: The posttraumatic stress disorder–major depression connection. *Biological Psychiatry, 48,* 902–909.

Breslau, N., Kilbey, M., & Andreski, P. (1991). Nicotine dependence, major depression, and anxiety in young adults. *Archives of General Psychiatry, 48,* 1069–1074.

Brozek, J., Keyes, A., & Blackburn, H. (1966). Personality differences between potential coronary and non-coronary subjects. *Annals of the New York Academy of Sciences: Vol. 134* (pp. 1057–1064). New York: New York Academy of Sciences.

Byrne, A., & Byrne, D. G. (1993). The effect of exercise on depression, anxiety, and other mood states: A review. *Journal of Psychosomatic Research, 37,* 565–574.

Carney, R. M., Freedland, K. E., Eisen, S. A., Rich, M. W., Skala, J. A., & Jaffe, A. S. (1998). Adherence to a prophylactic medication regimen in patients with symptomatic versus asymptomatic ischemic heart disease. *Behavioral Medicine, 24,* 35–39.

Carney, R. M., Freedland, K. E., Stein, P. K., Skala, J. A., Hoffman, P., & Jaffe, A. S. (2000). Change in heart rate and heart rate variability during treatment for depression in patients with coronary heart disease. *Psychosomatic Medicine, 62,* 639–647.

Carney, R. M., Saunders, R. D., Freedland, K. E., Stein, P., Rich, M. W., & Jaffe, A. S. (1995). Association of depression with reduced heart rate variability in coronary artery disease. *American Journal of Cardiology, 76,* 562–564.

Carroll, B. J. (1986). Informed use of dexamethasone suppression test. *Journal of Clinical Psychiatry, 47*(Suppl. 1), 10–12.

Chang, P. P., Ford, D. E., Meoni, L. A., Wang, N. Y., & Klag, M. J. (2002). Anger in young men and subsequent premature cardiovascular disease: The Precursors Study. *Archives of Internal Medicine, 162,* 901–906.

Cohen, H., Benjamin, J., Geva, A. B., Matar, M. A., Kaplan, Z., & Kotler, M. (2000). Autonomic dysregulation in panic disorder and in post-traumatic stress disorder: Application of power spectrum analysis of heart rate variability at rest and in response to recollection of trauma or panic attacks. *Psychiatry Research, 96,* 1–13.

Cohen, H., Gibson, G., & Alderman, M. H. (2000). Excess risk of myocardial infarction in patients treated with antidepressant medications: Association with use of tricyclic agents. *American Journal of Medicine, 108,* 87–88.

Cooper-Patrick, L., Crum, R. M., Pratt, L. A., Eaton, W. W., & Ford, D. E. (1999). The psychiatric profile of patients with chronic diseases who do not receive regular medical care. *International Journal of Psychiatry in Medicine, 29*, 165–180.

Covey, L. S., Glassman, A. H., & Stetner, F. (1998). Cigarette smoking and major depression. *Journal of Addictive Disorders, 17*, 35–46.

Dembroski, T. M., MacDougall, J. M., Costa, P. T., & Grandits, G. A. (1989). Components of hostility as predictors of sudden death and myocardial infarction in the multiple risk factor intervention trial. *Psychosomatic Medicine, 51*, 514–522.

DiMatteo, M. R., Lepper, H. S., & Croghan, T. W. (2000). Depression is a risk factor for noncompliance with medical treatment: Meta-analysis of the effects of anxiety and depression on patient adherence. *Archives of Internal Medicine, 160*, 2101–2107.

Ellison, L. F., & Morrison, H. I. (2001). Low serum cholesterol concentration and risk of suicide. *Epidemiology, 12*, 168–172.

The ENRICHD Investigators. (2000). Enhancing recovery in coronary heart disease patients (ENRICHD): Study design and methods. *American Heart Journal, 139*, 1–9.

Everson, S. A., Goldberg, D. E., Kaplan, G. A., Cohen, R. D., Pukkala, E., Tuomilehto, J., et al. (1996). Hopelessness and risk of mortality and incidence of myocardial infarction and cancer. *Psychosomatic Medicine, 58*, 113–121.

Everson, S. A., Kauhanen, J., & Kaplan, G. A. (1997). Hostility and increased risk of mortality and acute myocardial infarction. *American Journal of Epidemiology, 146*, 142–152.

Everson, S. A., Roberts, R. E., Goldberg, D. E., & Kaplan, G. A. (1998). Depressive symptoms and increased risk of stroke mortality over a 29-year period. *Archives of Internal Medicine, 158*, 1133–1138.

Farmer, M. E., Locke, B. Z., Moscicki, E. K., Dannenberg, A. L., Larson, D. B., & Radloff, L. S. (1988). Physical activity and depressive symptoms: The NHANES I Epidemiologic Follow-up Study. *American Journal of Epidemiology, 128*, 1340–1351.

Ferketich, A. K., Schwartzbaum, J. A., Frid, D. J., & Moeschberger, M. L. (2000). Depression as an antecedent to heart disease among women and men in the NHANES I study. National Health and Nutrition Examination Survey. *Archives of Internal Medicine, 160*, 1261–1268.

Ford, D. E., Mead, L. A., Chang, P. P., Cooper-Patrick, L., Wang, N. Y., & Klag, M. (1998). Depression is a risk factor for coronary artery disease in men: The Precursors study. *Archives of Internal Medicine, 158*, 1422–1426.

Frasure-Smith, N., Lesperance, F., Juneau, M., Talajic, M., & Bourassa, M. G. (1999). Gender, depression, and one-year prognosis after myocardial infarction. *Psychosomatic Medicine, 61*, 26–37.

Frasure-Smith, N., Lesperance, F., & Talajic, M. (1995). Depression and 18-month prognosis after myocardial infarction. *Circulation, 91*, 999–1005.

Gillum, R., Leon, G. R., Kamp, J., & Becerra-Aldama, J. (2000). Prediction of cardiovascular and other disease onset and mortality from 30-year longitudinal MMPI data. *Journal of Consulting and Clinical Psychology, 48,* 405–406.

Glassman, A. H., Helzer, J. E., Covey, L. S., Cottler, L. B., Stetner, F., Tipp, J. E., et al. (1990). Smoking, smoking cessation, and major depression. *Journal of the American Medical Association, 264,* 1546–1549.

Glassman, A. H., O'Connor, C. M., Califf, R. M., Swedberg, K., Schwartz, P., Bigger, J. T., Jr., et al. (2002). Sertraline treatment of major depression in patients with acute MI or unstable angina. *Journal of the American Medical Association, 288,* 701–709.

Glassman, A. H., & Shapiro, P. A. (1998). Depression and the course of coronary artery disease. *American Journal of Psychiatry, 155,* 4–11.

Goldberg, E. L., Comstock, G. W., & Graves, C. G. (1980). Psychosocial factors and blood pressure. *Psychological Medicine, 10,* 243–255.

Goldberg, E. L., Comstock, G. W., & Hornstra, R. K. (1979). Depressed mood and subsequent physical illness. *American Journal of Psychiatry, 136,* 530–534.

Hearn, M. D., Murray, D. M., & Luepker, R. V. (1989). Hostility, coronary artery disease, and total mortality. *Behavioral Medicine, 12,* 105–121.

Helmer, D. C., Ragland, D. R., & Syme, S. L. (1991). Hostility and coronary artery disease, and total mortality. *American Journal of Epidemiology, 133,* 112–122.

Hemingway, H., & Marmot, M. (1999). Psychosocial factors in the aetiology and prognosis of coronary heart disease: Systematic review of prospective cohort studies. *British Medical Journal, 318,* 1460–1467.

Hippisley-Cox, J., Fielding, K., & Pringle, M. (1998). Depression as a risk factor for ischaemic heart disease in men: Population based case-control study. *British Medical Journal, 316,* 1714–1719.

Hippisley-Cox, J., Pringle, M., Hammersley, V., Crown, N., Wynn, A., Meal, A., et al. (2001). Antidepressants as risk factor for ischaemic heart disease: Case-control study in primary care. *British Medical Journal, 323,* 666–669.

Hurt, R. D., Sachs, D. P. L., Glover, E. D., Offord, K. P., Johnston, J. A., Dale, L. C., et al. (1997). A comparison of sustained-release bupropion and placebo for smoking cessation. *New England Journal of Medicine, 337,* 1195–1202.

Iribarren, C., Sidney, S., Bild, D., Liu, K., Markoviyz, J. H., Roseman, J. M., & Matthews, K. (2000). Association of hostility with coronary artery calcification in young adults: The CARDIA study. *Journal of the American Medical Association, 283,* 2546–2551.

Jacobs, D. R., Jr., Adachi, H., Mulder, I., Kromhout, D., Menotti, A., Nissinen, A., et al. (1999). Cigarette smoking and mortality risk: Twenty-five-year follow-up of the Seven Countries Study. *Archives of Internal Medicine, 159,* 733–740.

Jonas, B. S., Franks, P., & Ingram, D. D. (1997). Are symptoms of anxiety and depression risk factors for hypertension? *Archives of Family Medicine, 6,* 43–49.

Jorenby, D. E., Leischow, S. J., Nides, M. A., Rennard, S. I., Johnston, J. A., Hughes, A. R., et al. (1999). A controlled trial of sustained-release bupropion, a nicotine patch, or both for smoking cessation. *New England Journal of Medicine, 340,* 685–691.

Kahn, H. A., Medalie, J. H., Neufeld, H. N., Riss, E., & Goldbourt, U. (1972). The incidence of hypertension and associated factors: The Israel Ischemic Heart Disease study. *American Heart Journal, 84,* 171–182.

Kessler, D. C., Sonnega, A., Bromet, E., Hughes, M., & Nelson, C. B. (1995). Posttraumatic stress disorder in the National Comorbidity Survey. *Archives of General Psychiatry, 52,* 1048–1060.

Kleiger, R. E., Miller, I. P., Bigger, J. T., Jr., & Moss, A. J. (1987). Decreased heart rate variability and its association with increased mortality after acute myocardial infarction. *American Journal of Cardiology, 59,* 256–262.

Larson, S. L., Owens, P. L., Ford, D., & Eaton, W. (2001). Depressive disorders, dysthymia and risk of stroke: A thirteen-year follow-up from the Baltimore ECA. *Stroke, 32,* 1979–1983.

Liao, D., Cai, J., Rosamond, W. D., Barnes, R. W., Hutchinson, R. G., Whitsel, E. A., et al. (1997). Cardiac autonomic function and incident coronary heart disease: A population-based case-cohort study. *American Journal of Epidemiology, 145,* 696–706.

Mendes de Leon, C. F., Krumholz, H. M., Seeman, T. S., Vaccarino, V., Williams, C. S., Kasl, S. V., et al. (1998). Depression and risk of coronary heart disease in elderly men and women: New Haven EPESE, 1982–1991. Established Populations for the Epidemiologic Studies of the Elderly. *Archives of Internal Medicine, 158,* 2341–2348.

Miranda, J., Chung, J. Y., Green, B. L., Krupnick, J., Siddique, J., Revicki, D. A., et al. (2003). Treating depression in predominately low-income young minority women: A randomized controlled trial. *Journal of the American Medical Association, 290,* 57–65.

Mittleman, M. A., Maclure, M., Sherwood, J. B., Mulry, R. P., Tofler, G. H. Jacob, S. C., et al. (1996). Triggering of acute myocardial infarction onset by episodes of anger: Determinants of Myocardial Infarction Onset Study Investigators. *Circulation, 92,* 1720–1725.

Miyawaki, E., & Salzman, C. (1991). Autonomic nervous system tests in psychiatry: Implications and potential uses of heart rate variability. *Integrative Psychiatry, 7,* 21–28.

Murphy, J. M., Neff, R. K., Sobol, A. M., Rick, J. X., & Olivier, D. C. (1985). Computer diagnosis of depression and anxiety: The Stirling County Study. *Psychological Medicine, 15,* 99–112.

Musselman, D. L., Evans, D. L., & Nemeroff, C. B. (1998). The relationship of depression to cardiovascular disease. *Archives of General Psychiatry, 55,* 580–592.

Musselman, D. L., Marzec, U. M., Manatunga, A. K., Penna, S., Reemsnyder, A., Knight, B. T., et al. (2000). Platelet reactivity in depressed patients treated with paroxetine: Preliminary findings. *Archives of General Psychiatry, 57,* 875–882.

Musselman, D. L., Tomer, A., Manatunga, A. K., Knight, B. T., Porter, M. R., Kasey, S., et al. (1996). Exaggerated platelet reactivity in major depression. *American Journal of Psychiatry, 153,* 1313–1317.

Myrteck, M. (2001). Meta-analyses of prospective studies on coronary heart disease, Type A personality, and hostility. *International Journal of Cardiology, 79,* 245–251.

Nemeroff, C. B., Widerlov, E., Bissette, G., Walleus, H., Karlsson, I., Eklund, K., et al. (1984). Elevated concentrations of CSF corticotropin-releasing factor-like immunoreactivity in depressed patients. *Science, 226,* 1342–1344.

Odemuyiwa, O., Malik, M., Farrel, T., Basher, Y., Poloniecke, J., & Camm, J. (1991). Comparison of heart rate variability index and left ventricular ejection fraction for all cause mortality, arrhythmic events, and sudden death after acute myocardial infarction. *American Journal of Cardiology, 68,* 434–439.

Ohira, T., Hiroyasu, I., Satoh, S., Sankai, T., Tanigawa, T., Ogawa, Y., et al. (2001). Prospective study of depressive symptoms and risk of stroke among Japanese. *Stroke, 32,* 903–908.

Ostfeld, A. M., Lebovits, B. Z., Shekelle, R. B., & Paul, O. (1964). A prospective study of the relationship between personality and coronary heart disease. *Journal of Chronic Disease, 17,* 265–276.

Penninx, B. J. H., Beekman, A. T. F., Honig, A., Deeg, D. J. H., Schoevers, R. A., van Eijk, J. T. M., et al. (2001). Depression and cardiac mortality. *Archives of General Psychiatry, 58,* 221–227.

Pratt, L. A., Ford, D. E., Crum, R. M., Armenian, H. K., Gallo, J. J., & Eaton, W. W. (1996). Depression, psychotropic medication, and risk of myocardial infarction. *Circulation, 94,* 3123–3129.

Prochazka, A. V., Weaver, M. J., Keller, R. T., Fryer, G. E., Licari, P. A., & Lofaso, D. (1998). A randomized trial of nortriptyline for smoking cessation. *Archives of Internal Medicine, 158,* 2035–2039.

Rechlin, T., Weis, M., & Claus, D. (1994). Heart rate variability in depressed patients and differential effects of paroxetine and amitriptyline on cardiovascular autonomic functions. *Pharmacopsychiatry, 27,* 124–128.

Ritchie, J. C., Belkin, B. M., Krishnan, K. R., Nemeroff, C. B., & Carroll, B. J. (1990). Plasma dexamethasone concentrations and the dexamethasone suppression test. *Biological Psychiatry, 27,* 159–173.

Roy, A., Guthrie, S., Pickar, D., & Linnoila, M. (1987). Plasma NE responses to cold challenge in depressed patients and normal controls. *Psychiatry Research, 21,* 161–168.

Sauer, W. H., Berlin, J. A., & Kimmel, S. E. (2001). Selective serotonin reuptake inhibitors and myocardial infarction. *Circulation, 104,* 1894.

Schnurr, P. P., & Jankowski, M. K. (1999). Physical health and post-traumatic stress disorder: Review and synthesis. *Seminars in Clinical Neuropsychiatry, 4,* 295–304.

Schwartz, S., Anderson, W. M., Cole, S. R., Cornoni-Huntley, J., Hays, J. C., & Blazer, D. (1999). Insomnia and heart disease: A review of epidemiologic studies. *Journal of Psychosomatic Research, 47,* 313–333.

Shapiro, P. A., Lesperance, F., Frasure-Smith, N., O'Connor, C. M., Baker, B., Jiang, J. W., et al. (1999). An open-label preliminary trial of sertraline for treatment of major depression after acute myocardial infarction (the SADHAT Trial): Sertraline Anti-Depressant Heart Attack Trial. *American Heart Journal, 137,* 1100–1106.

Simons, L. A., McCallum, J., Friedlander, Y., & Simons, J. (1998). Risk factors for ischemic stroke: Dubbo study of the elderly. *Stroke, 29,* 1341–1346.

Simonsick, E. M., Wallace, R. B., Blazer, D. G., & Berkman, L. F. (1995). Depressive symptomatology and hypertension-associated morbidity and mortality in older adults. *Psychosomatic Medicine, 57,* 427–435.

Steegmans, P. H., Hoes, A. W., Bak, A. A., van der Does, E., & Grobbee, D. E. (2000). Higher prevalence of depressive symptoms in middle-aged men with low serum cholesterol levels. *Psychosomatic Medicine, 62,* 205–211.

Stewart, R. A., Sharples, K. J., North, F. M., Menkes, D. B., Baker, J., & Simes, J. (2000). Long-term assessment of psychological well-being in a randomized placebo-controlled trial of cholesterol reduction with pravastatin. The LIPID Study Investigators. *Archives of Internal Medicine, 160,* 3144–3152.

Tsuji, H., Venditti, F. J., Manders, E. S., Evans, J. C., Larson, M. G., Feldman, C. L., et al. (1994). Reduced heart rate variability and mortality risk in an elderly cohort. *Circulation, 90,* 878–883.

Turner-Cobb, J. M., Sephton, S. E., Koopman, C., Blake-Mortimer, J., & Spiegel, D. (2000). Social support and salivary cortisol in women with metastatic breast cancer. *Psychosomatic Medicine, 62,* 337–345.

Vogt, T., Pope, C., Mullooly, J., & Hollis, J. (1994). Mental health status as a predictor of morbidity and mortality: A 15-year follow-up of members of a health maintenance organization. *American Journal of Public Health, 84,* 227–231.

Wardle, J., Rogers, P., Judd, P., Taylor, M. A., Rapoport, L., Green, M., et al. (2000). Randomized trial of the effects of cholesterol-lowering dietary treatment on psychological function. *American Journal of Medicine, 108,* 547–553.

Wassertheil-Smoller, S., Applegate, W. B., Berge, K., Chang, C. J., Davis, B. R., Grimm, R., et al. (1996). Change in depression as a precursor of cardiovascular events. *Archives of Internal Medicine, 156,* 553–561.

Wulsin, L. R., Vaillant, G. E., & Wells, V. E. (1999). A systematic review of the mortality of depression. *Psychosomatic Medicine, 61,* 6–17.

Zilber, N., Schufman, N., & Lerner, Y. (1989). Mortality among psychiatric patients: The groups at risk. *Acta Psychiatrica Scandinavia, 79,* 248–256.

5

COPING AND HEALTH: A COMPARISON OF THE STRESS AND TRAUMA LITERATURES

CAROLYN M. ALDWIN AND LORIENA A. YANCURA

More than 20,000 articles on stress and coping processes have been published in the past 2 decades (Aldwin, 1999); about 1,000 articles of these specifically examined how individuals cope with trauma. Given the magnitude of this literature, we do not provide a full review, but we briefly outline the different theoretical and methodological approaches to coping (see Aldwin, 1999; Lazarus, 2000; Schwarzer & Schwarzer, 1996). We then examine the similarities and differences between coping with general problems and coping with trauma. Finally, we review the relationship between coping and health outcomes, and focus on whether coping strategies can affect both the psychological and physical outcomes of trauma.

Preparation of this chapter was supported by Hatch Funds from the University of California Cooperative Extension Service. We would like to thank Crystal Park for her helpful comments on an earlier version of this chapter.

THEORETICAL AND METHODOLOGICAL APPROACHES TO COPING

There are three basic theoretical and methodological approaches to coping. Psychoanalytic approaches focus on the use of defense mechanisms, whereas personality approaches focus on coping styles. Both of these assume that adaptation is primarily a function of personal characteristics. In contrast, the coping process approach draws on cognitive–behavioral models and is more likely to emphasize environmental demands and influences on coping.

Psychoanalytic Approaches

Research on how individuals adapt grew out of early psychoanalytic studies of defense mechanisms, which are unconscious ways of warding off anxiety. In the classical definition, defense mechanisms are designated *a priori* as maladaptive and are not consciously chosen.

Cramer (2000) compared the similarities and differences between defense mechanisms and coping processes. Defense mechanisms are unconscious, nonintentional, dispositional, hierarchical, and associated with pathology, whereas coping processes are conscious, used intentionally, situationally determined, nonhierarchical, and associated with normality. Individuals can be characterized by primary defensive styles that they are likely to exhibit in many circumstances. In contrast, coping processes are thought to be consciously chosen and are responsive to environmental demands. Rather than hierarchically ordered, their effectiveness is thought to vary as a function of environmental demands.

Defense mechanisms are traditionally studied using intensive interviews and case studies. A number of inventories have been developed to assess defense mechanisms via self-report, but their psychometric properties are questionable (Cramer, 1991; Davidson & MacGregor, 1998). As Cramer (2000) pointed out, there is a logical inconsistency in asking individuals to report on unconscious processes, and researchers are more likely to use observational methods or rely on qualitative research, coding interview, or projective materials. Nonetheless, the study of defense mechanisms set the stage for understanding how people cope with both stress and trauma.

Coping Styles

The conception of coping styles borrowed some of its language from psychoanalysis but focused more on how people process information. The earliest typology was repression-sensitization (Byrne, 1964). Repressors avoid or suppress information, whereas sensitizers seek or augment information. This dichotomy has reappeared in different guises, with approach–avoidance

(Roth & Cohen, 1986) being the current manifestations of the dichotomy. Approach-monitoring-vigilant coping styles have been shown to be associated with better outcomes in a variety of situations, whereas repression-avoidant-blunting styles are associated with poorer outcomes (Aldwin, 1999; Roth & Cohen, 1986).

Dichotomizing coping strategies into two broad modalities is psychometrically appealing. Endler and Parker (1990) have shown that the factor structure of coping style inventories, which currently focus primarily on problem- versus emotion-focused coping, are more stable than process measures, and often correlate reasonably well with psychological symptom inventories. However, early research by Lazarus and his colleagues showed that both types of coping were used in more than 80% of episodes, and often individuals in highly stressful situations alternate between approaching and avoiding the problem (Folkman & Lazarus, 1980; see also Horowitz, 1986). Particular emotion-focused coping strategies may be more consistent across time, suggesting that individuals may have characteristic ways of dealing with and expressing emotion (Aldwin, 1999).

Coping Processes

The coping processes approach, drawing on the cognitive–behavioral perspective, argues that coping is flexible and responsive to environmental demands, as well as personal preferences. In this model, how individuals cognitively appraise situations is the primary determinant of how they cope. The four primary appraisals are benign, threat, harm or loss, and challenge, and these are influenced both by environmental demands and individual beliefs, values, and commitments (Lazarus & Folkman, 1984). Rather than examining general coping styles, coping process approaches examine how individuals cope with a particular stressor.

Coping process approaches have come under attack from a variety of perspectives. Critics have charged that the factor structures for such inventories as the Ways of Coping and the COPE (Carver, Scheier, & Weintraub, 1989) are not stable, either across time or across samples (Endler & Parker, 1990; Schwarzer & Schwarzer, 1996). However, the factor structure for coping process measures may not be stable precisely *because* they are responsive to environmental demands (Schwartz & Daltroy, 1999). Coyne and Racioppo (2000) further criticized coping inventories as being too vague to generate clinically meaningful results, and argued for more situation-specific inventories (which, however, would also create problems of generalizability across situations).

Nonetheless, there is broad agreement concerning the types of coping strategies that exist. There are five general types: problem-focused coping, emotion-focused coping, social support, religious coping, and cognitive reframing. Coping strategies are not mutually exclusive, and even strategies that may seem orthogonal, such as suppressing and expressing emotions, may be used sequentially in the same situation. Within each type of coping strategy, there are several subtypes. Furthermore, terminology varies among studies, and some use somewhat idiosyncratic measures. We will strive for consistency in terminology, but that may not always be possible.

Problem-focused coping, often called *active* or *planful* coping, includes cognitions and behaviors that are directed at analyzing and solving a problem. It may include "chunking," or breaking a problem into more manageable pieces, seeking information, and considering alternatives as well as direct action. Sometimes delaying or suppressing action is seen as a separate problem-focused strategy. Delaying action or decisions may be used in circumstances in which people await more information, and suppressing action may be useful in avoiding specific actions that may make a problem worse.

Emotion-focused coping also involves different subtypes. Avoidance, withdrawal, and disengagement are different than expressing emotion. Suppression, or setting one's emotions aside in the service of a problem-solving effort, is clearly different from the use of substances to regulate emotion. These types of coping are usually associated with poor outcomes (Aldwin & Revenson, 1987).

Seeking social support and religious coping are strategies that involve elements of both problem-focused and emotion-focused coping. Support seeking includes asking for advice, concrete aid, emotional support, or justification for one's perceptions or actions (Thoits, 1986). Similarly, religious coping, which includes prayer, is generally considered a form of emotion-focused coping, but may involve asking for advice or even concrete aid. The study of religious coping strategies is in its infancy (Pargament, 1997). In general, religious coping may be most helpful with uncontrollable stressors (Aldwin, 1994) or people facing chronic stressors such as caregiving, especially those in lower socioeconomic status groups (Cupertino, Aldwin, & Schulz, 2000).

Social support, conceptualized as social integration (Berkman & Syme, 1994) or social disclosure (Smyth, 1998), is almost always associated with better mental and physical health outcomes. However, *seeking* social support is almost always associated with poorer outcomes (Monroe & Steiner, 1986). The reasons for this are not well understood, but may revolve around negative reactions from others (Rook, 1998). The act of seeking support may be indicative of poor networks or a catastrophizing coping style.

Finally, cognitive reframing is a strategy that is least understood. It involves trying to make sense of the problem, and is often called *making meaning*. It involves such strategies as "looking for the silver lining" or trying to perceive positive aspects of the current problem. Making meaning may be most often used in coping with extreme stressors, such as trauma or major losses (Mikulincer & Florian, 1996), and will be discussed in greater detail shortly.

An interesting development in the coping literature is the assessment of daily process coping. Respondents may fill out questionnaires every evening or use experience-sampling techniques. This approach may be especially useful for studies in which individuals are coping with a problem that extends over time (Tennen, Affleck, Armeli, & Carney, 2000). Schwarzer and Schwarzer (1996) have criticized the psychometric properties of daily process measures, as they are of necessity quite short and often consist of single items. There are interesting differences in the results of within-subject and between-subject (aggregated) analyses. For example, within-subject analyses of pain patients show a more protective effect of coping strategies on pain than between-subject analyses (Tennen & Affleck, 1996).

COPING WITH TRAUMA

It would be tempting to argue that the environmental press of trauma is so great that there are few individual differences in reaction to it. However, the trauma literature reveals marked individual differences in how people cope, although clearly environmental factors may constrain choices. Aldwin (1999) identified four ways in which the pattern of coping responses in traumatic situations differs from that in ordinary life events. First, individuals in traumatic situations may feel they have little control over their cognitions and behaviors. In naturalistic descriptions of people in traumatic situations, the use of defense mechanisms such as dissociation, repression, and denial are widespread (Ward, 1988).

Second, disclosure is particularly important in traumatic situations. Individuals who disclose to others typically do much better both in terms of short and long-term outcomes (Lee, Vaillant, Torrey, & Elder, 1995; Smyth, 1998). The reaction of others may moderate this relationship. Individuals who experience negative reactions may have worse outcomes than those who did not disclose (Silver, Holman, & Gil-Rivas, 2000; Stephens & Long, 2000).

Third, the process of coping with trauma is usually much more extended than is coping with general hassles or even life events, especially if an individual develops posttraumatic stress disorder (PTSD). The sequelae of major trauma have been shown to last for decades (Aldwin, Levenson, & Spiro, 1994; Kahana, 1992; Schnurr, Spiro, Aldwin, & Stukel, 1998). The process of reconstructing both lives and sense of identity may take years (Lomranz, 1990).

The fourth difference concerns *making meaning*. This strategy has particular utility in traumatic situations (Mikulincer & Florian, 1996). Making meaning may entail both reorganization of existing cognitive–motivational structures, as well as reappraisal or reinterpretation of not only the event but also the context of the event in a person's life. Loss events may also entail a search for meaning, especially if those events are sudden or traumatic (Wortman, Battle, & Lemkau, 1997). Although this search for meaning may be painful in and of itself, and sometimes fruitless, it may also set the stage of posttraumatic growth (Aldwin & Sutton, 1998; Tedeschi, Park, & Calhoun, 1998).

The most intriguing aspects of the coping with trauma literature are the hints that trauma may constitute a major avenue for personality change in adulthood (Epstein, 1991). For example, Schnurr, Rosenberg, and Friedman (1993) examined change in Minnesota Multiphasic Personality Inventory (MMPI) scores from college to midlife as a function of combat exposure. They found that MMPI scores were most likely to improve in men who had moderate levels of combat exposure, compared with those who had heavy exposure or none at all. More studies in this area are needed, and the possible mediating function of coping strategies merits further investigation (Aldwin, Sutton, & Lachman, 1996).

Another way in which studies of coping with trauma differ from general studies of coping with stress is that trauma studies sometimes focus on just one strategy. Examples of such strategies include self-blame (Davis, Lehman, Silver, Wortman, & Ellard, 1996; Delahanty et al., 1997), "undoing" (Davis, Lehman, Wortman, Silver, & Thompson, 1995), and "temporal orientation" (Holman & Silver, 1998). Whereas self-blame in everyday situations is generally associated with poor outcomes, in traumatic situations such as rape or automobile accidents, it may be associated with positive outcomes as it provides at least an illusion of control in uncontrollable situations (Janoff-Bulman, 1979; but see Frazier, 1990). Undoing is defined as the use of counterfactuals, for example, how the event could have been avoided ("if only I had not . . ."). Davis and colleagues (1995) found that the more often participants used undoing, the more distress they reported, even controlling for general rumination. This strategy may not be specific to trauma. It would be very interesting to see how often and under what circumstances this strategy is used in everyday coping.

The process of coping with trauma may be more important for mental health outcomes than the exposure to trauma itself (Mikulincer & Florian, 1996; Wolfe, Keane, Kaloupek, Mora, & Winde, 1993). This has been found both retrospectively (Fairbank, Hansen, & Fitterling, 1991; Zeidner & Hammer, 1992), as well as prospectively (Solomon, Mikulincer, & Avitzur, 1988; Solomon, Mikulincer, & Benbenishty, 1989). Problem-focused coping is associated with better outcomes, whereas emotion-focused strategies such as wishful thinking and denial are associated with more

PTSD symptoms. The effects of trauma on health may be mediated through the development of PTSD (Baum, Cohen, & Hall, 1993; Davidson & Baum, 1993; Schnurr, Spiro, & Paris, 2000; see also Green & Kimerling, chap. 2, this volume). However, more studies are needed specifically linking pathways between coping, the development of PTSD, and the adverse health effects of trauma.

COPING AND PHYSICAL HEALTH OUTCOMES

The literature on trauma and health outcomes is reviewed by Green and Kimerling (chap. 2, this volume); we are focusing on coping and physical health outcomes. The relationships detailed in this literature are highly complex, in part because it is largely atheoretical. Therefore, we organized this review by type of outcomes: self-reported health, biomedical indicators (cortisol, immune, cardiovascular reactivity, and lipids), and disease outcomes. Finally, we reviewed the coping intervention literature.

Our initial strategy was to further divide the literature by coping with stressors versus coping with trauma to provide meaningful contrasts, but the gaps in the literature did not permit this. For example, there were no laboratory studies on coping with trauma, and most of the field studies of coping and neuroendocrine outcomes involved only traumatic situations. Thus, we combined both stressor and trauma studies in the same categories, noting differences and similarities where appropriate.

We identified four models of the relationship between coping and physical health outcomes.

1. *Direct effects* refer to simple correlations between coping strategies and outcomes. This model assumes a direct relationship between coping strategies and outcomes, regardless of context.
2. In the *moderated effects* model, coping is thought to moderate or buffer the effects of stress; that is, the effect may vary as a function of degree of stress.
3. The *mediated effects* model suggests that the effects of coping are mediated through other variables, especially affect. That is, coping relates to outcome variables only to the extent that it modifies affect.
4. The *contextual effects* model hypothesizes that the effects of coping vary as a function of context or by the reaction of other individuals in the context.

We will use these models to understand the relations between coping and health outcomes.

Coping and Self-Reported Health Outcomes

Whereas there is an extensive literature on coping and mental health outcomes (Aldwin, 1999; Lazarus & Folkman, 1984; Zeidner & Saklofske, 1996), there are surprisingly few studies of coping and self-reported physical health symptoms in general populations. A recent meta-analysis of the Ways of Coping measures and self-report outcomes found that 26 out of the 34 studies (76%) used clinical samples; most focused on mental health. Only nine examined physical health outcomes, but idiosyncratic rather than standardized measures were typically used (Penley, Tomaka, & Wiebe, 2002). They concluded that health was positively associated with problem-focused coping and negatively associated with emotion-focused coping but that these relationships were moderated by situational characteristics and varied by type of outcome.

This pattern is repeated in studies that use other types of coping measures. Eriksen and Ursin (1999) found that individual coping styles were more important for subjective health complaints than were either control or organizational factors. Specifically, coping moderated the effects of job stress: individuals with low demands and high coping skills had the fewest health complaints, whereas those with high demands and low coping reported the most. In contrast, Pisarski, Bohle, and Callan (1998) found direct, mediated, and contextual effects, depending on the type of coping strategies used. Both problem-focused and disengagement (avoidant) coping strategies had direct (and opposite) effects on physical symptoms, but emotional expression showed mediated effects that varied by type of context. In work situations, emotional expression led to increased conflict and concomitant psychological symptoms, which in turn increased physical symptoms. Used in the family context, however, emotional expression increased family support, which in turn decreased physical symptoms. Thus, the effect of coping varied by the context in which it was used.

Coping and Biomedical Outcomes

There are hundreds of studies in humans showing that stress affects both the neuroendocrine and immune systems, and there is a general agreement that there are individual differences in the effects of stress (Biondi & Picardi, 1999; Cohen & Herbert, 1996; Olff, 1999). However, it is difficult to demonstrate a relationship between coping strategies and biomedical outcomes, in part because there are surprisingly few published studies. Although Biondi and Picardi, in their otherwise excellent review of stress and neuroendocrine factors, state that "There is a large body of evidence that coping strategies may significantly influence hormonal responses to both laboratory stressors and real life stress situations" (p. 133), closer examination reveals that they based this conclusion on only four published studies. Furthermore, most reviews focus on a particular biomedical outcome, and we felt that an overview of several outcomes might prove instructive.

Laboratory Studies

Most laboratory studies examining the effect of coping on neuroendocrine outcomes rely on assessments of defenses or coping styles. In these often unpublished studies, defensiveness, avoidance, and repression are typically associated with higher cortisol levels (Biondi & Picardi, 1999), but other studies find no relationship between coping styles and cortisol (Bossert et al., 1988; Van Eck, Nicholson, Berkhof, & Sulon, 1996). Bohnen, Nicholson, Sulon, and Jolles (1991) found that "comforting cognitions," a type of cognitive reframing, was negatively associated with cortisol response.

A handful of studies examined coping and cardiovascular outcomes. Tomaka, Blascovich, and Kelsey (1992) found no association between repressive coping and psychophysiological reactivity to stress, once the effect of social desirability was controlled. However, Vitaliano, Russo, Paulsen, and Bailey (1995) examined cardiovascular recovery from laboratory stressors in older adults, and found that avoidance coping was positively related to diastolic blood pressure and heart rate. That laboratory had similar findings among caregivers of Alzheimer patients (Vitaliano, Russo, Bailey, Young, & McCann, 1993; Vitaliano, Russo, & Niaura, 1995). Controlling for standard risk factors, avoidance coping was associated with higher levels of cardiovascular reactivity.

Individuals with the highest levels of cardiovascular reactivity also show the greatest immune system disturbances to stress (Herbert, Coriell, & Cohen, 1994). Although there is a growing literature on stress and immune functioning (Cohen & Herbert, 1996; Kiecolt-Glaser & Glaser, 1995), we located no laboratory studies that examined induced stressors, coping, and immune outcomes. This is surprising in view of the fact that the immune response to stressors occurs in minutes (Eriksen, Olff, Murison, & Ursin, 1999), even before cortisol responses, and thus the immediate impact of coping on immune function could be relatively easily studied. Carefully constructed laboratory studies could clear up some of the conflicting findings in field studies.

Field Studies

Although studies have shown that coping styles are linked to neuroendocrine profiles in feral animals (Koolhaas et al., 1999), there are a limited number of field studies assessing this link in humans. Perhaps the most consistent finding is between urinary cortisol and the effectiveness of defenses. Vickers (1988) reviewed five field studies with stressors ranging from military training to having a fatally ill child, each of which found that individuals with effective psychological defenses had lower levels of urinary cortisol.

Studies of coping strategies and neuroendocrine outcomes yielded mixed results. An early study by Schaeffer and Baum (1984) showed that stress associated with the nuclear power plant disaster at Three Mile Island was related to urinary cortisol, as were psychological and physical symptoms, but that coping styles were not. However, coping styles were related to lower levels of distress (Baum, Fleming, & Singer, 1983). Distress levels should have some effect, albeit indirect, on cortisol and catecholamines outcomes, although this mediational model has not been tested. Arnetz and colleagues (1991) found emotion-focused coping was indirectly related to cortisol via its effect on mastery: that is, feelings of being in control of one's environment or oneself.

Control may also moderate this relationship. Street noise levels were associated with urinary norepinephrine levels in women who were not able to eliminate this noise by closing a window, but not in women who could exercise this control (Babisch, Fromme, Beyer, & Ising, 2001).

Avoidance coping is also related to cardiovascular outcomes. Cross-sectional studies have shown a direct relationship between coping and various cholesterol fractions, such as triglycerides and low-density lipoproteins (LDLs), which are associated with cardiovascular disease (CVD), whereas high-density lipoproteins (HDLs) may be protective against CVD. In a study of caregivers, avoidance coping was associated with higher levels of triglycerides and LDLs, but with lower levels of HDLs (Vitaliano, Russo, & Niaura, 1995). Aldwin, Levenson, Spiro, and Ward (1994) found that instrumental action was positively associated with HDLs and negatively with triglycerides, whereas self-blame showed the opposite pattern. However, more studies are needed to show a consistent effect, as well as to determine causal directionality.

A few studies have examined coping and immune system outcomes, which are typically divided into humoral (antibody) and cellular components (white blood cells). Humoral functioning is assessed by antibody titers (amounts), often in response to a stimulus such as concanavalin (ConA) or phytohemagglutinin (PHA). Cellular immunity is divided into nonspecific and specific immunity. Nonspecific cells include phagocytes that can engulf invaders (e.g., monocytes) and others (e.g., eosophinils) that are involved in allergic and anaphylactic reactions. Specific immunity cells include helper (CD4+) and suppressor (CD8+) cells, as well as many others, which regulate immune response.

Jamner, Schwartz, and Leigh (1988), in a study of outpatients with stress-related disorders, found that repressive coping was negatively related to monocyte counts but positively related to eosinophil counts. However, repressors were also more likely to be taking antihistamines for their allergies, so interpretation of this study is difficult. Repressive coping may suppress some aspects of immune function but overstimulate allergic reactions, or it may be that these repressive copers serendipitously had more allergies and thus higher eosinophil counts.

Among undergraduates, repressors had significantly higher antibody titers to Epstein-Barr virus, an indicator of a stressed immune system (Esterling, Antoni, Mahendra, & Schneiderman, 1990). However, this pattern was not found by Segerstrom and colleagues (1998) in a study of earthquake victims. Type C personality, an indicator of repressive coping, was unrelated to a variety of immune system outcomes, including lymphocyte counts, lymphoid cell mitogenesis, and natural killer cell cytotoxicity (NKCC). There was an interaction between generalized distress and life disruption, such that individuals with high levels of disruption who did not report being distressed had impaired immune functioning (lower levels of CD3+ and CD8+ T cells). The authors suggested that this was indirect support for the impact of repressive coping on immune function.

Stowell, Kiecolt-Glaser, and Glaser (2001) also reported a positive relationship between active (problem-focused) coping and antibody titers to ConA and PHA under high, but not low, stress environments. Conversely, students who coped by abusing substances were more likely to have inadequate antibody counts than those accepting the reality of stressful situations (Burns, Carroll, Ring, Harrison, & Drayson, 2002).

Problem focused coping was associated with higher levels of helper T (CD4+) cells (Goodkin, Fuchs, Feaster, Leeka, & Rishel, 1992), whereas venting emotions was associated with lower NKCCs. Although this study tested moderator effects, the results were inconclusive, because of a small sample size and problems with multicollinearity. Others have shown that person–environment fit moderates the relationship between job stress and antibody levels (IgA; Schaubroeck, Jones, & Xie, 2001).

Summary

Despite the hundreds of biomedical studies that have been done on stress and biomedical outcomes, relatively few studies have linked coping strategies with such indicators. Early laboratory studies relied primarily on trait measures of defenses; various indices of what could be seen as emotional repression were related to higher cortisol levels. In addition, avoidant and repressive coping are related to greater cardiovascular reactivity and impaired immune function. There is also some indication that positive coping is related to better outcomes. Problem-focused or active coping is related to higher NKCCs and CD4+ cell counts and higher HDL levels. These results are promising, but need more replication.

Besides its sparseness, a major limitation of this research is that most studies examine only main effects, and more sophisticated models should be analyzed. Baron and Kenny (1986) caution that valid examination of interaction effects for moderator models often require very large sample sizes, which may be problematic in the small samples typical of neuroendocrine and immune studies. A possible solution is for small sample studies to use jack-knife or bootstrap analyses which are ways of statistically resampling different combinations of data points and provide more accurate assessments of the standard errors in small samples, which are common in psychoneuroimmunology (PNI) studies (Aldwin, Spiro, Clark, & Hall, 1991).

Coping and Disease Outcomes

There is a much more extensive literature on coping and disease outcomes. Several studies have examined pain and symptoms for individuals with chronic illnesses such as rheumatoid arthritis, the progression of serious illnesses such as AIDS and cancer, and even mortality. For reviews of these studies, see Garssen and Goodkin (1999), Tennen and Affleck (1996), and Zautra and Manne (1992); these reviews often highlight the complex relationship between coping and outcomes.

A variety of personal and contextual factors may moderate the effects of coping on health outcomes. A review of studies on coping with rheumatoid arthritis (Zautra & Manne, 1992) showed that coping strategies were significantly associated with outcomes such as pain, but the results were often inconsistent across studies. Zautra and Manne argued that the relationship between coping strategies and outcomes depended on coping efficacy, family environments, and personality dispositions. For example, relying on others has different effects depending on the severity of illness. It led to increased psychological distress among women with rheumatoid arthritis in relatively good health, but lower levels of distress for women in poorer health (Reich & Zautra, 1995). Similarly, participating in social support groups had the most positive effect on physical functioning for breast cancer patients who lacked natural support or had fewer personal resources, but were harmful for women who had high levels of support (Helgeson, Cohen, Schulz, & Yasko, 2000).

The effects of coping may vary by type of disease. Affleck and colleagues (1999) found that emotion-focused coping was associated with increased pain in rheumatoid arthritis patients, but decreased pain in osteoarthritis patients. The emotion-focused coping coded in this study involved seeking support and venting to others. The authors suggested that the differences between these two groups were due to the caregiver's response. Osteoarthritis pain is specific to movement and thus may be more understandable, whereas the pain involved in rheumatoid arthritis (swollen joints and fatigue) is more global and may evoke less sympathetic responses. This parallels the trauma literature previously reviewed, in which the effects of social disclosure were also moderated by the response of others in the social environment.

There is also evidence that coping may have indirect or mediated effects on outcomes. Billings, Folkman, Acree, and Moskowitz (2000) showed that coping affected positive and negative affect among men providing care for AIDS patients. Social support coping predicted an increase in positive affect, which in turn was related to fewer physical symptoms. Avoidant coping, however, was related to an increase in negative affect, which was related to higher levels of physical symptoms.

Coping may also be related to the progression of AIDS. A prospective study of a sample of asymptomatic HIV-positive men and women also reported that avoidance and passive coping were positively correlated with development of symptoms, whereas planful (problem-focused) coping was negatively related to progression of HIV symptoms (Vassend, Eskild, & Halvorsen, 1997). A cross-sectional study also found that individuals diagnosed with AIDS were lower in planful problem solving than HIV-negative individuals (Krikorian, Kay, & Liang, 1995). Active confrontational coping predicted slower disease progression in HIV-positive men over the course of a year (Mulder, Antoni, Duivenvoorden, & Kauffmann, 1995). A follow-up study also showed that individuals who used avoidant coping had a more rapid deterioration of CD4+ cell counts over 7 years (Mulder, de Vroome, van Griensven, Antoni, & Sandfort, 1999).

Although there is at best weak evidence for the relationship between coping and the development of cancer (Garssen & Goodkin, 1999), coping strategies may affect the response to cancer treatments. Women who used confrontive coping reported fewer side effects from chemotherapy than those who used avoidant strategies (Shapiro et al., 1997). A few studies have directly looked at coping and the progression of cancer, primarily breast cancers. A series of British studies showed that women who used active coping styles lived longer, especially if they had early, nonmetastatic cancer (Greer, 1991; Greer & Morris, 1975; Morris, Greer, Pettingale, & Watson, 1981). Conversely, a study of women with breast cancer showed that repressors had elevated levels of mortality, with a risk ratio of 3.7 (Weihs, Enright, Simmens, & Reiss, 2000). Buddeberg and colleagues (1996) found modest associations between coping and death from breast cancer. Individuals using problem-focused coping (tackling and self-encouragement) were less likely to die, whereas those expressing distrust and pessimism were more likely to die. However, Petticrew, Bell, and Hunter (2002) cautioned that the results of coping and cancer survival studies are often inconsistent.

In summary, it is not surprising that coping skills and strategies should affect disease progression, especially in those diseases such as AIDS and cancer that have very arduous treatment regimens. Individuals who are good planful problem solvers may be more able to handle these regimens and have better outcomes, whereas avoidant copers may have a more problematic adherence and thus have worse outcomes. Problem solving may also provide a sense of control and decrease negative affect, whereas avoidant copers may be simply overwhelmed by anxiety and depression, which have also been linked with poor outcomes. But it must be remembered that there really is no "silver bullet" in coping research, and a variety of personal and contextual factors may moderate the relationship between coping and health outcomes. The effectiveness of coping strategies may vary by the stage and type of the illness, as well as the responsiveness of others in the environment. This suggests that interventions need to be very specifically tailored to individuals and their contexts.

Intervention Studies

One of the simplest coping interventions in the literature is a written emotional expression task with regard to stressful episodes, especially traumatic ones. In a review of this literature, Smyth (1998) found that disclosure led to significantly better health across a variety of biomedical outcomes, cardiovascular reactivity and risk factors, immune outcomes, physiological functioning, and health behaviors. No studies on neuroendocrine outcomes were included in this review. A drawback of these studies is that they use primarily undergraduate populations, and their utility varies as a function of duration of the writing task. Although single episode interventions can have significant effects, these tend to be weaker than interventions with multiple writing episodes because narratives tend to become more focused and coherent over time. It is also unclear whether this is due to cognitive processing or the reversal of emotional repression. A review by Esterling, L'Abate, Murray, and Pennebaker (1999) suggested that both mechanisms may be used, but for different types of outcomes. Cognitive processing is predictive for emotional well-being, but the reversal of emotional repression may be important for neuroendocrine and immune system outcomes.

A large number of coping interventions in the behavioral medicine literature consist of psychoeducational interventions (Compas, Haaga, Keefe, Leitenberg, & Williams, 1998). The most dramatic and consistent results are seen with pain interventions. In a meta-analysis of 191 studies, Devine (1992) found that statistically reliable, albeit modest, effects were found on recovery, postoperative pain, and psychological outcomes. Nearly all (79%) of these studies found a shorter length of hospitalization in those who received pain management interventions. Interestingly, adding specific coping skills training to standard pain management treatment programs greatly improved pain control (Kole-Snijders et al., 1999).

Perhaps the most dramatic of interventions studies was conducted by Fawzy and his colleagues (Fawzy, Cousins, Fawzy, Kemeny, & Morton, 1990; Fawzy et al., 1993; Fawzy & Fawzy, 1994; Fawzy, Kemeny, et al., 1990), who did specific coping skills interventions with patients who had melanoma. This was a 6-week, structured program with multiple components, including health education, psychological support, and training in both problem solving and stress management. Short-term, the experimental participants were more likely to use active behavior coping than the control groups, and they also had more positive affect. Differences in immune functioning were evident between the two groups at the 6-month assessment. Specifically, experimental participants had a greater percentage of large granular lymphocytes, more natural killer (NK) cells, and better NK cytotoxicity. Although coping strategies were not directly associated with immune cell changes, they were correlated with affect, which in turn was associated with immune functioning. This supports our supposition that the effects of coping on biomedical outcomes may be mediated through affect. At a 5-year follow-up, a third of the control group had died, compared with less than 10% of the experimental group. Longer survival was associated with more active coping.

Coping interventions are surprisingly successful. They have been shown to change psychosocial outcomes, physiological outcomes, the rate of disease progression, and even mortality. What appear to be missing, however, are published accounts of coping interventions for PTSD.

TOWARD A THEORETICAL MODEL

The literature reviewed here suggests that the different models described in this chapter apply to different types of outcome measures. Table 5.1 represents our attempt to summarize this literature and indicates which models were supported for different coping strategies by outcomes. Given the wide variety of coping measures used, we chose to group strategies roughly, using common scale names instead of the more generic terms referred to earlier in this chapter. Instrumental action is a specific problem-focused scale. The two emotion-focused scales used most often include avoidance (including escapism, wishful thinking, and self-isolation) and self-blame. Social support includes emotional expression and disclosure, whereas cognitive reframing includes meaning making. Surprisingly, we were unable to locate any studies of physiological outcomes that assessed religious coping.

We did try to differentiate between process and styles measures, although the distinction was not always clear from the studies. However, most of the measures summarized in Table 5.1 were process measures; coping

TABLE 5.1
Summary of Research on Coping and Health Outcomes

Outcome	Coping	Direct	Moderated	Mediated	Contextual
Self-reported symptoms	Instrumental action	→			
	Avoidant	↑			
	Social support			X	X
Neuroendocrine (catecholamines & cortisol)	Cognitive reframing	→			
	Avoidant style	→		X	
Cardiovascular reactivity	Avoidant	↑			
Lipids (HDL/LDL)	Instrumental action	↑ →			
	Avoidant	← ↑			
	Self-blame	← ↑			
Immune (CD4+ & NKCC)	Instrumental action	← →	?		
	Social support	→		X	
Disease outcomes	Instrumental action	→ ↑		X	
	Avoidant	←			
	Social support	→	X		

Note. All coping measures are process measures, unless otherwise indicated. For direct effects, downward arrows indicate negative correlations, whereas upward arrows indicate positive correlations. For mediated, moderated, and contextual models, an X indicates that the effect exists. Question marks indicate contradictory or inconsistent findings. *HDL* and *LDL* = high and low density lipoproteins, respectively. CD4+ = helper T cells. NKCC = natural killer cell count.

styles are indicated by the use of the term *style*. Unless otherwise noted, the direct effects of instrumental action, cognitive reframing, and meaning making are assumed to decrease or be associated with lower levels of health problems (indicated by a downward arrow), whereas avoidant and self-blame strategies are assumed to increase or be associated with higher levels of health problems (indicated by an upward arrow). Tests for other types of models are indicated simply with an X. Question marks indicate contradictory or inconsistent findings.

All of the studies of self-reported physical health symptoms reviewed here examined coping with ordinary stressors, not with trauma (see Table 5.1). Instrumental action is generally associated with fewer symptoms, and avoidant styles with higher symptoms. However, the effects of social support appear to be contextual. The one study that examined a mediated model found contradictory pathways: Emotional expression increased coworker conflict, but also increased family support. Thus, the effect is contextual: That is, emotional expression in the workplace may increase stress and therefore increase symptoms, but venting to family and friends may increase support and therefore decrease symptoms.

Given the vast literature on stress and neuroendocrine function, it is surprising that the coping results were so inconsistent. Although some early studies found that those with "effective defenses" had lower catecholamine levels, it was not clear exactly what this meant, so they were omitted from the table. More recent laboratory studies were just as likely to find no effects of coping styles in general or avoidant styles in particular as they were to find any effects, and none of the field studies found direct effects of coping on neuroendocrine function. However, both the trauma and stress literatures suggest that the effects may be mediated through affect.

Given the strength of the findings in the animal literature, it is surprising that stronger effects of coping on neuroendocrine function were not found. Our first inclination was to attribute this to the problem of timing in field studies. Catecholamines are very rapid responses to stress; it is unlikely that the time periods for data collection of the coping behaviors and urine collection adequately overlapped. If the coping resulted in long-term changes in affect, then mediated effects might be seen. However, Stanford's (1993) review of stress and catecholamines suggested an alternative hypothesis. In individuals adapting to stress, anxiety is associated with high levels of catecholamines, whereas depression is associated with low levels. Failure to differentiate between the reactions might well lead to the contradictory findings in the literature. In other words, avoidant coping may lead to depression or anxiety, that is, to lower or higher levels of catecholamines. Thus, the relationship between coping and catecholamine levels is complex, and mediated not only by level of negative affect but by type as well.

Only a handful of studies have examined coping and biomedical outcomes, and only one was in the context of coping with trauma. Avoidant strategies are associated with higher levels of cardiovascular reactivity. Similarly, instrumental action is associated with higher levels of HDL and lower levels of LDL and triglycerides, whereas the emotion-focused strategies of avoidance and self-blame show the opposite pattern.

The early studies on coping and immune outcomes are very difficult to interpret, given poor coping measures, specialized samples, and inconsistent results. Tentatively, instrumental action appears to be associated with higher levels of CD4+ and NKCC, whereas social support, in the form of emotional venting, was associated with lower levels of NKCC. Clearly there is a huge gap in the literature. More studies are needed on the effects of coping on biomedical outcomes, especially in the context of trauma, and more sophisticated models need to be examined.

Finally, a more extensive and consistent literature exists on coping and disease outcomes. Nearly every study has found that instrumental action is associated with slower disease progression, fewer side effects of treatment, and fewer symptoms, whereas avoidant coping shows the opposite pattern. Given the importance of adherence to medical regimens and dietary restrictions in coping with chronic illnesses, it is not surprising that problem-focused coping leads to better outcomes, and avoidant coping to poorer ones. However, Billings and colleagues (2000) suggested that all of the effects of coping (at least on physical symptoms in AIDS patients) are mediated through affect. Problem-focused coping is related to positive affect, which in turn is inversely related to physical symptoms, and avoidant coping is associated with negative affect, which in turn increases physical symptoms. More studies are needed that examine the mediators of coping on disease outcomes, especially vis-à-vis adherence and affect.

The effect of social support on disease outcomes presents a more sobering picture. It is clear that the effects of support are contextual, and vary depending on the type of illness, reactions of others, and needs of the individual. If individuals are severely disabled or socially isolated, provision of positive support may be very beneficial. However, if the primary caretaker is unresponsive to genuine expressions of need or creates dependency if support is not needed, then use of social support can have harmful effects.

CONCLUSIONS AND FUTURE DIRECTIONS

More research is needed to understand the effects of coping on physical outcomes, whether in the context of everyday stressors, chronic illness, or trauma. The trauma literature is especially deficient with regard to the effect of coping on biomedical outcomes. Although most studies have simply examined direct effects, there are hints in the literature that reality is much more complicated. In particular, it is likely that nearly all of the effects of coping on biomedical and disease outcomes are mediated through affect, and, in the context of chronic illness, to adherence to medical regimes. The effects of social support, as noted, are highly contextual. Given that nearly all of the theoretical models posit coping as a stress buffer, it is extremely surprising that almost no one bothers to test this. Despite these gaps, the evidence indicates that how individuals cope with problems does have an effect on their physiology, and coping interventions can sometimes have dramatic effects on disease outcomes.

A number of clinical implications follow from this research. If patients engage in avoidant behaviors, clinicians need to help them to develop better ways of managing their negative affect so that they can better comply with medical regimes. Helgeson and Mickelson (2000) remind us that there is a difference between denial of illness and denial of consequences. Avoidant coping that leads to a denial of illness can result in death, but maintaining hope for more positive outcomes may result in better compliance. At some point, however, clinicians may need to help patients make reasoned decisions whether to comply with further treatment. Terminal patients may choose to avoid additional procedures to enhance their quality of life rather than to endure aggressive medical treatment with severe and painful side effects. Thus, avoidance is a complicated coping strategy that may be useful under certain conditions.

Clinicians should also evaluate the patient's context. In truth, chronic illness affects the whole family and not just the patient. The best problem solving may be ineffective if it receives a hostile response from significant others. Different stages of illness may also require different coping strategies. Active problem solving may be especially helpful at early stages of an illness, but eventually a patient may need to learn how to accept dependency and help from others. Thus, clinicians need to tailor interventions to individual needs and requirements, and be sensitive to the personal, social, and situational factors that may alter the effectiveness of coping strategies.

REFERENCES

Affleck, G., Tennen, H., Keefe, F. J., Lefebvre, J. C., Kashikar-Zuck, S., Wright, K., et al. (1999). Everyday life with osteoarthritis or rheumatoid arthritis: Independent effects of disease and gender on daily pain, mood, and coping. *Pain, 83,* 601–609.

Aldwin, C. M. (1994, August). *The California Coping Inventory.* Paper presented at the annual meeting of the American Psychological Association, Los Angeles, CA.

Aldwin, C. M. (1999). *Stress, coping, and development: An integrative approach*. New York: Guilford.

Aldwin, C. M., Levenson, M. R., & Spiro, A., III. (1994). Vulnerability and resilience to combat exposure: Can stress have lifelong effects? *Psychology and Aging, 9*, 33–44.

Aldwin, C. M., Levenson, M. R., Spiro, A., III, & Ward, K. (1994). Hostility, stress, coping, and serum lipid levels [Abstract]. *The Gerontologist, 34*, 333.

Aldwin, C. M., & Revenson, T. A. (1987). Does coping help? A reexamination of the relationship between coping and mental health. *Journal of Personality and Social Psychology, 53*, 337–348.

Aldwin, C. M., Spiro, A., III, Clark, G., & Hall, N. (1991). Thymic hormones, stress and psychological symptoms in older men: A comparison of different statistical techniques for small samples. *Brain, Behavior, and Immunity, 5*, 206–218.

Aldwin, C. M., & Sutton, K. J. (1998). A developmental perspective on posttraumatic growth. In R. G. Tedeschi & C. L. Park (Eds.), *Posttraumatic growth: Positive changes in the aftermath of crisis* (pp. 43–63). Mahwah, NJ: Erlbaum.

Aldwin, C. M., Sutton, K. J., & Lachman, M. (1996). The development of coping resources in adulthood. *Journal of Personality, 64*, 837–871.

Arnetz, B. B., Brenner, S. O., Levi, L., Hjelm, R., Petterson, I. L., Wasserman, J., et al. (1991). Neuroendocrine and immunologic effects of unemployment and job insecurity. *Psychotherapy and Psychosomatics, 55*, 76–80.

Babisch, W., Fromme, H., Beyer, A., & Ising, H. (2001). Increased catecholamine levels in urine in subjects exposed to road traffic noise: The role of stress hormones in noise research. *Environment International, 26*, 475–481.

Baron, R. M., & Kenny, D. A. (1986). The mediator–moderator variable distinction in social psychological research: Conceptual, strategic, and statistical considerations. *Journal of Personality and Social Psychology, 51*, 1173–1182.

Baum, A., Cohen, L., & Hall, M. (1993). Control and intrusive memories as possible determinants of chronic stress. *Psychosomatic Medicine, 55*, 274–286.

Baum, A., Fleming, R., & Singer, J. (1983). Coping with victimization by technological disaster. *Journal of Social Issues, 39*, 117–138.

Berkman, L., & Syme, S. L. (1994). Social networks, host resistance, and mortality: A nine year follow-up study of Alameda County residents. In A. Steptoe & J. Wardle (Eds.), *Psychosocial processes and health: A reader* (pp. 43–67). Cambridge: Cambridge University.

Billings, D. W., Folkman, S., Acree, M., & Moskowitz, J. T. (2000). Coping and physical health during caregiving: The roles of positive and negative affect. *Journal of Personality and Social Psychology, 79*, 131–142.

Biondi, M., & Picardi, A. (1999). Psychological stress and neuroendocrine function in humans: The last two decades of research. *Psychotherapy and Psychosomatics, 68*, 114–150.

Bohnen, N., Nicholson, N., Sulon, J., & Jolles, J. (1991). Coping style, trait anxiety and cortisol reactivity during mental stress. *Journal of Psychosomatic Research, 35,* 141–147.

Bossert, S., Berger, M., Krieg, J. C., Schrieber, W., Junker, M., & von Zerssen, S. (1988). Cortisol response to various stressful situations: Relationship to personality variables and coping styles. *Neuropsychobiology, 20,* 36–42.

Buddeberg, C., Sieber, M., Wolf, C., Laudolt-Ritter, C., Richter, D., & Steiner, R. (1996). Are coping strategies related to disease outcome in early breast cancer? *Journal of Psychosomatic Research, 40,* 255–264.

Burns, V. E., Carroll, D., Ring, C., Harrison, L. K., & Drayson, M. (2002). Stress, coping, and hepatitis B antibody status. *Psychosomatic Medicine, 64,* 287–293.

Byrne, D. (1964). Repression-sensitization as a dimension of personality. In B. A. Maher (Ed.), *Progress in experimental personality research, Vol. 1* (pp. 169–220). New York: Academic Press.

Carver, C. S., Scheier, M. F., & Weintraub, J. K. (1989). Assessing coping strategies: A theoretically-based approach. *Journal of Personality and Social Psychology, 56,* 267–283.

Cohen, S., & Herbert, T. (1996). Health psychology: Physiological factors and physical disease from the perspective of human psychoneuroimmunology. *Annual Review of Psychology, 47,* 113–142.

Compas, B. E., Haaga, C. A. F., Keefe, F. J., Leitenberg, H., & Williams, D. A. (1998). Sampling of empirically supported psychological treatments from health psychology: Smoking, chronic pain, cancer, and bulimia nervosa. *Journal of Consulting and Clinical Psychology, 66,* 89–112.

Coyne, J. C., & Racioppo, M. (2000). Never the twain shall meet? Closing the gap between coping research and clinical intervention research. *American Psychologist, 55,* 655–664.

Cramer, P. (1991). Anger and the use of defense mechanisms in college students. *Journal of Personality, 59,* 39–55.

Cramer, P. (2000). Defense mechanisms in psychology today: Further processes for adaptation. *American Psychologist, 55,* 637–646.

Cupertino, A. P., Aldwin, C. M., & Schulz, R. (2000, August). *Socioeconomic status differences in religiosity and the perceived benefits of caregiving.* Paper presented at the annual meeting of the American Psychological Association, Washington, DC.

Davidson, K., & MacGregor, M. (1998). A critical appraisal of self-report defense mechanism measures. *Journal of Personality, 66,* 965–992.

Davidson, L. M., & Baum, A. (1993). Predictors of chronic stress among Vietnam veterans: Stress exposure and intrusive recall. *Journal of Traumatic Stress, 6,* 195–212.

Davis, C. G., Lehman, D. R., Silver, R. C., Wortman, C. B., & Ellard, E. H. (1996). Self-blame following a traumatic event: The role of perceived avoidability. *Personality and Social Psychology Bulletin, 22,* 557–567.

Davis, C. G., Lehman, D. R., Wortman, C. B., Silver, R. C., & Thompson, S. C. (1995). The undoing of traumatic life events. *Personality and Social Psychology Bulletin, 21,* 109–124.

Delahanty, D. L., Herberman, H. B., Craig, K. H., Hayward, M. C., Fullerton, C. S., Ursano, R. J., et al. (1997). Acute and chronic distress and posttraumatic stress disorder as a function of responsibility for serious motor vehicle accidents. *Journal of Consulting and Clinical Psychology, 65,* 560–567.

Devine, E. C. (1992). Effects of psychoeducational care for adult surgical patients: A meta-analysis of 191 studies. *Patient Education and Counseling, 19,* 129–142.

Endler, N. S., & Parker, J. D. (1990). Multidimensional assessment of coping: A critical evaluation. *Journal of Personality and Social Psychology, 58,* 844–854.

Epstein, S. (1991). The self-concept, the traumatic neurosis, and the structure of personality. In D. Ozer, J. H. Healy, & A. J. Stewart (Eds.), *Perspectives in personality: Vol. 3* (pp. 63–98). Bristol, PA: Jessica Kingsley Publishers.

Eriksen, H. R., Olff, M., Murison, R., & Ursin, H. (1999). The time dimension in stress responses: Relevance for survival and health. *Psychiatry Research, 85,* 39–50.

Eriksen, H. R., & Ursin, H. (1999). Subjective health complaints: Is coping more important than control? *Work and Stress, 13,* 238–252.

Esterling, B. A., Antoni, M. H., Mahendra, K., & Schneiderman, N. (1990). Emotional repression, stress disclosure responses, and Epstein Barr viral capsid antigen titers. *Psychosomatic Medicine, 52,* 397–410.

Esterling, B. A., L'Abate, L., Murray, E. J., & Pennebaker, J. W. (1999). Empirical foundations for writing in prevention and psychotherapy: Mental and physical health outcomes. *Clinical Psychology Review, 19,* 79–96.

Fairbank, J. A., Hansen, D. J., & Fitterling, J. M. (1991). Patterns of appraisal and coping across different stressor conditions among former prisoners of war with and without posttraumatic stress disorder. *Journal of Consulting and Clinical Psychology, 59,* 274–281.

Fawzy, F. I., Cousins, N., Fawzy, N. W., Kemeny, M., & Morton, D. I. (1990). A structured psychiatric intervention for cancer patients: I. Changes over time in methods of coping and affective disturbance. *Archives of General Psychiatry, 47,* 720–725.

Fawzy, F. I., & Fawzy, N. W. (1994). Psychoeducational interventions and health outcomes. In R. Glaser & J. K. Kiecolt-Glaser (Eds.), *Handbook of human stress and immunity* (pp. 365–402). San Diego: Academic Press.

Fawzy, F. I., Fawzy, N. W., Hyun, C., Elashoff, R., Guthrie, D., Fahey, J. L., et al. (1993). Malignant melanoma: Effects of an early structured psychiatric intervention, coping, and affective state on recurrence and survival six years later. *Archives of General Psychiatry, 50,* 681–689.

Fawzy, F. I., Kemeny, M., Fawzy, N. W., Elashoff, R., Morton, D., Cousins, N., et al. (1990). A structured psychiatric intervention for cancer patients: II. Changes over time in immunological measures. *Archives of General Psychiatry, 47,* 729–735.

Folkman, S., & Lazarus, R. (1980). An analysis of coping in a middle-aged community sample. *Journal of Health and Social Behavior, 21*, 219–239.

Frazier, P. A. (1990). Victim attributions and post-rape trauma. *Journal of Personality and Social Psychology, 59*, 298–304.

Garssen, B., & Goodkin, K. (1999). On the role of immunological factors as mediators between psychosocial factors and cancer progression. *Psychiatry Research, 85*, 51–61.

Goodkin, K., Fuchs, I., Feaster, D., Leeka, J., & Rishel, L. (1992). Life stressors and coping style are associated with immune measures in HIV-1 infection: A preliminary report. *International Journal of Psychiatry in Medicine, 22*, 155–172.

Greer, S. (1991). Psychological response to cancer and survival. *Psychological Medicine, 21*, 43–49.

Greer, S., & Morris, T. (1975). Psychological attributes of women who develop breast cancer. *Journal of Psychosomatic Research, 19*, 147–153.

Helgeson, V. S., Cohen, S., Schulz, R., & Yasko, J. (2000). Group support interventions for women with breast-cancer: Who benefits from what? *Health Psychology, 19*, 107–114.

Helgeson, V. S., & Mickelson, K. (2000). Coping with chronic illness among the elderly: Maintaining self-esteem. In S. B. Mauck, R. Jennings, B. S. Rabin, & A. Baum (Eds.), *Behavior, health, and aging* (pp. 153–178). Mahwah, NJ: Erlbaum.

Herbert, T. B., Coriell, M., & Cohen, S. (1994). Analysis of lymphocyte proliferation data: Do different approaches yield the same results? *Brain, Behavior, and Immunity, 8*, 153–162.

Holman, E. A., & Silver, R. C. (1998). Getting "stuck" in the past: Temporal orientation and coping with trauma. *Journal of Personality and Social Psychology, 74*, 1146–1163.

Horowitz, M. J. (1986). *Stress response syndromes* (2nd ed.). Northvale, NJ: Jason Aronson.

Jamner, L. D., Schwartz, G. E., & Leigh, H. (1988). The relationship between repressive and defensive coping styles and monocyte, eosinophile, and serum glucose levels: Support for the opioid peptide hypothesis of repression. *Psychosomatic Medicine, 50*, 567–575.

Janoff-Bulman, R. (1979). Characterological versus behavioral self-blame: Inquiries into depression and rape. *Journal of Personality and Social Psychology, 37*, 1798–1809.

Kahana, B. (1992). Late-life adaptation in the aftermath of extreme stress. In M. Wykel, E. Kahana, & J. Kowal (Eds.), *Stress and health among the elderly* (pp. 5–34). New York: Springer.

Kiecolt-Glaser, J. K., & Glaser, R. (1995). Psychoneuroimmunology and health consequences: Data and shared mechanisms. *Psychosomatic Medicine, 57*, 269–274.

Kole-Snijders, A. M. J., Vlaeyen, J. W. S., Goossens, M. E. J. B., Rutten-van Moelken, M. P. M. H., Heuts, P. H. T. G., van Breukelen, G., et al. (1999). Chronic low-back pain: What does cognitive coping skills training add to operant behavioral treatment? Results of a randomized clinical trial. *Journal of Consulting and Clinical Psychology, 67,* 931–944.

Koolhaas, J. M., Korte, S. M., DeBoer, S. F., Van Der Vegt, B. J., Van Reenen, C. G., Hopster, H., et al. (1999). Coping styles in animals: Current status in behavior and stress-physiology. *Neuroendocrine and Biobehavioral Reviews, 23,* 925–935.

Krikorian, R., Kay, J., & Liang, W. M. (1995). Emotional distress, coping, and adjustment in human immunodeficiency virus infection and acquired immune deficiency syndrome. *Journal of Nervous and Mental Disease, 183,* 293–298.

Lazarus, R. (2000). Toward better research on stress and coping. *American Psychologist, 55,* 665–673.

Lazarus, R., & Folkman, S. (1984). *Stress, appraisal, and coping.* New York: Springer.

Lee, K. A., Vaillant, G. E., Torrey, W. C., & Elder, G. H., Jr. (1995). A 50-year prospective study of the psychological sequelae of World War II combat. *American Journal of Psychiatry, 152,* 516–522.

Lomranz, J. (1990). Long-term adaptation to traumatic stress in light of adult development and aging perspectives. In M. A. P. Stephens, J. H. Crowther, S. E. Hobfoll, & D. L. Tennenbaum (Eds.), *Stress and coping in later-life families* (pp. 99–124). New York: Hemisphere.

Mikulincer, M., & Florian, V. (1996). Coping and adaptation to trauma and loss. In M. Zeidner & N. S. Endler (Eds.), *Handbook of coping: Theory, research, applications* (pp. 554–572). New York: John Wiley.

Monroe, S. M., & Steiner, S. C. (1986). Social support and psychopathology: Interrelations with preexisting disorder, stress, and personality. *Journal of Abnormal Psychology, 95,* 29–39.

Morris, T., Greer, S., Pettingale, K. W., & Watson, M. (1981). Patterns of expression of anger and their psychological correlates in women with breast cancer. *Journal of Psychosomatic Research, 25,* 111–117.

Mulder, C. L., Antoni, M. H., Duivenvoorden, H. J., & Kauffmann, R. H. (1995). Active confrontational coping predicts decreased clinical progression over a one-year period in HIV-infected homosexual men. *Journal of Psychosomatic Research, 39,* 957–965.

Mulder, C. L., de Vroome, E. M. M., van Griensven, G. J. P., Antoni, M. H., & Sandfort, T. G. M. (1999). Avoidance as a predictor of the biological course of HIV infection over a 7-year period in gay men. *Health Psychology, 18,* 107–113.

Olff, M. (1999). Stress, depression and immunity: The role of defense and coping styles. *Psychiatry Research, 85,* 7–15.

Pargament, K. (1997). *The psychology of religion and coping: Theory, research, and practice.* New York: Guilford.

Penley, J. A., Tomaka, J., & Wiebe, J. S. (2002). The association of coping to physical and psychological health outcomes: A meta-analytic review. *Journal of Behavioral Medicine, 25,* 551–603.

Petticrew, M., Bell, R., & Hunter, D. (2002). Influence of psychological coping on survival and recurrence in people with cancer: Systematic review. *British Medical Journal, 325,* 1066–1075.

Pisarski, A., Bohle, P., & Callan, V. J. (1998). Effects of coping strategies, social support and work–nonwork conflict on shift worker's health. *Scandinavian Journal of Work, Environment, and Health, 24*(Suppl. 3), 141–145.

Reich, J. W., & Zautra, A. J. (1995). Other-reliance encouragement effects in female rheumatoid arthritis patients. *Journal of Social and Clinical Psychology, 14,* 119–133.

Rook, K. S. (1998). Investigating the positive and negative sides of personal relationships: Through a lens darkly? In B. H. Spitzberg & W. R. Cupach (Eds.), *The dark side of close relationships* (pp. 369–393). Mahwah, NJ: Erlbaum.

Roth, S., & Cohen, L. J. (1986). Approach, avoidance, and coping with stress. *American Psychologist, 41,* 813–819.

Schaeffer, M. A., & Baum, A. (1984). Adrenal response at Three Mile Island. *Psychosomatic Medicine, 46,* 227–237.

Schaubroeck, J., Jones, J. R., & Xie, J. L. (2001). Individual differences in utilizing control to cope with job demands: Effects on susceptibility to infectious disease. *Journal of Applied Psychology, 86,* 265–278.

Schnurr, P. P., Rosenberg, S., & Friedman, M. (1993). Change in MMPI scores from college to adulthood as a function of military service. *Journal of Abnormal Psychology, 102,* 288–296.

Schnurr, P. P., Spiro, A., III, Aldwin, C. M., & Stukel, T. A. (1998). Symptom trajectories following trauma exposure: Longitudinal findings from the Normative Aging Study. *Journal of Nervous and Mental Disease, 186,* 522–528.

Schnurr, P. P., Spiro, A., III, & Paris, A. H. (2000). Physician diagnosed medical disorders in relation to PTSD symptoms in older male military veterans. *Health Psychology, 17,* 91–97.

Schwartz, C. E., & Daltroy, L. H. (1999). Learning from unreliability: The importance of inconsistency in coping dynamics. *Social Science and Medicine, 48,* 619–631.

Schwarzer, R., & Schwarzer, C. (1996). A critical survey of coping instruments. In M. Zeidner & N. S. Endler (Eds.), *Handbook of coping: Theory, research, and applications* (pp. 107–132). New York: John Wiley.

Segerstrom, S. C., Solomon, G. F., Kemeny, M., & Fahey, J. L. (1998). Relationship of worry to immune sequelae of the Northridge earthquake. *Journal of Behavioral Medicine, 21,* 433–450.

Shapiro, D. E., Boggs, S. R., Rodrigue, J. R., Urrya, H. L., Algina, J. J., Hellman, R., et al. (1997). Stage II breast cancer: Differences between four coping patterns in side effects during chemotherapy. *Journal of Psychosomatic Research, 43,* 143–157.

Silver, R. C., Holman, E. A., & Gil-Rivas, V. (2000, December). *Social responses to discussion of traumatic life events*. Paper presented at the University of California Intercampus Health Psychology Conference, Lake Arrowhead, CA.

Smyth, J. M. (1998). Written emotional expression: Effect sizes, outcome types, and moderating variables. *Journal of Consulting and Clinical Psychology, 66*, 174–184.

Solomon, Z., Mikulincer, M., & Avitzur, E. (1988). Coping, locus of control, social support, and combat-related posttraumatic stress disorder: A prospective study. *Journal of Personality and Social Psychology, 55*, 279–285.

Solomon, Z., Mikulincer, M., & Benbenishty, R. (1989). Combat stress reaction: Clinical manifestations and correlates. *Military Psychology, 1*, 35–47.

Stanford, S. C. (1993). Monoamines in response and adaptation to stress. In S. C. Stanford & P. Salmon (Eds.), *Stress: From synapse to syndrome* (pp. 282–332). San Diego: Academic Press.

Stephens, C., & Long, N. (2000). Communication with police supervisors and peers as a buffer of work-related traumatic stress. *Journal of Organizational Behavior, 21*, 407–424.

Stowell, J. R., Kiecolt-Glaser, J. K., & Glaser, R. (2001). Perceived stress and cellular immunity: When coping counts. *Journal of Behavioral Medicine, 24*, 323–339.

Tedeschi, R. G., Park, C. L., & Calhoun, L. G. (1998). Posttraumatic growth: Conceptual issues. In R. G. Tedeschi, C. L. Park, & L. G. Calhoun (Eds.), *Posttraumatic growth: Positive changes in the aftermath of crisis* (pp. 1–22). Mahwah, NJ: Erlbaum.

Tennen, H., & Affleck, G. (1996). Daily processes in coping with chronic pain: Methods and analytic strategies. In M. Zeidner & N. S. Endler (Eds.), *Handbook of coping: Theory, research, and applications* (pp. 151–177). New York: John Wiley.

Tennen, H., Affleck, G., Armeli, S., & Carney, M. A. (2000). A daily process approach to coping: Linking theory research and practice. *American Psychologist, 55*, 626–636.

Thoits, P. (1986). Social support as coping assistance. *Journal of Consulting and Clinical Psychology, 54*, 416–423.

Tomaka, J., Blascovich, J., & Kelsey, R. M. (1992). Effects of self-deception, social desirability, and repressive coping on psychophysiological reactivity to stress. *Personality and Social Psychology Bulletin, 18*, 616–624.

Van Eck, M. M., Nicholson, A. A., Berkhof, H., & Sulon, J. (1996). Individual differences in cortisol responses to a laboratory speech task and their relationship to responses to stressful daily events. *Biological Psychology, 43*, 69–84.

Vassend, O., Eskild, A., & Halvorsen, R. (1997). Negative affectivity, coping, immune status, and disease progression in HIV infected individuals. *Psychology and Health, 12*, 375–388.

Vickers, R. R. (1988). Effectiveness of defenses: A significant predictor of cortisol excretion under stress. *Journal of Psychosomatic Research, 32*, 21–29.

Vitaliano, P. P., Russo, J., Bailey, S. L., Young, H. M., & McCann, B. S. (1993). Psychosocial factors associated with cardiovascular reactivity in older adults. *Psychosomatic Medicine, 55,* 164–177.

Vitaliano, P. P., Russo, J., & Niaura, R. D. (1987). Locus of control, type of stressor, and appraisal within a cognitive-phenomenological model of stress. *Journal of Research in Personality, 21,* 224–237.

Vitaliano, P. P., Russo, J., & Niaura, R. (1995). Plasma lipids and their relationships with psychosocial factors in older adults. *Journals of Gerontology: Series B, Psychological Sciences and Social Sciences, 50,* P18–P24.

Vitaliano, P. P., Russo, J., Paulsen, V. M., & Bailey, S. L. (1995). Cardiovascular recovery from laboratory stress: Biopsychosocial concomitants in older adults. *Journal of Psychosomatic Research, 39,* 361–377.

Ward, C. (1988). Stress, coping, and adjustment in victims of sexual assault: The role of psychological defense mechanisms. *Counseling Psychology Quarterly, 1,* 165–178.

Weihs, K. L., Enright, T. M., Simmens, S. J., & Reiss, D. (2000). Negative affectivity, restriction of emotions, and site of metastases predict mortality in recurrent breast cancer. *Journal of Psychosomatic Research, 49,* 59–68.

Wolfe, J., Keane, T. M., Kaloupek, D. G., Mora, C. A., & Winde, P. (1993). Patterns of positive readjustment in Vietnam combat veterans. *Journal of Traumatic Stress, 6,* 179–191.

Wortman, C. B., Battle, E. S., & Lemkau, J. P. (1997). Coming to terms with the sudden, traumatic death of a spouse or child. In R. C. Davis & A. J. Lurigio (Eds.), *Victims of crime* (2nd ed., pp. 108–133). Thousand Oaks, CA: Sage.

Zautra, A. J., & Manne, S. L. (1992). Coping with rheumatoid arthritis: A review of a decade of research. *Annals of Behavioral Medicine, 14,* 31–39.

Zeidner, M., & Hammer, A. L. (1992). Coping with missile attack: Resources, strategies, and outcomes. *Journal of Personality, 6,* 709–746.

Zeidner, M., & Saklofske, D. (1996). Adaptive and maladaptive coping. In M. Zeidner & N. S. Endler (Eds.), *Handbook of coping: Theory, research, and applications* (pp. 505–531). New York: John Wiley.

III

BIOLOGICAL MECHANISMS LINKING TRAUMA AND HEALTH

6

PSYCHONEUROIMMUNOLOGY AND TRAUMA

ANGELA LIEGEY DOUGALL AND ANDREW BAUM

In this chapter we review research suggesting that stress-related changes in immune system function mediate many associations between traumatic stressors and infectious illness, cancer, HIV disease progression, and other aspects of physical health. It is widely accepted that reliable changes in immune activity are seen in the wake of exposure to stressors, but the extent to which observed stress-related changes affect susceptibility to disease or infection is not yet resolved. Brief discussion of relationships between stressors and immune system regulation and consideration of potential health effects of these relationships will include direct effects of stress on the immune system and indirect effects mediated through stress-related changes in other physiological, psychological, and behavioral pathways that also affect immunity (e.g., neuroendocrines, psychosocial variables, and health behaviors). Stress-related immune components of illness or related events are considered as well. We identify major gaps in the literature and examine future directions for research and practice.

Psychoneuroimmunology (PNI) is a multidisciplinary specialty that studies stress and immunity in the context of bidirectional interactions among psychological, neuroendocrine, and other central nervous system events or responses and the immune system. The study of stress reactions as a factor in regulation of the immune system as well as underlying neuroendocrine mechanisms have been a key focus of PNI investigation. Much of this research has been on immune alterations to acute stressors and commonplace chronic stressors such as examinations and caregiving. Recently, attention has turned to effects of extreme stressors and sequelae of psychological trauma.

The Immune System

A full review of the immune system is beyond the scope of this chapter. This system is highly complex, serving regulatory and sensory functions as well as providing the body's primary defenses against infection and disease. It constantly surveys the body to detect and eliminate infectious and noninfectious agents and to heal resulting damage. It also communicates with regulatory systems (e.g., nervous and endocrine systems) and participates in overall preservation of homeostasis.

Standard measures of immune system activity used in clinical and research settings are the numbers of immune cells present in circulation or storage sites (e.g., spleen) and measures of their functioning (e.g., their ability to replicate, fight off infection, or respond to a specific pathogenic challenge). The most common immune indices are listed in Table 6.1 and include enumerative and functional measures of T lymphocytes (T cells), B lymphocytes (B cells), and natural killer cells (NK cells). These lymphocytes are important defensive agents against infection and diseases such as

TABLE 6.1
Summary of Commonly Measured Immune Cells
and Their Functional Measures

Immune cell	Type of immunity	Functional measure(s)
B lymphocyte	Humoral acquired immunity	• Lymphocyte proliferation • Antibody titers
T lymphocyte (T cell) • Helper T cell • Cytotoxic T cell	Cell-mediated acquired immunity	• Lymphocyte proliferation • Cytotoxic activity • Antibody titers to latent viruses • Cutaneous cell-mediated immunity multitest scores
Natural killer cell	Natural immunity	• Cytotoxic activity

cancer, but the numbers of these cells in circulation or most assays of functional capacity are not complete indicators of host resistance. Furthermore, most research has examined immune responses to acute controlled stressors or to more chronic naturalistic stressors. Relatively little research has focused directly on immune changes following traumatic events.

Acute Stressors and Alterations in Immunity

Transient and immediate immune changes are observed during and following acute stressor exposure. Numbers of some peripheral lymphocytes consistently increase in response to acute stressors, most notably NK cells and cytotoxic T cells (Breznitz et al., 1998; Herbert et al., 1994; Naliboff et al., 1991). These changes are thought to reflect a redistribution of cells from storage in the lymphoid organs (e.g., lymph nodes, spleen) into the peripheral blood during stress (Benschop, Rodriguez-Feuuerhahn, & Schedlowski, 1996). One hypothesis is that these cells are traveling through the blood to reach areas, such as the skin or gastrointestinal tract, where they combat wounds or infection (Dhabhar, 1998). However, these additional lymphocytes appear to be inhibited in some way and produce a weaker response to stimulation (Bachen et al., 1992). In vitro proliferation responses of peripheral blood lymphocytes are usually suppressed during or after acute stressor exposure (Herbert et al., 1994). This means that lymphocyte replication in the face of challenge is suppressed, theoretically limiting immune defense. In contrast, functional measures of NK cell activity appear to covary with changes in NK cell numbers. Both numbers of NK cells and overall cytotoxicity increase during acute stressor exposure and then decrease to below baseline levels after stressor termination (Breznitz et al., 1998; Delahanty, Wang, Maravich, Forlenza, & Baum, 2000). Changes in NK cell numbers appear to be the principal stressor-related alteration, mediating the concomitant changes in NK cell cytotoxicity (Delahanty et al., 2000). Although acute stressor paradigms are useful for examining the mechanisms underlying immune changes, acute stressors usually last from 5 to 30 minutes, and changes in immunity in this time frame tell us little about the effects of major stressors or effects on disease susceptibility.

Chronic Stressors and Alterations in Immunity

Chronic, day-to-day stressors (e.g., caregiving, marital stress, bereavement) have been characterized by suppression of immune cell numbers and immune function. The same lymphocytes that show the largest increases during or shortly after exposure to acute stressors (e.g., cytotoxic T cells and NK cells) show the largest decreases during chronic stress (see Herbert & Cohen, 1993). Cell proliferation and NK cell cytotoxicity are usually diminished (Kiecolt-Glaser et al., 1987) and antibody titers for latent viruses such as Epstein-Barr are elevated (suggesting breakdown of cellular immunity that maintains latency of these viruses; Jenkins & Baum, 1995; Kiecolt-Glaser et al., 1987). In addition, chronic stress alters responses to acute stressors, blunting typical immune changes such as increases in T cells and NK cell cytotoxicity (Brosschot et al., 1994; Pike et al., 1997). Because posttraumatic stress has been characterized as a special case of a chronic stress condition (Baum, Cohen, & Hall, 1993; Baum, O'Keeffe, & Davidson, 1990), these studies are relevant to understanding effects of traumatic stressors on immunity and associated illnesses.

Traumatic Stressors and Alterations in Immunity

Relatively few studies have examined immune alterations following traumatic stressors. Only 15 published studies have examined immune function and psychological trauma, and this handful of studies has produced mixed findings. Eight found immune system changes similar to those associated with acute stressors (Boscarino & Chang, 1999; Burges Watson, Muller, Jones, & Bradley, 1993; Delahanty, Dougall, Craig, Jenkins, & Baum, 1997; Kemeny as cited in Solomon, Segerstrom, Grohr, Kemeny, & Fahey, 1997; Laudenslager et al., 1998; Sabioncello et al., 2000; Spivak et al., 1997; Weiss et al., 1996). Of these, four evaluated posttraumatic stress disorder (PTSD) and four studied exposure to a traumatic stressor. Five studies found immune responses more consistent with reactions to chronic stressors (DeBellis, Burke, Trickett, & Putnam, 1996; Inoue-Sakurai, Maruyama, & Morimoto, 2000; Ironson et al., 1997; McKinnon, Weisse, Reynolds, Bowles, & Baum, 1989; Mosnaim et al., 1993). Of these studies, three used diagnosis of PTSD as a predictor of immunity. Two reports from one study describe both types of changes (Segerstrom, Solomon, Kemeny, & Fahey, 1998; Solomon et al., 1997). Several explanations for these mixed findings can be proposed.

Timing of the Stressor

One important possibility is the timing of the immune measures relative to the traumatic event. Traumatic events can be time-limited (e.g., hurricane, airplane crash) or they can be repeated or ongoing (e.g., abuse, war combat). In addition, victims may need to deal with secondary stressors such as relocation, financial hardship, or reminders of the event after a traumatic event is over. Most trauma research assesses victims after the actual event has ended, sometimes even decades later. One could expect posttraumatic stress to be manifested as either acute stress, chronic stress, or as a combination of both depending on the type of event and the timing of the assessment.

Two studies assessed victims during ongoing traumatic events (Sabi-oncello et al., 2000; Weiss et al., 1996). Both studied civilians affected by an ongoing war and reported immune alterations that were similar to observations of acute stress response, including increases in T cells and NK cells and increases in overall NK cell cytotoxicity. Kemeny's unpublished study examined immune responses immediately after an earthquake (cited in Solomon et al., 1997). Again, consistent with studies of acute laboratory challenges, numbers of T cells and NK cells were higher immediately after the earthquake than they were at 6 weeks and 1 year later.

Recovery and Persistent Effects

Although most people who experience psychological trauma recover rapidly during the ensuing year (e.g., Blanchard et al., 1997), subsets of victims continue to experience significant distress years or decades afterwards. It is possible that changes in immune function could reflect this same pattern, with most people exhibiting a return to "normal" in the year following the trauma but with some showing larger or more persistent effects. Two of the studies that examined victims during or immediately after a psychological trauma found evidence of recovery 4–8 weeks after the trauma had ended (i.e., Kemeny cited in Solomon et al., 1997; Weiss et al., 1996). However, because of the nature of traumatic events, most studies do not begin assessment until the victims have already started to recover. In addition, most of these studies do not study PTSD but rather consider less specific or milder syndromes. Although most victims appear to recover quickly, some show more chronic alterations. Delahanty and colleagues (1997) found increased NK cell cytotoxicity among rescue and recovery workers at an airplane crash site (consistent with an acute response) within 2 months of a horrific air disaster. These effects dissipated quickly and were not evident 4 months later. Higher levels of NK cell cytotoxicity at the first assessment were positively correlated with posttraumatic stress measured as event-related intrusive thoughts. In contrast, Ironson and colleagues (1997) found higher numbers of NK cells but lower levels of NK cell cytotoxicity and numbers of T cells 2–4 months after a major hurricane. Lower levels of NK cell cytotoxicity were associated with higher levels of posttraumatic stress. De-Bellis and colleagues (1996) also found evidence of long-term immune suppression consistent with a chronic stress response when they studied girls who were sexually abused for an average duration of 23 months ($SD = 25$ months) with a range of 1–84 months. Abused girls had higher levels of plasma antinuclear antibodies than healthy adult women.

Solomon and colleagues (1997) also reported evidence of general recovery but some persistent effects, finding an overall decrease in NK and T cell numbers and activity over 4 months after a major earthquake. Low earthquake-specific distress at the first assessment (i.e., 11–24 days after the earthquake) was associated with larger decreases over time. In contrast, high general distress and disruption at the first assessment were associated with lower numbers of T cells, and high earthquake-specific distress at the first assessment was associated with increases over time in T cell and B cell numbers and poorer proliferation to the mitogen phytohemagglutinin (PHA) at all time points. When these data were examined by dividing the earthquake victim sample into high and low worry groups, the high worry group had lower numbers of NK cells at all time points than did the low worry group or the laboratory control values (Segerstrom et al., 1998). However, because the worry measure was not specific to the earthquake, it was not clear whether worry moderated the effects of the earthquake or whether worry was independently related to NK cell numbers. Another study examined victims 14–18 months after an earthquake and found that those victims with the highest number of PTSD symptoms had lower levels of NK cell cytotoxicity than those victims who did not report any symptoms of PTSD (Inoue-Sakurai et al., 2000).

Six more studies investigated persistent symptoms years after the traumatic event had ended. Most of them measured PTSD as opposed to the experience of a traumatic stressor (Boscarino & Chang, 1999; Burges Watson et al., 1993; Laudenslager et al., 1998; McKinnon et al., 1989; Mosnaim et al., 1993; Spivak et al., 1997) and examined victims who had psychiatric diagnoses. Only two examined victims who were not in psychiatric treatment (Boscarino & Chang, 1999; McKinnon et al., 1989). In McKinnon et al.'s study, residents who lived near the Three Mile Island (TMI) nuclear reactor accident had lower numbers of NK, T, and B cells and higher antibody titers to herpes simplex virus (HSV) than people who lived 80 miles away, and these alterations were associated with stress responses such as catecholamine production and distress. These changes were found 6 years after the TMI incident and suggested chronic immune system changes in these victims. However, it is difficult to say anything about timing in this group of studies because five of the six compared PTSD versus no PTSD.

Additionally, the five studies that examined combat veterans with PTSD are difficult to compare because of differences across studies in psychiatric treatments and type of immune measures. Mosnaim and colleagues (1993) measured NK cell cytotoxicity in Vietnam War veterans with PTSD after 10 days of substance abuse detoxification treatment and found no differences in NK cell cytotoxicity compared with four different control groups. However, if patients were used as their own controls, the PTSD group had lower NK cell cytotoxicity following stimulation with methionine-enkephalin (MET) than without stimulation, suggesting trauma-related inhibition of response to stimulation of NK cells. However, another study of Vietnam veterans with PTSD undergoing substance abuse detoxification found that NK cell cytotoxicity was higher in the patients with PTSD and substance abuse problems than in patients who only had substance abuse problems (Laudenslager et al., 1998). Small group sizes and the lack of a PTSD group without substance use make resolution of these findings difficult.

The remaining three studies reported evidence of increases in some indices of immune system activity (Boscarino & Chang, 1999; Burges Watson et al., 1993; Spivak et al., 1997). Burges Watson and colleagues found higher Cutaneous Cell-mediated Immunity (CMI) Multitest scores in Vietnam veterans with PTSD than in civilian control groups. Depending on how the CMI Multitest was scored, noncombat servicemen either did not differ from veterans with PTSD or had lower scores. The larger responses in the PTSD group suggested some immune enhancement and were consistent with findings from the acute stress literature (cf. Dhabhar, 1998). Spivak and colleagues (1997), studying Israeli war patients with PTSD who were free from any comorbid diagnoses, found that patients with PTSD had higher levels of interleukin-1β (IL-1β) than healthy control participants. Interleukin-1β levels were positively correlated with the duration of PTSD. These findings suggest greater activity of the mononuclear phagocytes that produce IL-1β. However, neither study measured the numbers of peripheral blood lymphocytes or their activities, limiting comparison of these findings to the studies mentioned previously.

Boscarino and Chang (1999) measured numbers of lymphocytes and responses to the CMI Multitest in Vietnam veterans with and without PTSD, with and without an anxiety disorder (presumably excluding PTSD), or with and without depression. After controlling for sociodemographic factors and health behaviors (e.g., drug use and alcohol consumption), differences were found only between the veterans with and without PTSD. Veterans with PTSD had more white blood cells, total lymphocytes, and T cell counts than veterans without PTSD. However, there were no group differences in CMI Multitest scores, inconsistent with results from Burges Watson and colleagues (1993).

These studies suggest that immune responses during or immediately following trauma exposure most closely resemble those observed after an acute stressor (e.g., increases in numbers of T and NK cells and increases in NK cell cytotoxicity). As people recover from trauma, immune profiles increasingly resemble those for unexposed individuals. However, because of the difficulties in predicting the occurrence of traumatic events, no studies have been able to obtain true baseline data. Additionally, there appear to be subgroups of victims who experience chronic reactions related to psychological trauma and who exhibit evidence of immunosuppression. In victims who are still plagued by symptoms of PTSD and other comorbid disorders decades after a trauma, there is evidence of both increases and decreases in quantitative and qualitative aspects of immune activity, highlighting the need for further study of individual difference factors in immune response to trauma (see Friedman & McEwen, chap. 7, this volume).

POTENTIAL MEDIATORS OF TRAUMA-RELATED IMMUNE ALTERATIONS

In addition to the type of traumatic event experienced and the timing of the assessments, several variables may influence a victim's immune response to trauma. Stress responding is a whole body response that affects not only the immune system but other physiological systems, psychological processes, and behaviors (Dougall & Baum, 2001). There are extensive bidirectional relationships among these stress response pathways, and immune alterations and disease processes following trauma are likely the products of these interactions.

Neuroendocrine Factors

Immune cells secrete cytokines that act on other immune cells and travel through the body, affecting cells in the periphery and in the central nervous system. These transmitters and messengers evoke bodily responses, including tiredness, depressed mood, decreased activity, fever, and inflammation. These symptoms of sickness are consequences of immune system activation rather than illness per se (Maier & Watkins, 1998). Immune cells, in turn, are affected by the release of central and peripheral neuroendocrine factors such as catecholamines and cortisol.

There is extensive innervation of immune organs and tissue by the autonomic nervous system, and, because most immune cells display receptors for neuroendocrines, it is likely that immune system activation is mediated by neuroendocrine activity (Esquifino & Cardinali, 1994; Yehuda, Boisoneau, Lowy, & Giller, 1995). Exogenous administration of epinephrine and norepinephrine produce immune system changes that are consistent with responses to acute stressors, including increases in numbers of cytotoxic T cells and NK cells, increases in NK cell cytotoxicity, and decreases in cell replication (Crary et al., 1983). Additionally, adrenergic blockade with drugs such as labetalol and propranolol attenuates stress-related changes in immunity (Bachen et al., 1995; Benschop, Jacobs, et al., 1996).

Glucocorticoids have been used for decades to reduce inflammation by suppressing immune functioning in diseases such as rheumatoid arthritis, asthma, and multiple sclerosis (Katzung, 1992). In contrast to the large immunosuppressive effects of pharmacological doses of glucocorticoids, physiological doses have been found to shift the immune response from primarily cell-mediated to B-cell-mediated humoral activity (Daynes, Araneo, Henne-bold, Enioutina, & Mu, 1995).

Both the sympathetic nervous system (SNS; e.g., catecholamines, blood pressure, heart rate) and the hypothalamic–pituitary–adrenal (HPA) axis (e.g., glucocorticoids) increase activity in response to stress (Weiner, 1992). Acute stressors initiate increases in SNS arousal that are correlated with increases in T cell and NK cell numbers, decreases in cell proliferation, and biphasic response of NK cell cytotoxicity (Delahanty et al., 2000; Manuck, Cohen, Rabin, Muldoon, & Bachen, 1991). However, acute stress alterations in HPA axis activity (e.g., increases in serum cortisol) have not been reliably associated with immune changes in humans (Zakowski, 1995).

Less research attention has focused on the relationship between the immune system and neuroendocrine arousal following exposure to a trau-matic stressor (i.e., Laudenslager et al., 1998; McKinnon et al., 1989; Sabi-oncello et al., 2000; Spivak et al., 1997). In the study of the TMI area 6 years after the nuclear reactor accident, high levels of urinary epinephrine were inversely related to numbers of NK cells and total lymphocytes and positively correlated with higher HSV titers, immunoglobulin G (IgG) levels, and numbers of neutrophils (McKinnon et al., 1989). Urinary norepi-nephrine was associated with lower numbers of NK cells and cytotoxic T cells, but urinary cortisol was not associated with these immune indices. The remaining three studies did not measure SNS arousal, focusing on HPA axis activation, cortisol, prolactin, dehydroepiandrosterone (DHEA), growth hormone, and β-endorphin (Laudenslager et al., 1998; Sabioncello et al., 2000; Spivak et al., 1997). In two studies of victims many years after their trauma (Laudenslager et al., 1998; Spivak et al., 1997), none of these hormones were associated with immune indices, corroborating McKinnon and colleagues' finding (1989) that HPA axis activation was not a strong predictor of immune measures. However, in the one study that examined victims of an ongoing war, serum cortisol levels were positively correlated with numbers of helper T cells (CD4) and activated lymphocytes (CD71), and β-endorphin levels were positively correlated with the percentage of spontaneously proliferating blood lymphocytes (Sabioncello et al., 2000). These results are contradictory to previous findings that cortisol suppresses cell-mediated immunity (Daynes et al., 1995).

Both the Laudenslager and colleagues (1998) and Spivak and colleagues (1997) studies were of trauma victims who had developed PTSD. Changes in the activation of the SNS system and the HPA axis in patients with PTSD have been documented and appear to vary on the basis of tonic versus phasic activation (see Friedman & McEwen, chap. 7, this volume). Although there remains some debate about associations between PTSD and cortisol levels or rhythms, there is little disagreement about SNS arousal as a component of PTSD (Yehuda, Southwick, Giller, Ma, & Mason, 1992).

Sympathetic activation appears to be a key component of acute and chronic stress and an important mediator of stress effects on immunity. Neuroendocrine alterations following trauma appear to be one pathway through which immune alterations occur. However, they do not account for all changes in immune functioning, leaving substantial variability that may be accounted for by other factors such as psychological and behavioral variables.

Psychosocial Variables

Psychosocial variables such as perceived control, predictability, personality variables, coping, and social support are commonly associated with the severity of stressors or their effects and are related to immune outcomes. Unpredictable stressors have been associated with decreases in cell proliferation not observed after exposure to a predictable stressor (Zakowski, 1995). Like predictability, controllability of the stressor is an important moderator of immune responding, but stressor controllability and immune responding do not vary in a linear fashion (Shea, Clover, & Burton, 1991). Low perceptions of control have been associated with decreases in immune functioning, specifically decreases in helper T cell numbers and decreases in NK cell cytotoxicity (Brosschot et al., 1998; Sieber et al., 1992). High perceived control has been linked with decreases in proliferation and percentages of monocytes and increases in B cell numbers (Brosschot et al., 1998; Weisse et al., 1990). The variability in these findings may be attributable to other individual difference factors, such as personality. Sieber and colleagues (1992) found that optimism and the desire to control one's experience exacerbated stressor effects on immune responding after exposure to an uncontrollable stressor. Independently, pessimism has been associated with decreases in NK cell cytotoxicity, proliferation, and numbers of T cells, increases in illness reporting, and decreases in survival of cancer and HIV-positive patients, making it an important variable for study (Byrnes et al., 1998; Lin & Peterson, 1990; Reed, Kemeny, Taylor, Wang, & Visscher, 1994; Schulz, Bookwala, Knapp, Scheier, & Williamson, 1996).

Social support also has independent effects on well-being and can be a potent buffer of stress (see Uchino, Cacioppo, & Kiecolt-Glaser, 1996). More social support has been consistently linked with less self-reported distress, lower heart rate and blood pressure, lower catecholamine levels, use of more adaptive coping strategies, and better immune functioning. Social support is also positively associated with better health, recovery from illness, and survival (see Reifman, 1995; Schwarzer & Leppin, 1989). However, seeking social support, which may reflect inadequate real or perceived support, has been associated with more negative outcomes (see Aldwin & Yancura, chap. 5, this volume).

Although relatively little research has examined the interrelationships among traumatic stressors, psychosocial variables, and immune functioning, psychosocial variables constitute one pathway through which individual differences in immune changes may emerge following a traumatic stressor. They are important targets of future research because they are more amenable to change than neuroendocrine response and could have important implications for interventions designed to alleviate posttraumatic stress. Health behaviors are also individual difference factors that have important implications for both immune functioning and disease morbidity following trauma.

Health Behaviors

Use of licit and illicit drugs, diet, and exercise are affected by perceptions of stress and are often used as a form of coping. They have also been linked with health outcomes independently and in conjunction with stress (see Rheingold, Acierno, & Resnick, chap. 9, this volume). These health behaviors have important effects on the immune system as well. Chronic use of drugs such as alcohol, marijuana, opiates, nicotine, caffeine, and cocaine has been linked with immunosuppression and increased risk for disease (Eisenstein & Hilburger, 1998; Klein, Friedman, & Specter, 1998; McAllister-Sistilli et al., 1998; Pellegrino & Bayer, 1998; Rosenthal, Taub, Moors, & Blank, 1992; Watson, Eskelson, & Hartmann, 1984). Habitual use or abuse of these substances may potentiate changes in immune system functioning following trauma, placing victims who are chronic users at an increased risk for illnesses. Additionally, victims who use these substances to cope with psychological trauma may experience further impairments in immune functioning and be at an even greater risk for developing illnesses.

Other health behaviors such as diet and exercise also affect the immune system and can alter immunological changes following stress. When people are coping with a great deal of stress, their diets tend to decrease in nutritional value and they engage in less physical exercise (Rosenbloom & Whittington, 1993; Willis, Thomas, Garry, & Goodwin, 1987). Changes in the type and quantity of food eaten can result in metabolic changes that are associated with changes in the immune system (Chandra & Chandra, 1986; Shronts, 1993). Deficiencies in protein, vitamins A, E, B_6, and folate, as well as excesses in fat, iron, and vitamin E have been linked to immunosuppression (Chandra & Chandra, 1986; Rasmussen, Kiens, Pedersen, & Richter, 1994). Obesity has also been linked with immune system alterations, specifically increases in numbers of leukocytes and lymphocytes with the exception of NK cells and cytotoxic T cells, and decreases in cell proliferation and NK cell cytotoxicity (Moriguchi, Oonishi, Kato, & Kishino, 1995; Nieman et al., 1999). Both poor nutritional status and obesity are associated with higher risk of disease susceptibility and morbidity (Shronts, 1993; Wolf & Colditz, 1996). Therefore, trauma victims who are obese or have nutritional imbalances in their diets may be at a greater risk for immune changes following trauma and disease onset or exacerbation. Similarly, victims may experience changes in eating patterns that make them more susceptible to immunosuppression and related consequences.

Moderate bouts of exercise are associated with increases in immune functioning similar to changes following an acute psychological stressor (Perna, Schneiderman, & LaPerriere, 1997). In fact, exercise is used as a "stressor" in many laboratory studies and is a useful model for examining neuroendocrine and metabolic mechanisms of immune reactivity to stress (Goebel & Mills, 2000). Exercise training increases fitness levels, improves mood and overall general health, and is associated with sustained increases in immune system functioning (Galloway & Jokl, 2000; LaPerriere et al., 1997; Paluska & Schwenk, 2000). This heightened immune system activity appears to reduce immune reactivity to stress, countering its deleterious effects (LaPerriere et al., 1990). Therefore, exercise training should be beneficial to someone who experiences a traumatic event. However, people who are experiencing chronic stress tend to decrease physical exercise (Rosenbloom & Whittington, 1993). For these victims, beneficial effects of exercise may dissipate as victims forgo usual exercise routines to deal with stressors and psychological trauma.

IMMUNE ALTERATIONS AS MECHANISMS FOR TRAUMATIC STRESS EFFECTS ON HEALTH AND DISEASE OUTCOMES

The relationship between illness symptoms and traumatic stressors is reviewed in detail elsewhere in this volume (see Green & Kimerling, chap. 2). Although there are many mechanisms through which traumatic stressors can alter disease processes, the current discussion focuses on the role of stress-related alterations in immunity (either suppression or enhancement) in the onset, management, and recovery of acute and chronic diseases such as infections, injuries, cancer, arthritis, diabetes, and chronic fatigue syndrome.

Infectious Illness

One of the immune system's principal responsibilities is to seek, control, and destroy infectious agents such as viruses and bacteria. If immune system activity is suppressed during periods of stress, there may be less resistance to infectious illnesses. Research in both controlled and natural settings supports the conventional wisdom that stress makes a person more susceptible to infectious illness (see Biondi & Zannino, 1997; Kiecolt-Glaser &

Glaser, 1995). Correlational studies have shown that increases in stress often precede the onset of illnesses (Kasl, Evans, & Niederman, 1979; Stone, Reed, & Neale, 1987). More controlled studies in which healthy participants are exposed to known amounts of a virus and then quarantined for 5 or more days have shown that people with high levels of life stress are more likely to become infected and exhibit symptoms than are people with lower levels of stress (Cohen et al., 1998). Rates of both viral infection and illness symptoms increase in a dose–response fashion with the amount of life stress the participants reported (Cohen et al., 1998).

Only a few studies have examined immune measures as potential mechanisms, but neither cell counts, NK cell cytotoxicity, nor cell proliferation have been associated with illness (Cohen et al., 1998; Lee, Meehan, Robinson, Mabry, & Smith, 1992). These studies may not have assessed the "right" immune mediators or failed to measure them at the "right" time. Given the route of entry of infectious agents, immune factors in the mucosal lining may be better targets for study. However, antibody levels in the saliva (i.e., immunoglobulin A) were not correlated with illness episodes following medical examinations in one sample (Deinzer & Schüller, 1998).

More evidence for immune system mediators of illness has been found in the trauma literature. Although symptom reports 6 months after work at an airplane crash site were not associated with trauma exposure, NK cell cytotoxicity was negatively correlated with the number of colds, number of days ill, presence of allergies, and presence of asthma reported during the preceding 6-month time frame (Delahanty et al., 1997). Similarly, an increase in illness symptoms after a hurricane was negatively associated with NK cell cytotoxicity and positively associated with numbers of NK cells and white blood cells (Ironson et al., 1997). Reports of poorer health following the hurricane were associated with lower NK cell cytotoxicity and higher white blood cell counts. Hurricane victims reported an almost twofold increase in illness symptoms following the hurricane. Although these findings are suggestive, other variables could be responsible for observed outcomes and there were no true baseline rates of illness and immunity established.

In general, immune changes of the type associated with psychological trauma are thought to affect immune system surveillance for disease-causing pathogens, providing an opportunity for infectious agents to gain a foothold in susceptible tissue. First-line defenses do not appear to be as impaired as more complex secondary reactions. Initial responses to the detection of a pathogen in the body are by innate immune agents such as neutrophils, which attack and phagocytize (engulf and destroy) these pathogens. Some studies suggest that stress increases numbers of neutrophils, possibly because of steroid-related stimulation of bone marrow to release stored cells (e.g., McKinnon et al., 1989). Monocytes, macrophages, and natural killer cells are also involved in this initial defense against incursion by infectious agents and although relatively little is known about monocyte and macrophage activity after stressor exposure, natural killer cell numbers are increased acutely but appear to decrease rapidly with continued exposure or elimination of the stressor (e.g., Breznitz et al., 1998; Delahanty et al., 2000). Because these cells are more central to defense against viruses (neutrophils are particularly useful against bacteria), stressor exposure could heighten but then weaken viral defense. Longer-term stress exposure or stressful experience should reduce most components of acquired immunity and may increase inflammation, heightening possibilities for infection and tissue damage. Therefore, immune alterations following trauma may place a victim at greater risk for developing infectious illnesses. Similarly, studies of wound healing suggest that stress impairs healing processes and that reduction of IL-1β plays an important role in this effect (Marucha, Kiecolt-Glaser, & Favagehi, 1998). However, these findings are far from definitive and more research needs to examine the interrelationships among trauma, immunity, and infection. Expanding the types of immunological markers that are examined as well as making multiple assessments may help to clarify these relationships.

Latent Viruses

A large percentage of the population has been exposed to viruses that lay dormant in their bodies, kept in check by their immune systems. These viruses occasionally escape containment and reactivate, causing symptoms that include cold sores, shingles, and genital rashes. The immune system responds by increasing production of antibody titers specific to the virus. Antibody titers to these viruses are elevated in people undergoing chronic stressors, such as caregiving for family members and academic stress (Glaser et al., 1987; Kasl et al., 1979). Consistent with these findings, residents of Three Mile Island 6 years after the nuclear accident had higher antibody titers to HSV than people living more than 80 miles away (McKinnon et al., 1989).

The human immunodeficiency virus (HIV) invades helper T cells (CD4+) and can remain latent in the form of proviruses. Progression of HIV disease occurs when the virus replicates and starts destroying the host cells, leading to the progressive degeneration of the immune system. Rapid progression is associated with decreases in numbers of naive helper T cells and decreases in NK cell number and activity (Bruunsgaard, Pedersen, Skinhoj, & Pedersen, 1997; Ullum et al., 1997). Therefore, stress-related immunosuppression following exposure to psychological trauma could be harmful to patients with HIV, but research needs to test this hypothesis.

Cancer

Cancer develops over years or decades and is the result of several different processes. The immune system normally acts to detect and eliminate mutagenic cells, but poorer repair of damaged DNA, alterations in apoptosis, and other processes are also important (see Kiecolt-Glaser & Glaser, 1999). Stress-related immune alterations could affect neoplastic growth by inhibiting immunosurveillance for nascent tumor growth, affecting progression from benign to malignant tumor growth and metastatic spread. However, the chronic nature of cancer development has made studies of stress, immunity, and cancer difficult. Most have focused on alterations in NK cell numbers and activity (Kiecolt-Glaser & Glaser, 1999) with a smaller body of evidence linking stress to DNA repair capabilities and alterations in apoptosis (Kiecolt-Glaser, Stephens, Lipetz, Speicher, & Glaser, 1985; Tomei, Kiecolt-Glaser, Kennedy, & Glaser, 1990). NK cells are important in the elimination of metastatic cancer cells (Whiteside & Herberman, 1989). Decreases in NK cell cytotoxicity have been linked to cancer patients' reports of stress, to poorer immune function, and to poorer disease prognosis (Levy, Herberman, Lippman, & D'Angelo, 1987). Additionally, some stress-reducing psychological interventions for cancer patients appear to bolster immune system activity and extend survival (e.g., Fawzy et al., 1993). At this time, however, evidence linking stress, immunity, and cancer course is neither definitive nor complete.

Autoimmune Diseases

Autoimmune diseases such as rheumatoid arthritis (RA) and diabetes mellitus type I are chronic conditions that result when the immune system mounts an attack against self-cells. Immune alterations following stress can exacerbate or ameliorate symptoms of these diseases and may play a role in their onset. For example, most cases of rheumatoid arthritis are the result of helper T cell mediated immune responses that cause joint inflammation and destruction (Janeway & Travers, 1994). Some cases also involve the production of self-antibodies (rheumatoid factor). Increases in immune system activity (as in response to acute stressors) should be associated with symptom flare-ups whereas chronic immunosuppression should be associated with an improvement in symptoms. Some evidence supports these differential relationships. Minor daily stressors are associated with exacerbation of RA, whereas major life events are associated with decreases in disease activity (Potter & Zautra, 1997). However, there is a subset of patients with RA whose disease symptoms are not affected by stress; among people who are seropositive for the autoantibody rheumatoid factor, stressful life events are not related to disease activity. Among seronegative patients, these life events are associated with increases in disease activity and with the onset of the disease (Stewart, Knight, Palmer, & Highton, 1994). This suggests that some RA patients will experience exacerbation of disease symptoms during or immediately following traumatic events. If the resulting trauma is sufficient to cause chronic PTSD, this may suppress disease activity. One study of RA patients found more disease flare-ups and more disease progression following a hurricane or an earthquake than among patients not exposed to a disaster (Grady et al., 1991).

In insulin-dependent or Type I diabetes mellitus, immune cells attack the insulin-producing cells in the pancreas, slowing insulin production and decreasing the amount of glucose that can be used by cells (Bosi & Sarugeri, 1998; Schranz & Lernmark, 1998). Because Type I diabetes is an autoimmune disease, stress should affect it in much the same way as RA. Acute exposure should lead to increases in immune activity and disease symptoms whereas chronic stress should be associated with immunosuppression and possibly improvement of symptoms. Very little research has examined the relationship between stress and diabetes. However, evidence suggests that repetitive or persistent stressors may make individuals more susceptible to the onset of both Type I and Type II diabetes (American Diabetes Association, 1997; Ionescu-Tirgoviste, Simion, Mariana, Dan, & Iulian, 1987) and can interfere with symptom management by interfering with glycemic control (Murphy, Thompson, & Morris, 1997). Most of this research has focused on the direct effects of stress on the release of large quantities of glucose as well as health behaviors that can impair self-care and result in abnormal glucose levels. Stress may lead to persistent increases in glucose levels that the body cannot properly handle (Surwit & Wiliams, 1996). In extreme cases, these alterations may lead to ketoacidosis and diabetic coma (Guyton, 1991).

Chronic Fatigue Syndrome

Chronic fatigue syndrome (CFS) is characterized by severe fatigue present for at least 6 months and accompanied by symptoms of sore throat, painful lymph nodes, arthralgia, cognitive deficits, headaches, postexertional malaise, and sleep disturbances (Fukuda et al., 1994). Despite its debilitating effects, the etiology of CFS is unknown. Acute infections, especially viral infections, appear to modulate disease onset in some patients (Glaser & Kiecolt-Glaser, 1998). Subgroups of CFS patients have elevated antibody titers to latent viruses, including Epstein-Barr virus (EBV) and strains of HSV (Sairenji, Yamanishi, Tachibana, Bertoni, & Kurata, 1995). Additionally, there is a dysregulation of the immune and neuroendocrine systems in some CFS patients (Evengård, Schacterle, & Komaroff, 1999). Most notably, there is evidence for decreased HPA activity, decreased NK cell cytotoxicity, and decreased T cell proliferation (Caligiuri et al., 1987; Demitrack et al., 1991; Straus, Fritz, Dale, Gould, & Strober, 1993). There is also evidence of decreased sensitivity of the immune system to exogenous administration of glucocorticoids, suggesting a breakdown in the neuroendocrine–immune communication pathways (Kavelaars, Kuis, Knook, Sinnema, & Heijnen, 2000).

Stress has been implicated in the onset and exacerbation of CFS (Glaser & Kiecolt-Glaser, 1998). Patients often report that the onset of their CFS symptoms was preceded by stressful events (Chalder, Power, & Wessely, 1996). Additionally, patients' daily reports of CFS symptoms are correlated with daily stressful experiences (Dougall, Baum, & Jenkins, 1998). There are several possible mechanisms through which stress may influence CFS symptomatology (Glaser & Kiecolt-Glaser, 1998). As discussed earlier, chronic stress is associated with decreases in NK cell cytotoxicity and cell proliferation similar to the alterations seen in CFS. Stress is also associated with reactivation of latent viruses. Traumatic stressors may be particularly detrimental to CFS patients. One study examined CFS patients who were affected by Hurricane Andrew and found an exacerbation of CFS symptoms that was positively associated with the amount of posttraumatic stress they experienced (Lutgendorf et al., 1995). Anecdotal evidence also suggests that traumatic stressors may be precipitating factors in CFS, possibly interacting with viral infections (Chalder et al., 1996). Although the relationships among stress, immunity, and CFS are not clear, researchers are working to unravel the mystery of CFS.

CONCLUSIONS AND FUTURE DIRECTIONS

Traumatic stressors appear to affect vulnerability to illness and have effects on the immune system that may mediate heightened susceptibility to infectious illnesses and exacerbation of disease symptoms. Although the directions of effects are not always consistent nor immediately explained, it is likely that the point at which people are studied after psychological trauma and whether they develop PTSD or another psychiatric disorder contribute to this seeming inconsistency. Because stress responses following such traumatic exposure are probably not consistent and regular, but rather episodic and of varying intensities, immune measures collected in studies of trauma victims may not always reflect the same things. Studies that target a long-distant stressor may initiate stressful thoughts about it and precipitate an acute episode of distress in a generally quiescent individual. This kind of experience would be expected to generate different immune sequelae than would more consistent, unvarying distress associated with an inability to adjust to life circumstances. At the same time, the interplay of direct effects of stress and of indirect effects of behaviors that are responses to stress may contribute complexity to this picture. Some of the consequences of increased tobacco or alcohol use, for example, may interact with direct stressor effects to produce paradoxical or potentially misleading effects on immune system activity. Future research should address these and other possibilities as we learn more about the physical health impact of traumatic stressors.

Investigation of traumatic stressors and immune system activity is important because stress responding and trauma-related outcomes are likely mediators of physical and mental health. In particular, PTSD may mediate the impact of stressful or traumatic events on disease vulnerability and progression (chap. 2 and chap. 10, this volume; Friedman & Schnurr, 1995; Schnurr & Jankowski, 1999). If these relationships hold, and the hormonal and immunological sequelae of PTSD are reliable outcomes of psychological trauma, they may explain some instances of disease onset or progression. It is unlikely that the impact of routine, day-to-day stressors are sufficient to disrupt normal bodily defenses and render people more susceptible to infection or illness. The cumulative burden of these stressors may predict vulnerability in some cases, but it is more likely that severe stressors that can cause psychological trauma and consequent disruptions of normal bodily functioning over prolonged time are associated with increased susceptibility to disease processes. PTSD, as a principal mental health outcome of exposure to severe stressors, reflects profound and integrated behavioral and biological changes that may together represent an important intervening step between environmental events and health. Similarly, any interventions that are designed to alleviate symptoms of posttraumatic stress should also counteract the resultant immunological changes. This is supported by findings from studies on stress management interventions designed to reduce distress in populations such as patients with cancer, patients with HIV, and community samples that have shown concomitant effects on stress-related immunological changes (Antoni et al., 2000; Fawzy et al., 1993; Kiecolt-Glaser, Glaser, et al., 1985).

The recognition of immune system and physical health effects of traumatic stressors adds a sense of urgency and heightened importance to studying them, although no additional significance is needed to pursue investigation and treatment of psychological trauma syndromes. Knowing that traumatic stressors have particular effects may be useful in diagnosing posttrauma conditions, may help to refine or broaden treatment approaches to address mechanisms underlying observed immune system effects, and may help us understand the nature of mind–body determination of a range of outcomes following trauma. This literature will also help us to manage the health sequelae of psychological trauma, an increasingly important and studied area. Much remains to be done as we continue to apply what we know about traumatic stressors and psychoneuroimmunology to the study and treatment of victimized people.

REFERENCES

American Diabetes Association. (1997). *American Diabetes Association complete guide to diabetes*. Alexandria, VA: Author.

Antoni, M. H., Cruess, D. G., Cruess, S., Lutgendorf, S. K., Kumar, M., Ironson, G., et al. (2000). Cognitive–behavioral stress management intervention effects on anxiety, 24-hour urinary norepinephrine output, and T-cytotoxic/suppressor cells over time among symptomatic HIV-infected gay men. *Journal of Consulting and Clinical Psychology, 68,* 31–45.

Bachen, E. A., Manuck, S. B., Cohen, S., Muldoon, M. F., Raible, R., Herbert, T. B., et al. (1995). Adrenergic blockade ameliorates cellular immune responses to mental stress in humans. *Psychosomatic Medicine, 57,* 366–372.

Bachen, E. A., Manuck, S. B., Marsland, A. L., Cohen, S., Malkoff, S. B., Muldoon, M. F., et al. (1992). Lymphocyte subset and cellular immune response to a brief experimental stressor. *Psychosomatic Medicine, 54,* 673–679.

Baum, A., Cohen, L., & Hall, M. (1993). Control and intrusive memories as possible determinants of chronic stress. *Psychosomatic Medicine, 55,* 274–286.

Baum, A., O'Keeffe, M. K., & Davidson, L. M. (1990). Acute stressors and chronic response: The case of traumatic stress. *Journal of Applied Social Psychology, 20,* 1643–1654.

Benschop, R. J., Jacobs, R., Sommer, B., Schurmeyer, T. H., Raab, J. R., Schmidy, R. E., et al. (1996). Modulation of the immunologic response to acute stress in humans by beta-blockade or benzodiazepines. *FASEB Journal, 10,* 517–524.

Benschop, R. J., Rodriguez-Feuuerhahn, M., & Schedlowski, M. (1996). Catecholamine-induced leukocytosis: Early observations, current research, and future directions. *Brain, Behavior, and Immunity, 10,* 77–91.

Biondi, M., & Zannino, L. (1997). Psychological stress, neuroimmunomodulation, and susceptibility to infectious diseases in animals and man: A review. *Psychotherapy and Psychosomatics, 66,* 3–26.

Blanchard, E. B., Hickling, E. J., Forneris, C. A., Taylor, A. E., Buckley, T. C., Loos, W. R., et al. (1997). Prediction of remission of acute posttraumatic stress disorder in motor vehicle accident victims. *Journal of Traumatic Stress, 10,* 215–234.

Boscarino, J. A., & Chang, J. (1999). Higher abnormal leukocyte and lymphocyte counts 20 years after exposure to severe stress: Research and clinical implications. *Psychosomatic Medicine, 61,* 378–386.

Bosi, E., & Sarugeri, E. (1998). Advances and controversies in etiopathogenesis of Type 1 (insulin-dependent) diabetes mellitus. *Journal of Pediatric Endocrinology and Metabolism, 11*(Suppl. 2), 293–305.

Breznitz, S., Ben-Zur, H., Berzon, Y., Weiss, D. W., Levitan, G., Tarcic, N., et al. (1998). Experimental induction and termination of acute psychological stress in human volunteers: Effects on immunological, neuroendocrine, cardiovascular, and psychological parameters. *Brain, Behavior, and Immunity, 12*, 34–52.

Brosschot, J. F., Benschop, R. J., Godaert, G. L. R., Olff, M., De Smet, M., Heijnen, C. J., et al. (1994). Influence of life stress on immunological reactivity to mild psychological stress. *Psychosomatic Medicine, 56*, 216–224.

Brosschot, J. F., Godaert, G. L. R., Benschop, R. J., Olff, M., Ballieux, R. E., & Heijnen, C. J. (1998). Experimental stress and immunological reactivity: A closer look at perceived uncontrollability. *Psychosomatic Medicine, 60*, 359–361.

Bruunsgaard, H., Pedersen, C., Skinhoj, P., & Pedersen, B. K. (1997). Clinical progression of HIV infection: Role of NK cells. *Scandinavian Journal of Immunology, 46*, 91–95.

Burges Watson, I. P., Muller, H. K., Jones, I. H., & Bradley, A. J. (1993). Cell-mediated immunity in combat veterans with posttraumatic stress disorder. *Medical Journal of Australia, 159*, 513–516.

Byrnes, D. M., Antoni, M. H., Goodkin, K., Efantis-Potter, J., Asthana, D., Simon, T., et al. (1998). Stressful events, pessimism, natural killer cell cytotoxicity, and cytotoxic/suppressor T cells in HIV+ Black women at risk for cervical cancer. *Psychosomatic Medicine, 60*, 714–722.

Caligiuri, M., Murray, C., Buchwald, D., Levine, H., Cheney, P., Peterson, D., et al. (1987). Phenotypic and functional deficiency of natural killer cells in patients with chronic fatigue syndrome. *Journal of Immunology, 139*, 3306–3313.

Chalder, T., Power, M. J., & Wessely, S. (1996). Chronic fatigue in the community: A question of attribution. *Psychological Medicine, 26*, 791–800.

Chandra, S., & Chandra, R. K. (1986). Nutrition, immune response, and outcome. *Progress in Food and Nutrition Science, 10*, 1–65.

Cohen, S., Frank, E., Doyle, W. J., Skoner, D. P., Rabin, B. S., & Gawltney, J. M., Jr. (1998). Types of stressors that increase susceptibility to the common cold in healthy adults. *Health Psychology, 17*, 214–223.

Crary, B., Borysenko, D. C., Sutherland, D. C., Kutz, I., Borysenko, J. Z., & Benson, H. (1983). Decrease in mitogen responsiveness of mononuclear cells from peripheral blood after epinephrine administration in humans. *Journal of Immunology, 130*, 694–697.

Daynes, R. A., Araneo, B. A., Hennebold, J., Enioutina, E., & Mu, H. H. (1995). Steroids as regulators of the mammalian immune response. *Journal of Investigative Dermatology, 105*(Suppl. 1), 14S–19S.

DeBellis, M. D., Burke, L., Trickett, P. K., & Putnam, F. W. (1996). Antinuclear antibodies and thyroid function in sexually abused girls. *Journal of Traumatic Stress, 9*, 369–378.

Deinzer, R., & Schüller, N. (1998). Dynamics of stress-related decrease of salivary immunoglobulin A (sIgA): Relationship to symptoms of the common cold and studying behavior. *Behavioral Medicine, 23*, 161–169.

Delahanty, D. L., Dougall, A. L., Craig, K. J., Jenkins, F. J., & Baum, A. (1997). Chronic stress and natural killer cell activity after exposure to traumatic death. *Psychosomatic Medicine, 59,* 467–476.

Delahanty, D. L., Wang, T., Maravich, C., Forlenza, M., & Baum, A. (2000). Time-of-day effects on response of natural killer cells to acute stress in men and women. *Health Psychology, 19,* 39–45.

Demitrack, M. A., Dale, J. K., Straus, S. E., Laue, L., Listwak, S. J., Kruesi, M. J., et al. (1991). Evidence for impaired activation of the hypothalamic-pituitary-adrenal axis in patients with chronic fatigue syndrome. *Journal of Clinical Endocrinology and Metabolism, 73,* 1224–1234.

Dhabhar, F. S. (1998). Stress-induced enhancement of cell-mediated immunity. *Annals of the New York Academy of Sciences: Vol. 840* (pp. 359–372). New York: New York Academy of Sciences.

Dougall, A. L., & Baum, A. (2001). Stress, health, and illness. In A. Baum, T. A. Revenson, & J. E. Singer (Eds.), *Handbook of health psychology* (pp. 321–337). Mahwah, NJ: Lawrence Erlbaum.

Dougall, A. L., Baum, A., & Jenkins, F. J. (1998). Daily fluctuation in chronic fatigue syndrome severity and symptoms. *Journal of Biobehavioral Research, 3,* 12–28.

Eisenstein, T. K., & Hilburger, M. E. (1998). Opioid modulation of immune responses: Effects on phagocytes and lymphoid cell populations. *Journal of Neuroimmunology, 83,* 36–44.

Esquifino, A. I., & Cardinali, D. P. (1994). Local regulation of the immune response by the autonomic nervous system. *Neuroimmunomodulation, 1,* 265–273.

Evengård, B., Schacterle, R. S., & Komaroff, A. L. (1999). Chronic fatigue syndrome: New insights and old ignorance. *Journal of Internal Medicine, 246,* 455–469.

Fawzy, F. I., Fawzy, N. W., Hyun, C. S., Guthrie, D., Fahey, J. L., & Morton, D. (1993). Malignant melanoma: Effects of an early structured psychiatric intervention, coping, and affective state on recurrence and survival six years later. *Archives of General Psychiatry, 50,* 681–689.

Friedman, M. J., & Schnurr, P. P. (1995). The relationship between PTSD, trauma, and physical health. In M. J. Friedman, D. S. Charney, & A. Y. Deutch (Eds.), *Neurobiological and clinical consequences of stress: From normal adaptation to PTSD* (pp. 507–527). Philadelphia: Lippincott-Raven.

Fukuda, K., Straus, S. E., Hickie, I., Sharpe, M. C., Dobbins, J. G., Komaroff, A., et al. (1994). The chronic fatigue syndrome: A comprehensive approach to its definition and study. *Annals of Internal Medicine, 121,* 953–959.

Galloway, M. T., & Jokl, P. (2000). Aging successfully: The importance of physical activity in maintaining health and function. *Journal of the American Academy of Orthopaedic Surgeons, 8,* 37–44.

Glaser, R., & Kiecolt-Glaser, J. K. (1998). Stress-associated immune modulation: Relevance to viral infections and chronic fatigue syndrome. *American Journal of Medicine, 105,* 35S–42S.

Glaser, R., Rice, J., Sheridan, J., Fertel, R., Stout, J., Speicher, C., et al. (1987). Stress-related immune suppression: Health implications. *Brain, Behavior, and Immunity, 1*, 7–20.

Goebel, M. U., & Mills, P. J. (2000). Acute psychological stress and exercise and changes in peripheral leukocyte adhesion molecule expression and density. *Psychosomatic Medicine, 62*, 664–670.

Grady, K. E., Reisine, S. T., Fifield, J., Lee, N. R., McVay, J., & Kelsey, M. E. (1991). The impact of Hurricane Hugo and the San Francisco earthquake on a sample of people with rheumatoid arthritis. *Arthritis Care and Research, 4*, 106–110.

Guyton, A. C. (1991). *Textbook of medical physiology* (8th ed.). Philadelphia: W. B. Saunders.

Herbert, T. B., & Cohen, S. (1993). Stress and immunity in humans: A meta-analytic review. *Psychosomatic Medicine, 55*, 364–379.

Herbert, T. B., Cohen, S., Marsland, A. L., Bachen, E. A., Rabin, B. S., Muldoon, M. F., et al. (1994). Cardiovascular reactivity and the course of immune response to an acute psychological stressor. *Psychosomatic Medicine, 56*, 337–344.

Inoue-Sakurai, C., Maruyama, S., & Morimoto, K. (2000). Posttraumatic stress and lifestyles are associated with natural killer cell activity in victims of the Hanshin-Awaji Earthquake in Japan. *Preventive Medicine, 31*, 467–473.

Ionescu-Tirgoviste, C., Simion, P., Mariana, C., Dan, C. M., & Iulian, M. (1987). The signification of stress in the aetiopathogenesis of Type-sub-2 diabetes mellitus. *Stress Medicine, 3*, 277–284.

Ironson, G., Wynings, C., Schneiderman, N., Baum, A., Rodriguez, M., Greenwood, D., et al. (1997). Posttraumatic stress symptoms, intrusive thoughts, loss and immune function after Hurricane Andrew. *Psychosomatic Medicine, 59*, 128–141.

Janeway, C. A., Jr., & Travers, P. (1994). *Immunobiology: The immune system in health and disease.* New York: Garland Publishing.

Jenkins, F. J., & Baum, A. (1995). Stress and reactivation of latent herpes simplex virus: A fusion of behavioral medicine and molecular biology. *Annals of Behavioral Medicine, 17*, 116–123.

Kasl, S. V., Evans, A. S., & Niederman, J. C. (1979). Psychosocial risk factors in the development of infectious mononucleosis. *Psychosomatic Medicine, 41*, 445–466.

Katzung, B. G. (1992). Introduction to autonomic pharmacology. In B. G. Katzung (Ed.), *Basic and clinical pharmacology* (5th ed., pp. 69–81). Norwalk, CT: Appleton & Lange.

Kavelaars, A., Kuis, W., Knook, L., Sinnema, G., & Heijnen, C. J. (2000). Disturbed neuroendocrine-immune interactions in chronic fatigue syndrome. *Journal of Clinical Endocrinology and Metabolism, 85*, 692–696.

Kiecolt-Glaser, J. K., Fisher, L. D., Ogrocki, P., Stout, J. C., Speicher, C. E., & Glaser, R. (1987). Marital quality, marital disruption, and immune function. *Psychosomatic Medicine, 49,* 13–34.

Kiecolt-Glaser, J. K., & Glaser, R. (1995). Psychoneuroimmunology and health consequences: Data and shared mechanisms. *Psychosomatic Medicine, 57,* 269–274.

Kiecolt-Glaser, J. K., & Glaser, R. (1999). Psychoneuroimmunology and cancer: Fact or fiction? *European Journal of Cancer, 35,* 1603–1607.

Kiecolt-Glaser, J. K., Glaser, R., Williger, D., Stout, J., Messick, G., Sheppard, S., et al. (1985). Psychosocial enhancement of immunocompetence in a geriatric population. *Health Psychology, 4,* 25–41.

Kiecolt-Glaser, J. K., Stephens, R. E., Lipetz, P. D., Speicher, C. E., & Glaser, R. (1985). Distress and DNA repair in human lymphocytes. *Journal of Behavioral Medicine, 8,* 311–320.

Klein, T. W., Friedman, H., & Specter, S. (1998). Marijuana, immunity and infection. *Journal of Neuroimmunology, 83,* 102–115.

LaPerriere, A., Antoni, M. H., Schneiderman, N., Ironson, G., Klimas, N., Caralis, P., et al. (1990). Exercise intervention attenuates emotional distress and natural killer cell decrements following notification of positive serologic status for HIV-1. *Biofeedback and Self-Regulation, 15,* 229–242.

LaPerriere, A., Klimas, N., Fletcher, M. A., Perry, A., Ironson, G., Perna, F., et al. (1997). Change in CD4+ cell enumeration following aerobic exercise training in HIV-1 disease: Possible mechanisms and practical applications. *International Journal of Sports Medicine, 18*(Suppl.), S56–S61.

Laudenslager, M. L., Aasal, R., Adler, L., Berger, C. L., Montgomery, P. T., Sandberg, E., et al. (1998). Elevated cytotoxicity in combat veterans with long-term post-traumatic stress disorder: Preliminary observations. *Brain, Behavior, and Immunity, 12,* 74–79.

Lee, D. J., Meehan, R. T., Robinson, C., Mabry, T. R., & Smith, M. L. (1992). Immune responsiveness and risk of illness in U.S. Air Force Academy cadets during basic cadet training. *Aviation Space and Environmental Medicine, 63,* 517–523.

Levy, S., Herberman, R., Lippman, M., & D'Angelo, T. (1987). Correlation of stress factors with sustained depression of natural killer cell activity and predicted prognosis in patients with breast cancer. *Journal of Clinical Oncology, 5,* 348–353.

Lin, E. H., & Peterson, C. (1990). Pessimistic explanatory style and response to illness. *Behaviour, Research, and Therapy, 28,* 243–248.

Lutgendorf, S. K., Antoni, M. H., Ironson, G., Fletcher, M. A., Penedo, F., Baum, A., et al. (1995). Physical symptoms of chronic fatigue syndrome are exacerbated by the stress of Hurricane Andrew. *Psychosomatic Medicine, 57,* 310–323.

Maier, S. F., & Watkins, L. R. (1998). Cytokines for psychologists: Implications for bidirectional immune-to-brain communication for understanding behavior, mood, and cognition. *Psychological Review, 105,* 83–107.

Manuck, S. B., Cohen, S., Rabin, B. S., Muldoon, M. F., & Bachen, E. A. (1991). Individual differences in cellular immune response to stress. *Psychological Science, 2*, 111–115.

Marucha, P. T., Kiecolt-Glaser, J. K., & Favagehi, M. (1998). Mucosal wound healing is impaired by examination stress. *Psychosomatic Medicine, 60*, 362–365.

McAllister-Sistilli, C. G., Cagiula, A. R., Knopf, S., Rose, C. A., Miller, A. L., & Donny, E. C. (1998). The effects of nicotine on the immune system. *Psychoneuroendocrinology, 23*, 175–187.

McKinnon, W., Weisse, C. S., Reynolds, C. P., Bowles, C. A., & Baum, A. (1989). Chronic stress, leukocyte subpopulations, and humoral response to latent viruses. *Health Psychology, 8*(4), 389–402.

Moriguchi, S., Oonishi, K., Kato, M., & Kishino, Y. (1995). Obesity is a risk factor for deteriorating cellular immune functions with aging. *Nutrition Research, 1995*, 151–160.

Mosnaim, A. D., Wolf, M. E., Maturana, P., Mosnaim, G., Puente, J., Kucuk, O., et al. (1993). In vitro studies of natural killer cell activity in posttraumatic stress disorder patients. Response to methionine-enkephalin challenge. *Immunopharmacology, 25*, 107–116.

Murphy, L. M. B., Thompson, R. J., Jr., & Morris, M. A. (1997). Adherence behavior among adolescents with Type 1 insulin-dependent diabetes mellitus: The role of cognitive appraisal processes. *Journal of Pediatric Psychology, 22*, 811–825.

Naliboff, B. D., Benton, D., Solomon, G. F., Morley, J. E., Fahey, J. L., Bloom, E. T., et al. (1991). Immunological changes in young and old adults during brief laboratory stress. *Psychosomatic Medicine, 53*, 121–132.

Nieman, D. C., Henson, D. A., Nehlsen-Canarella, S. L., Ekkens, M., Utter, A. C., Butterworth, D. E., et al. (1999). Influence of obesity on immune function. *Journal of the American Dietetic Association, 99*, 294–299.

Paluska, S. A., & Schwenk, T. L. (2000). Physical activity and mental health: Current concepts. *Sports Medicine, 29*, 167–180.

Pellegrino, T., & Bayer, B. M. (1998). In vivo effects of cocaine on immune cell function. *Journal of Neuroimmunology, 83*, 139–147.

Perna, F. M., Schneiderman, N., & LaPerriere, A. (1997). Psychological stress, exercise and immunity. *International Journal of Sports Medicine, 18*(Suppl. 1), S78–83.

Pike, J. L., Smith, T. L., Hauger, R. L., Nicassio, P. M., Patterson, T. L., McClintick, J., et al. (1997). Chronic life stress alters sympathetic, neuroendocrine, and immune responsivity to an acute psychological stressor in humans. *Psychosomatic Medicine, 59*, 447–457.

Potter, P. T., & Zautra, A. J. (1997). Stressful life events' effects on rheumatoid arthritis disease activity. *Journal of Consulting and Clinical Psychology, 65*, 319–323.

Rasmussen, L. B., Kiens, B., Pedersen, B. K., & Richter, E. A. (1994). Effect of diet and plasma fatty acid composition on immune status in elderly men. *American Journal of Clinical Nutrition, 59,* 572–577.

Reed, G. M., Kemeny, M. E., Taylor, S. E., Wang, H. J., & Visscher, B. R. (1994). "Realistic acceptance" as a predictor of decreased survival time in gay men with AIDS. *Health Psychology, 13,* 299–307.

Reifman, A. (1995). Social relationships, recovery from illness, and survival: A literature review. *Annals of Behavioral Medicine, 17,* 124–131.

Rosenbloom, C. A., & Whittington, F. J. (1993). The effects of bereavement on eating behaviors and nutrient intakes in elderly widowed persons. *Journal of Gerontology, 48,* S223–S229.

Rosenthal, L. A., Taub, D. D., Moors, M. A., & Blank, K. J. (1992). Methylxanthine-induced inhibition of the antigen- and superantigen-specific activation of T and B lymphocytes. *Immunopharmacology, 24,* 203–217.

Sabioncello, A., Kocijan-Hercigonja, D., Rabatic, S., Tomasic, J., Jeren, T., Matijevic, L., et al. (2000). Immune, endocrine, and psychological responses in civilians displaced by war. *Psychosomatic Medicine, 62,* 502–508.

Sairenji, T., Yamanishi, K., Tachibana, Y., Bertoni, G., & Kurata, T. (1995). Antibody responses to Epstein-Barr virus, human herpesvirus 6 and human herpesvirus 7 in patients with chronic fatigue syndrome. *Intervirology, 38,* 269–273.

Schnurr, P. P., & Jankowski, M. K. (1999). Physical health and posttraumatic stress disorder: Review and synthesis. *Seminars in Clinical Neuropsychiatry, 4,* 295–304.

Schranz, D. B., & Lernmark, A. (1998). Immunology in diabetes: An update. *Diabetes-Metabolism Reviews, 14,* 3–29.

Schulz, R., Bookwala, J., Knapp, J. E., Scheier, M., & Williamson, G. M. (1996). Pessimism, age, and cancer mortality. *Psychology and Aging, 11,* 304–309.

Schwarzer, R., & Leppin, A. (1989). Social support and health: A meta-analysis. *Psychology and Health, 3,* 1–15.

Segerstrom, S. C., Solomon, G. F., Kemeny, M. E., & Fahey, J. L. (1998). Relationship of worry to immune sequelae of the Northridge earthquake. *Journal of Behavioral Medicine, 21,* 433–450.

Shea, J., Clover, K., & Burton, R. (1991). Relationships between measures of acute and chronic stress and cellular immunity. *Medical Science Research, 19,* 221–222.

Shronts, E. P. (1993). Basic concepts of immunology and its application to clinical nutrition. *Nutrition in Clinical Practice, 8,* 177–183.

Sieber, W. J., Rodin, J., Larson, L., Ortega, S., Cummings, N., Levy, S., et al. (1992). Modulation of human natural killer cell activity by exposure to uncontrollable stress. *Brain, Behavior, and Immunity, 6,* 141–156.

Solomon, G. F., Segerstrom, S. C., Grohr, P., Kemeny, M., & Fahey, J. (1997). Shaking up immunity: Psychological and immunological changes after a natural disaster. *Psychosomatic Medicine, 59,* 114–127.

Spivak, B., Shohat, B., Mester, R., Avraham, S., Gil-As, I., Bleich, A., et al. (1997). Elevated levels of serum interleukin-1β in combat-related posttraumatic stress disorder. *Biological Psychiatry, 42,* 345–348.

Stewart, M. W., Knight, R. G., Palmer, D. G., & Highton, J. (1994). Differential relationships between stress and disease activity for immunologically distinct subgroups of people with rheumatoid arthritis. *Journal of Abnormal Psychology, 103,* 251–258.

Stone, A. A., Reed, B. R., & Neale, J. M. (1987). Changes in daily event frequency precede episodes of physical symptoms. *Journal of Human Stress, 13,* 70–74.

Straus, S. E., Fritz, S., Dale, J. K., Gould, B., & Strober, W. (1993). Lymphocyte phenotype and function in the chronic fatigue syndrome. *Journal of Clinical Immunology, 13,* 30–40.

Surwit, R. S., & Williams, P. G. (1996). Animal models provide insight into psychosomatic factors in diabetes. *Psychosomatic Medicine, 58,* 582–589.

Tomei, L. D., Kiecolt-Glaser, J. K., Kennedy, S., & Glaser, R. (1990). Psychological stress and phorbol ester inhibition of radiation-induced apoptosis in human PBLs. *Psychiatric Research, 33,* 59–71.

Uchino, B. N., Cacioppo, J. T., & Kiecolt-Glaser, J. K. (1996). The relationship between social support and physiological processes: A review with emphasis on underlying mechanisms and implications for health. *Psychological Bulletin, 119,* 488–531.

Ullum, H., Lepri, A. C., Victor, J., Skinhoj, P., Phillips, A. N., & Pedersen, B. K. (1997). Increased losses of CD4⁺CD45RA⁺ cells in late stages of HIV infection is related to increased risk of death: Evidence from a cohort of 347 HIV-infected individuals. *AIDS, 11,* 1479–1485.

Watson, R. R., Eskelson, C., & Hartmann, B. B. (1984). Severe alcohol abuse and cellular immune functions. *Arizona Medicine, 41,* 665–668.

Weiner, H. (1992). *Perturbing the organism: The biology of stressful experience.* Chicago: University of Chicago Press.

Weiss, D. W., Hirt, R., Tarcic, N., Berzon, Y., Ben-Zur, H., Breznitz, S., et al. (1996). Studies in psychoneuroimmunology: Psychological, immunological, and neuroendocrinological parameters in Israeli civilians during and after a period of Scud missile attacks. *Behavioral Medicine, 22,* 5–14.

Weisse, C. S., Pato, C. N., McAllister, C. G., Littman, R., Breier, A., Paul, S. M., et al. (1990). Differential effects of controllable and uncontrollable acute stress on lymphocyte proliferation and leukocyte percentages in humans. *Brain, Behavior, and Immunity, 4,* 339–351.

Whiteside, T. T., & Herberman, R. (1989). The role of natural killer cells in human disease. *Clinical Immunology and Immunopathology, 53,* 1–23.

Willis, L., Thomas, P., Garry, P. J., & Goodwin, J. S. (1987). A prospective study of response to stressful life events in initially healthy elders. *Journal of Gerontology, 42,* 627–630.

Wolf, A. M., & Colditz, G. A. (1996). Social and economic effects of body weight in the United States. *American Journal of Clinical Nutrition, 63*(Suppl.), 466S–469S.

Yehuda, R., Boisoneau, D., Lowy, M. T., & Giller, E. L., Jr. (1995). Dose-response changes in plasma cortisol and lymphocyte glucocorticoid receptors following dexamethasone administration in combat veterans with and without posttraumatic stress disorder. *Archives in General Psychiatry, 52,* 583–593.

Yehuda, R., Southwick, S., Giller, E. L., Jr., Ma, X., & Mason, J. W. (1992). Urinary catecholamine excretion and severity of PTSD symptoms in Vietnam combat veterans. *Journal of Nervous and Mental Disease, 180,* 321–325.

Zakowski, S. G. (1995). The effects of stressor predictability on lymphocyte proliferation in humans. *Psychology and Health, 10,* 409–425.

7

POSTTRAUMATIC STRESS DISORDER, ALLOSTATIC LOAD, AND MEDICAL ILLNESS

MATTHEW J. FRIEDMAN AND BRUCE S. McEWEN

In this chapter we present a psychobiological conceptual framework that accounts for the mounting evidence that posttraumatic stress disorder (PTSD) is a risk factor for medical illness. First we describe the human response to stress to provide the context for the ensuing discussion. Then we summarize the extensive literature on the relationship of chronic stress syndrome to medical illness. Next we review the biological alterations associated with chronic PTSD and how these PTSD-related psychobiological abnormalities might increase the risk for medical illness among affected individuals. Then we introduce the allostatic load model (McEwen, 1998; McEwen & Stellar, 1993) and demonstrate how this theoretical approach enables us to understand the etiological significance of such abnormalities. Finally, we discuss how the allostatic load model helps us conceptualize resilience, prevention, and treatment.

This chapter was coauthored by an employee of the United States government as part of official duty and is considered to be in the public domain. Any views expressed herein do not necessarily represent the views of the United States government, and the author's participation in the work is not meant to serve as an official endorsement.

BACKGROUND AND CONCEPTUALIZATION

In 1995, Friedman and Schnurr (1995) observed that exposure to trauma was associated with poor health outcomes and proposed that this relationship was mediated by PTSD. They suggested that biological and psychological abnormalities associated with PTSD might increase the risk for medical illness among people experiencing this disorder. At the time of that review, there were limited data for evaluating this hypothesis. Four years later, Schnurr and Jankowski (1999) reported that recent empirical findings did indeed support an association between PTSD and poor health on the basis of self-reports, clinical utilization, and medical morbidity. After considering the various biological and behavioral factors that might promote such a relationship, they suggested that the McEwen and Stellar (1993; McEwen, 1998) model of allostasis and allostatic load appeared to provide a plausible mechanism through which stress in general, and PTSD in particular, might lead to medical illness. This chapter focuses on the elaboration and application of this model to trauma, PTSD, and health.

Allostasis, as originally proposed and elaborated (McEwen, 1998; McEwen & Stellar, 1993; Sterling & Eyer, 1988) is an organizing principle for understanding the biological basis of an organism's ability to achieve stability through change—that is, of maintaining homeostasis by expending and directing energy toward challenges. Allostasis, referring to the process of adaptation, incorporates the notion of stress but also includes the contributions of genetic factors, early life experiences, and features of lifestyle that determine the nature of the physiological responses to daily life events as well as to the situations that qualify as stressors.

Allostatic load is the cumulative cost to the organism of going through repeated cycles of allostasis or adaptation. This cost may accumulate from having to respond to repeated challenges or from misdirection of the physiological responses that constitute allostasis: for example, failure to shut off production of mediators like cortisol and catecholamines, or failure to habituate to repeated challenges of the same kind. Mismanagement also includes the failure to mount an adequate response to a challenge: for example, inadequate glucocorticoids leading to overproduction of inflammatory cytokines. Allostatic load may result from the sustained activity of mediators of allostasis, referred to as an *allostatic state*: for example, elevated blood pressure in hypertension, elevated inflammatory cytokine production when glucocorticoid levels are inadequate, or elevated diurnal production of glucocorticoids in major depressive illness that contribute to bone mineral loss, abdominal obesity and atrophy of brain structures (see McEwen, 1998). In other words, sustained allostatic load can lead to medical illness.

From the perspective of allostatic load, PTSD is extremely complex. This is because humans who fail to meet the demands of traumatic stressors use and perturb many key psychobiological mechanisms that have evolved for coping, adaptation, and preservation of the species (Friedman, 1999; Friedman, Charney, & Deutch, 1995). Thus, we propose that allostatic load is a rich heuristic model through which to understand the many complex psychobiological abnormalities associated with PTSD. As we attempt to demonstrate, it is also a useful context for understanding why these abnormalities make PTSD a risk factor for medical illness. We conclude that allostatic load provides a new framework for understanding PTSD and its comorbidities. We also propose a new term, *allostatic support*, to refer to mechanisms that confer resilience on individuals, making them more resistant to PTSD and other chronic illnesses.

THE HUMAN RESPONSE TO STRESS

The human stress system has evolved to maintain allostasis, especially in response to significant challenges that might be characterized as stressors. It consists of the central and peripheral nervous systems, the endocrine system, and the immunological system. The two major components of the stress system are the hypothalamic–pituitary–adrenocortical (HPA) axis and the locus coeruleus/norepinephrine-sympathetic system (LC/NE system).

Corticotropin releasing factor (CRF) might be considered the ignition switch for the human stress response because it has a key role in activating both HPA and LC/NE systems. In the HPA axis, CRF is secreted from the hypothalamus, after which it releases adrenocorticotropic hormone (ACTH) from the pituitary gland. ACTH then promotes the release of cortisol and other glucocorticoids from the cortex of the adrenal gland. Maintenance of the integrity of the HPA system is crucial for normal coping and adaptation (Selye, 1956). As discussed subsequently, this integrity is not maintained in PTSD. Indeed, a large body of evidence indicates that HPA abnormalities figure prominently in the pathophysiology of PTSD.

The second major system, the LC/NE system, includes adrenergic mechanisms in both the central nervous system (CNS) and the peripheral sympathetic nervous system (SNS). The LC/NE component of the stress response was first described by Cannon (1932) as the classic "fight-or-flight response." The two neurotransmitters in the adrenergic system, norepinephrine and epinephrine, are collectively called catecholamines because of their similar chemical structure. CRF also has a major role in the LC/NE system in which it functions as the principal neurotransmitter that activates the locus coeruleus, a midbrain structure that contains the majority of the brain's adrenergic neurons (Aston-Jones, Valentino, Van Bockstaele, & Meyerson, 1994). There is abundant evidence that the LC/NE system also functions abnormally in PTSD.

BIOLOGICAL ABNORMALITIES ASSOCIATED WITH
CHRONIC STRESS

The human stress response evolved as an acute reaction for coping with a significant challenge or threat. The effectiveness of such a reaction is measured not only by the efficiency with which it mobilizes physiological, neurohormonal, and immunological mechanisms, but also by how quickly organismic function can return to prestress homeostatic and allostatic levels. Indeed, recovery of the baseline steady state is as important a part of coping, adaptation, and resilience as is the capacity to mount an effective stress response in the first place (Dienstbier, 1989; McEwen, 1998).

Sometimes recovery does not occur or cannot be achieved. This may happen because the stressor itself continues to persist for a protracted period of time. At other times, return to homeostasis or allostasis is impossible because the organism lacks the capacity to implement those mechanisms needed for recovery. Under such circumstances, psychobiological alterations designed for a time-limited reaction persist as chronic stress syndrome, which we shall consider from the perspective of allostatic load. For now, we focus on specific alterations in biological function.

Chronic stress syndrome (Chrousos, 1998; McEwen, 1998) is associated with sustained abnormalities in key biological systems. Persistent elevation in CRF secretion promotes increased HPA, SNS, LC/NE, and opioid function. Table 7.1 (Column 2) shows that activation of HPA function is associated with higher ACTH and cortisol and reduced dehydroepiandrosterone (DHEA) levels. Physiological and LC/NE enhancement is associated with increased SNS and adrenergic reactivity as well as elevations in tonic (steady state) function. Endogenous opioid mechanisms are also enhanced during chronic stress. A major consequence of CRF-induced increased activity in these systems is a reduction of activity in others. As shown in Table 7.1, reproductive, growth, and immunological mechanisms in particular exhibit significant deficits in function as part of chronic stress syndrome. Readers seeking more information are referred to comprehensive reviews on this subject by Chrousos (1998) and McEwen (1998).

MEDICAL ABNORMALITIES ASSOCIATED WITH
CHRONIC STRESS SYNDROME

Biological abnormalities that comprise chronic stress syndrome may have adverse health consequences leading to medical illness. More detailed review of this important and complex topic may be found elsewhere (Chrousos, 1998; McEwen, 1998). Table 7.2 (Column 2) summarizes some of the most prominent medical problems addressed in those comprehensive

TABLE 7.1
Biological Abnormalities Associated With Chronic Stress Syndrome and PTSD

System	Chronic stress syndrome	PTSD
HPA	Increased HPA activity ↑CRF, ↑Cortisol, ↓DHEA ?↓GR sensitivity	HPA dysregulation ↑CRF ?↓/↑Cortisol ?↑GR sensitivity
Physiological (SNS)	↑SNS reactivity ↑Tonic SNS activity Disrupted sleep	↑SNS reactivity, ↑Tonic SNS arousal ↑Startle response Disrupted sleep
LC/NE (Adrenergic)	↑Adrenergic reactivity ↑Catecholamine levels	↑Adrenergic reactivity ↑Tonic adrenergic activity Downregulation α_2/β receptors Blunted NPY activity
Opioids	↑Endogenous opioids (↑β endorphin)	↓/↑Endogenous opioids (tonic dysregulation) Phasic hyperactivity
Thyroid	↓TSH, ↓T3 ↓T3/T4 ratio	↑T3, ↑T4 ↑T3/T4 ratio
Reproductive	↓GnRH men: ↓LH, ↓testosterone women: ↓LH, ↓FSH, estradiol	?↓/↑testosterone
Growth	↓GH ↓Growth factors (IGF-1)	Normal GH levels ↓GH activation by clonidine or levodopa (in abused boys)
Metabolic	Metabolic syndrome X (see Table 7.2)	Osteopenia
Immunologic	Immunosuppression ↑Inflammatory cytokines (IL-1, IL-2, IL-6, TNFs)	Immunosuppression ↑Inflammatory cytokines

Note. HPA = hypothalamic–pituitary–adrenocortical; CRF = corticotropin releasing factor; DHEA = dehydroepiandrosterone; GR = glucocorticoid receptor; SNS = sympathetic nervous system; TSH = thyroid stimulating hormone; T3 = triiodothyronine; T4 = thyroxine; GnRH = gonadotropin releasing hormone; LH = luteinizing hormone; FSH = follicle stimulating hormone; GH = growth hormone; IGH = insulin-like growth factor; IL = interleukin; TNF = tissue necrosis factor.

reviews. It can be seen that SNS and LC/NE system dysregulation may result in a variety of cardiovascular changes that are clinically significant including atherosclerosis, hypertension, cardiac arrhythmias, compromised coronary function, and increased risk for myocardial infarction and stroke. Immunological consequences range from impaired immunological capacity (e.g., immunosuppression) to episodic inflammatory and autoimmune disorders. Hormonal suppression may affect all aspects of reproductive function as well as normal growth and development. Metabolic syndrome X is a

TABLE 7.2
Medical Problems Associated With Chronic Stress Syndrome and PTSD

System	Chronic stress syndrome	PTSD
HPA	Hypercortisolism and Cushing's Disease, as well as endocrine, reproductive, metabolic, and immunological problems (shown below)	?Hypo- or Hypercortisolism, as well as endocrine, reproductive, metabolic, and immunological problems (shown below)
SNS/LC/NE	*Cardiovascular abnormalities* Atherosclerosis Hypertension Cardiac arrhythmias EKG abnormalities Damaged myocardium Myocardial infarction Stroke Increased coronary vascular tone Increased coronary turbulence and shearing forces Increased platelet aggregation	*Cardiovascular abnormalities* Angina ↓ Effort tolerance Peripheral vascular illness EKG abnormalities
Opioids	*Chronic* Hyperalgesia Pain syndromes Headaches	*Chronic pain syndromes* Hyperalgesia
Thyroid	Hyperthyroidism	?Hyperthyroidism
Reproductive	*Reproductive abnormalities* Infertility, spontaneous abortion, ectopic pregnancy, preterm contractions, excessive fetal growth Possible *Congenital abnormalities* Conotruncal heart defects Neural tube defects Cleft lip with or without cleft palate	Reproductive abnormalities (one study)
Growth	Possible interference with normal growth and development (especially during critical periods)	No research
Metabolic	*Metabolic Syndrome X* Dyslipidemia, visceral adiposity, insulin resistance, Type II diabetes, hypertension, excessive clotting or deficient fibrinolysis Osteopenia and osteoporosis	Osteopenia (one study) No other research
Immunological	*Immunosuppression* Increased disease susceptibility Delayed wound healing Retarded immunization response Suppressed delayed-type hypersensitivity	*Immunosuppression* ↑ Disease susceptibility (one study)

(continued)

System	Chronic Stress Syndrome	PTSD
	Inflammatory and autoimmune disorders	*Inflammatory and autoimmune disorders*
	Irritable bowel syndrome	Stress-induced
	Rheumatoid arthritis	exacerbation of
	Type I diabetes	chronic fatigue
	Chronic fatigue syndrome	syndrome (one
	Fibromyalgia	study)
	Temperomandibular disorders	
	Tension headaches	
	Dysmenorrhea	
	Irritable bladder syndrome	
	Multiple chemical sensitivity	

complex cluster of symptoms resulting from HPA suppression of growth hormone, gonadal steroids, and bone production; the clinical manifestations are Type II diabetes, visceral adiposity, and atherosclerosis (from insulin resistance and carbohydrate intolerance, abnormal lipid metabolism, and excessive blood clotting or deficient fibrinolysis). Osteoporosis is another manifestation of metabolic syndrome X that affects women more than men (because suppression of estrogen impairs bone growth).

In the following sections, we consider biological abnormalities and medical problems associated with PTSD. We compare PTSD-related biological abnormalities with those previously discussed with regard to chronic stress syndrome. In addition, we consider empirical observations concerning medical problems associated with PTSD and see how they compare with medical consequences due to chronic stress syndrome. It should be noted that other chapters in this book provide thorough reviews of the published literature on PTSD and health status (Green & Kimerling, chap. 2), cardiovascular illness (Ford, chap. 4), and immune function (Dougall & Baum, chap. 6).

BIOLOGICAL ABNORMALITIES ASSOCIATED WITH PTSD

As shown in Table 7.1 (Column 3), there are a number of biological abnormalities that have been detected among people with PTSD that are reviewed more extensively elsewhere (Friedman, 1999; Friedman, Charney, & Deutch, 1995; Yehuda & McFarlane, 1997). These include hyperreactivity in several physiological systems, an excessive startle reflex, and disrupted sleep. Major psychobiological systems that mediate the human response to stress are also dysregulated. Empirical research has detected significant alterations in neurotransmitter and neuroendocrine activity involving the

HPA system, adrenergic mechanisms, neuropeptide Y (NPY), endogenous opioids, the hypothalamic–pituitary–thyroid (HPT) axis, the hypothalmic–pituitary–gonadotropic (HPG) axis, and the immune system (with respect to both humoral and cell-mediated mechanisms). In many respects, PTSD-related abnormalities are similar to those found in chronic stress syndrome. But there are intriguing differences and there are many gaps in our knowledge.

Hypothalamic–Pituitary–Adrenocortical System

A large body of evidence indicates that HPA abnormalities figure prominently in the pathophysiology of PTSD. Investigations have focused mostly on CRF release, cortisol levels, and glucocorticoid receptor sensitivity. There also appear to be important gender-related differences in HPA function.

Corticotropin Releasing Factor

As stated previously, CRF is the ignition switch for the cascade of reactions that constitute the human stress response. It initiates both the HPA and LC/NE systems as well as other neurotransmitter, neurohormonal, metabolic, and immunological responses. Studies with male combat veterans and premenopausal survivors of childhood sexual abuse have detected elevated cerebrospinal fluid, CRF levels, and enhanced hypothalamic release of CRF, among people with PTSD compared to those without PTSD (Baker et al., 1999; Bremner, Licinio, et al., 1997; Yehuda et al., 1996). Mixed results have been found with respect to the ACTH response to CRF (Heim, Newport, Bonsall, Miller, & Nemeroff, 2001; Smith et al., 1989). This suggests that CRF function is dysregulated in people with PTSD.

Cortisol Levels

Findings on urinary free cortisol levels are mixed. Earlier studies with male combat veterans and elderly male and female Holocaust survivors generally found reduced 24-hour urinary cortisol levels in those with PTSD compared to trauma survivors without PTSD. Other studies with male veterans have shown no difference. More recent investigations, mostly with premenopausal women and traumatized children, have found the opposite (i.e., elevated urinary cortisol levels) among those with PTSD (see reviews by Heim, Ehlert, & Hellhammer, 2000; Rasmusson & Friedman, 2002; Rasmusson et al., 2001; Yehuda, 1999).

It is not clear how to explain such variable findings. Some investigators have cited methodological differences (Rasmusson et al., 2001; Yehuda,

1999). Rasmusson has also suggested that gender differences may account for some of this variability (see Rasmusson & Friedman, 2002).

Finally, the question of tonic versus phasic HPA abnormalities in PTSD must be considered carefully. Mason, Giller, Kosten, and Wahby (1990) measured urinary cortisol levels in hospitalized combat veterans with PTSD at admission, midpoint, and discharge. Remarkable fluctuations were seen throughout the hospitalization. Many veterans with low urinary cortisol at admission exhibited high levels several weeks later during that phase of the hospitalization that included therapeutic reexposure of patients to stressful traumatic memories of the Vietnam War. After more weeks had passed, these same veterans reexhibited low urinary cortisol prior to discharge. The investigators proposed that baseline HPA function can fluctuate dramatically in response to external (stressful) circumstances and, therefore, that it must be monitored longitudinally if we ever hope to understand its complex expression in PTSD.

Glucocorticoid Receptor Sensitivity

HPA allostasis is maintained by a negative feedback system. CRF produces ACTH secretion, which promotes cortisol release from the adrenal cortex. The hypothalamus monitors the amount of circulating cortisol through its glucocorticoid receptors. If a sufficient number of these receptors are occupied by cortisol, CRF secretion is inhibited. This negative feedback mechanism prevents blood cortisol levels from getting too high. If cortisol levels are too low, however, and an insufficient number of hypothalamic glucocorticoid receptors are occupied, CRF is released until the proper blood cortisol level is achieved.

An important theory concerning HPA function in PTSD, derived mostly from Yehuda's work (see Yehuda, 1997, 1999), is that there is an allostatic equilibrium marked by low cortisol, an increase in the number (e.g., up-regulation) of glucocorticoid receptors, and enhanced negative feedback of the HPA system due to supersensitivity of these same glucocorticoid receptors. The paradox of this elegant model is that despite lower cortisol levels, the system may act as if there were excessive HPA activity because of the supersensitivity of the glucocorticoid receptors. Indeed, many of the research findings presented below are consistent with the hypothesis that HPA activity is elevated, not reduced, in PTSD.

To summarize, HPA function appears to be dysregulated in PTSD, although variable experimental findings make it impossible to specify a unitary pattern of abnormalities at this time. Many findings suggest enhanced HPA activity due to some combination of elevated CRF activity, glucocorticoid receptor sensitivity, and, in some cases, elevated cortisol levels. Reports vary regarding whether hypocortisolism in PTSD (and other stress-related disorders) is or is not associated with glucocorticoid receptor supersensitivity. Such variability may reflect tonic (e.g., baseline) as well as phasic (e.g., stress-induced episodic) HPA abnormalities, the magnitude of an individual's stress response at the time of measurement, methodological issues regarding the collection and assay of urinary samples, or gender-related differences in neurohormonal factors affecting CRF, cortisol levels, or glucocorticoid receptor sensitivity.

Physiological Abnormalities in PTSD

Sympathetic Nervous System (SNS) Hyperreactivity

The other major mediator of the stress response is the sympathetic nervous system. One of the oldest and most robust findings in all PTSD research is the excessive SNS reactivity of people with PTSD to stimuli related to the traumatic event. Such stimuli may be auditory (Blanchard, Kolb, Prins, Gates, & McCoy, 1991), pictorial (Keane et al., 1998), or narrative descriptions of the traumatic experience (Pitman, Orr, Forgue, de Jong, & Clairborn, 1987). Participants with PTSD are distinguishable from trauma exposed non-PTSD comparison participants by a markedly greater SNS response to such traumamimetic (or threatening) stimuli, manifested by increased cardiovascular (e.g., systolic–diastolic, heart rate), skin conductance, and electromyographic (EMG) responses.

Increased Startle Response

The excessive startle response (or "jumpiness") observed in patients with PTSD was first reported by Kardiner (1941) in his landmark book on World War I veterans. Laboratory research has confirmed Kardiner's clinical observations by using a protocol that examines the physiological response evoked by loud and unexpected acoustic stimuli. The most common measure has been the eyeblink response to such bursts of sound, although cardiovascular indices have also been monitored. In general, the startle response among individuals with PTSD has been significantly greater than that among exposed individuals without the disorder (Pitman, Orr, Shalev, Metzger, & Mellman, 1999; Shalev, Orr, Peri, Schreiber, & Pitman, 1992).

Disrupted Sleep

Insomnia and traumatic nightmares have long been recognized as hallmarks of PTSD. Polysomnographic studies consistently show increased awakenings, reduced sleep time, and increased motor activity during sleep among those with PTSD. Some studies also suggest disrupted rapid eye movement (REM) sleep continuity, but this latter finding remains controversial (Mellman, Kulick-Bell, Ashlock, & Nolan, 1995; Pitman et al., 1999).

Traumatic nightmares appear to be unique events that differ significantly from Stage IV Night Terrors and REM Dream Anxiety Attacks (Friedman, 1981; Ross, Ball, Sullivan, & Caroff, 1989).

Tonic Physiological Arousal

The aforementioned observations, especially those concerning SNS hyperreactivity and the increased startle response, are clear indications of *phasic* abnormalities following exposure to discrete stimuli among individuals with PTSD. It appears that individuals with PTSD also exhibit excessive physiological manifestations at rest, or *tonic* abnormalities. A recent meta-analytic examination of basal cardiovascular activity indicated that individuals with PTSD have a higher resting heart rate and blood pressure in comparison with both trauma-exposed and nonexposed controls (Buckley & Kaloupek, 2001).

Adrenergic Abnormalities in PTSD

Given the physiological alterations mentioned previously and the crucial role of adrenergic mechanisms in the human stress response (Cannon, 1932), one might expect that PTSD would be associated with both tonic and phasic alterations of catecholaminergic function.

Tonic Adrenergic Activity

Evidence suggesting altered baseline catecholamine activity in PTSD is based on studies with 24-hour urinary levels and investigations of platelet and lymphocyte adrenergic receptors. Twenty-four hour urinary norepinephrine and epinephrine have been measured in male combat veterans, male and female Holocaust survivors, and female sexual abuse victims. Results have generally shown elevated catecholamine levels among individuals with PTSD compared with both trauma exposed–no-PTSD and nonexposed controls (see Southwick et al., 1999 for references).

It would be expected that increased catecholamine levels would produce a compensatory reduction (or down-regulation) of adrenergic receptors. This has been shown in research on both alpha-2 and beta adrenergic receptors. Two studies (with combat veterans and traumatized children, respectively) have shown reduced platelet alpha-2 binding sites among individuals with PTSD compared with controls (Perry, 1994; Perry, Giller, & Southwick, 1987). In addition, there is evidence that beta receptors are also down-regulated (Lerer, Gur, Bleich, & Newman, 1994).

Phasic Adrenergic Activity

As with the physiological findings, a variety of challenge studies have consistently demonstrated excessive phasic adrenergic responses among individuals with PTSD. In addition to physiological hyperreactivity, exposure to psychological stressors has been associated with abrupt elevations in plasma epinephrine and norepinephrine, respectively, in two studies with combat veterans with PTSD (Blanchard et al., 1991; McFall, Murburg, Ko, & Veith, 1990).

Yohimbine, an alpha-2 adrenergic receptor antagonist, has been an important pharmacological probe in studies on phasic adrenergic activity. Yohimbine enhances adrenergic activity by blocking the inhibitory presynaptic alpha-2 receptor, thereby enhancing presynaptic release of norepinephrine. An investigation with Vietnam combat veterans found that among the participants with PTSD, yohimbine elicited panic attacks, combat-related flashbacks, and elevated brain adrenergic metabolism in contrast to veterans without PTSD who did not exhibit such abnormalities (Bremner, Innis, et al., 1997; Southwick et al., 1993).

Thus, studies on both physiological and catecholamine function indicate that the major adrenergic abnormality in PTSD is a hyperreactive phasic response, although alterations in tonic activity have also been detected.

Neuropeptide Y

NPY is a neuropeptide found in adrenergic neurons in the brain or SNS that is released along with norepinephrine during intense activation of the adrenergic system by yohimbine or excessive exercise (Pernow, 1988; Rasmusson et al., 2000). It apparently enhances the efficiency of adrenergic transmission in the SNS (Colmers & Bleakman, 1994) and appears to have a profound anxiety-reducing effect (Kask, Rago, & Harro, 1996). Of particular relevance to our previous discussion of HPA function, anxiolytic doses of NPY also antagonize the anxiogenic and other actions of CRF, making NPY a potential major moderator of the intensity of the human stress response (Britton et al., 1997). NPY is, therefore, an important neuropeptide to consider in PTSD because it is released during intense phasic activation of the adrenergic system and because it is a potent antagonist of CRF.

Veterans with PTSD exhibited significantly lower baseline NPY levels as well as a blunted NPY response to yohimbine in comparison to non-PTSD controls (Rasmusson et al., 2000). This is consistent with animal studies showing reduced NPY inhibition of adrenergic function following chronic stress (Corder, Castagne, Rivet, Mormede, & Gaillard, 1992). Indeed, it is possible that hypoactive NPY function contributes both to adrenergic hyperreactivity and increased CRF activity in PTSD (Rasmusson & Friedman, 2002).

Endogenous Opioids

CRF also activates the opioid peptide beta endorphin, which recipro-cally inhibits both the adrenergic and HPA components of the human stress response. The little research on opioid activity in PTSD suggests that there may be both tonic and phasic abnormalities. Abnormal baseline opioid function has been detected among individuals with PTSD although the specifics of such findings have varied from study to study. Elevated cerebro-spinal fluid beta endorphin levels were observed in male combat veterans with PTSD (Baker et al., 1997). Studies on plasma beta endorphin show mixed results: higher levels among Croatian women with PTSD due to the trauma of war (Sabioncello et al., 2000); normal levels in male combat veterans (Baker et al., 1997); and lower levels in a different cohort of combat veterans with PTSD (Hoffman, Burges Watson, Wilson, & Montgomery, 1989). There is also evidence that exposure of people with PTSD to relevant trauma-related stimuli (e.g., Vietnam veterans with PTSD viewing combat scenes) produces an abrupt phasic elevation in circulating opioid levels (Pitman, van der Kolk, Orr, & Greenberg, 1990).

Hypothalamic–Pituitary–Thyroid Axis

The HPA system has an important impact on HPT function. CRF and cortisol suppress both secretion of thyroid stimulating hormone (TSH) from the pituitary and conversion of thyroxine (T4) to the more metaboli-cally active triiodothyronine (T3). Studies with combat veterans have dem-onstrated elevations in both T3 and T4. Such increases were positively associated with PTSD severity (Mason et al., 1995; Wang & Mason, 1999). Furthermore, unpublished observations on women with PTSD related to childhood sexual abuse (CSA), show higher T3 in comparison with female CSA survivors without PTSD (Friedman et al., 2001). Such findings suggest that chronic PTSD differs from chronic stress syndrome where TSH and T3 levels are reduced.

Hypothalamic–Pituitary–Gonadal Axis

Increased HPA activity suppresses all aspects of HPG function includ-ing secretion of gonadotropin-releasing hormone from the hypothalamus, follicle stimulating and luteinizing hormones from the pituitary, and estradiol and testosterone from the reproductive organs. Conflicting findings have been reported in two studies in which testosterone was measured in people with PTSD. Elevated serum (Mason et al., 1990), in contrast to reduced cerebrospinal fluid (Mulchahey et al., 2001), testosterone levels were detected among male combat veterans with PTSD.

Growth Axis

Increased HPA activity interferes with growth axis function through inhibition of growth hormone release as well as through suppression of growth at target tissues. Vietnam combat veterans with and without PTSD showed no difference in growth hormone levels (Laudenslager et al., 1998). Another study, in which PTSD was not measured, may be relevant here. Sexually and physically abused boys (not assessed for PTSD) exhibited a blunted growth hormone response to both clonidine and levodopa, in contrast to nonabused control participants.

Metabolic Axis

Metabolic syndrome X (defined earlier) is a complex cluster of symptoms resulting from suppression of growth hormone, sex steroids, and bone production. The only research on this syndrome among individuals with PTSD has focused on osteopenia, a reflection of bone metabolism, which is an osteoporotic condition marked by a significant reduction in bone density. Among 140 male American naval aviators previously held as prisoners of war, those with PTSD exhibited greater frequency of osteopenia than those without PTSD, who were more likely to show normal bone density (Sausen, Moore, Ambrose, Wells, & Mitchell, 2001).

The Immune System

Because blood levels of lymphocyte or NK cells vary according to the dynamics of catecholamine and glucocorticoid secretion, we limit this brief review to functional measures of immunological activity such as NK cytotoxicity per cell, assays of cell proliferation, and the cytokine response to specific antigens (Dhabhar & McEwen, 1997). More comprehensive reviews can be found elsewhere (see Dougall & Baum, chap. 6, this volume; Schnurr & Jankowski, 1999). The results in people with chronic PTSD are mixed. Extrapolating from findings associated with chronic stress syndrome (shown in Table 7.1) one would expect to observe immunosuppression in individuals with chronic PTSD. Surprisingly, enhanced immunological function has actually been found more often than immunosuppression. Three studies on veterans with chronic PTSD observed higher cutaneous, cell-mediated immunity and higher cytokine levels among those with PTSD compared with a non-PTSD group (Burges Watson, Muller, Jones, & Bradley, 1993; Laudenslager et al., 1998; Spivak et al., 1997). In a fourth report, however, immunological activation by antigens was no different among veterans with PTSD than among controls (Boscarino & Chang, 1999). Finally, Boscarino (1997) found that male Vietnam combat veterans with PTSD appeared to have reduced immunological function because they reported higher prevalence of nonsexually transmitted infectious disease than non-PTSD veterans.

Given the complexity of the immune system and given that both tonic and phasic abnormalities have been found in people with PTSD in most biological systems investigated, one way to reconcile these diverse findings is to postulate that there is both a tonic state of immunosuppression as well as an episodic or phasic state characterized by enhanced immunological function.

Comparison of Biological Abnormalities Associated With Chronic Stress Syndrome and PTSD

As with chronic stress syndrome, PTSD appears to be associated with significant alterations in function of the same key biological systems. Current evidence (shown in Table 7.1) suggests that specific abnormalities detected in these two pathological states may be quite similar in some respects and quite different in others. Data on physiological and LC/NE mechanisms seem most comparable whereas the pattern of HPA dysregulation may be most different. Research with opioids, HPT, HPG, growth and immunological systems is much too preliminary to invite serious speculation. Of greater importance is that allostatic load caused by the pathophysiology of both PTSD and chronic stress syndrome appears to increase the risk for medical illness. We explore the clinical consequences of these two pathological states in the following section.

HOW MIGHT PTSD-RELATED BIOLOGICAL ABNORMALITIES INCREASE THE RISK FOR MEDICAL ILLNESS?

Chronic stress syndrome is best understood as a cascade of reactions stimulated by CRF-induced actions on HPA, LC/NE, opioid, and immunological systems. Medical illnesses associated with this syndrome are well understood within such a conceptual framework (Chrousos, 1998; McEwen, 1998). As noted previously, the pathophysiology is less clear with respect to PTSD. Here, elevated CRF appears to produce a different pattern of HPA dysregulation marked by variable cortisol levels and alterations in glucocorticoid receptor sensitivity. For purposes of the present discussion, we propose that PTSD-related HPA dysregulation will generate clinically significant allostatic load that will increase the risk for medical illness. Tonic abnormalities, which will usually (but not always) promote increased HPA activity (through higher CRF activity and possibly through enhanced gluco-corticoid receptor sensitivity), are more likely to produce pathological changes similar to those associated with chronic stress syndrome. We further propose that phasic abnormalities are much more significant in PTSD and, therefore, more likely to produce the clinically significant allostatic load that distinguishes medical illnesses due to PTSD from those associated with chronic stress syndrome.

Physiological Abnormalities

We focus this discussion primarily on adrenergic abnormalities, re-viewed previously, because the most prominent physiological alterations in PTSD involve SNS activity (which is adrenergic). With respect to both SNS and adrenergic function in PTSD, dramatic hyperreactivity has been observed much more consistently than tonic abnormalities.

Schneiderman (1977) first proposed that the abrupt increase in blood pressure and heart rate caused by stress-induced recurrent activation of the SNS produces hemodynamic disturbances that might produce atherosclero-sis. He later proposed that heightened cardiovascular reactivity in response to psychological stressors might increase the risk for chronic heart disease (CHD) (Schneiderman, 1987). Other investigators have confirmed this prediction, showing that cardiovascular reactivity predicts the development of atherosclerosis (Everson et al., 1997). In addition, Shapiro (1988) found that cardiovascular reactivity to laboratory stressors predicts hypertension among (susceptible) individuals with a family history of this illness.

These findings concerning the risk for cardiovascular illness associated with chronic stress syndrome also apply to PTSD. Indeed, the risk may be even higher in PTSD, in which physiological and adrenergic hyperreactivity is such a prominent feature.

There are currently a few studies showing a positive relationship be-tween PTSD and cardiovascular abnormalities (also see Green & Kimerling, chap. 2, this volume). Such findings include higher rates of angina (Falger et al., 1992), lower cardiovascular effort tolerance on a laboratory treadmill test (Shalev, Bleich, & Ursano, 1990), earlier onset of arterial disorders (Schnurr, Spiro, & Paris, 2000), and electrocardiogram abnormalities show-ing arterioventricular conduction defects and a myocardial infarction pattern (Boscarino & Chang, 1999).

Pain Syndromes

Abnormalities in opioid function would be expected to be expressed clinically as altered pain perception. Indeed, lower pain thresholds have been observed among individuals with PTSD in comparison with nonaffected individuals (Perry, Cella, Falkenberg, Heidrich, & Goodwin, 1987; Shalev, Peri, Canetti, & Schreiber, 1996) and there are clinical reports of an association between chronic pain and PTSD (Benedikt & Kolb, 1986; Rapaport, 1987). Other pertinent literature has shown an association between trauma exposure and self-reported painful clinical complaints (see Friedman & Schnurr, 1995; Green & Kimerling, chap. 2, this volume), but such findings are only suggestive because PTSD was not diagnosed in most of these studies.

Endocrine, Metabolic, and Immunological Abnormalities

Clinical studies on the impact of PTSD on endocrine function are in their infancy. Laboratory studies, reviewed previously, have shown that individuals with PTSD have higher T3 compared with normal controls, although T3 levels for both groups were generally within the normal range. Although there are no data on thyroid abnormalities in PTSD, an interesting clinical report that is consistent with such laboratory findings, describes a marked increase in the number of documented cases ($n = 87$) of hyperthyroidism diagnosed in the same region of Bosnia during a 12-month period of war in contrast to the incidence of hyperthyroidism during the previous 12-month period of peacetime ($n = 54$). Without exception, wartime cases exhibited elevations in both T3 and T4 (Zubovic, Mikac, Biukovic, Skrobic, & Rajkovaca, 1993).

Because of the reciprocal relationship between HPA and HPG axes, one would predict that reproductive abnormalities would be more likely to occur among people with PTSD than among nonaffected individuals. This prediction was confirmed in the only published study on this question. After controlling for demographic and psychological factors, Seng and colleagues (2001) found that 455 women with PTSD had significantly higher odds of ectopic pregnancy, spontaneous abortion, preterm contractions, and excessive fetal growth, relative to 638 nonpsychiatric controls. This is consistent with other studies in which PTSD was not assessed, which have shown that women who experienced stressful life events around the time of conception or early gestation were more likely to deliver infants with certain congenital abnormalities (Carmichael & Shaw, 2000) and that domestic battering was associated with higher incidence of gynecological disorders and abortions that were not the direct result of injuries sustained during the physical abuse (Bergman & Brismar, 1991).

To date, there have not been any published clinical findings concerning the relationship between PTSD and the growth hormone axis. We predict that future research will show that normal growth and maturation can be adversely affected by exposure to traumatic stress, especially if such exposure occurs during critical developmental periods of childhood and adolescence.

We previously reviewed the cluster of medical problems, called metabolic syndrome X, associated with chronic stress syndrome. It consists of a cluster of symptoms resulting from excessive HPA-induced suppression of growth hormone, gonadal steroids, and bone growth (see Table 7.2). We also cited the one relevant study, in this regard, showing abnormalities in bone metabolism (e.g., osteopenia) associated with PTSD among U.S. Navy repatriated prisoners of war (Sausen et al., 2001). Consistent with our argument that tonic HPA abnormalities in PTSD will generally resemble those seen with chronic stress syndrome, we would predict that people with PTSD are more likely than non-PTSD individuals to develop other manifestations of metabolic syndrome X in addition to osteopenia.

There is evidence for both suppression and enhancement of immunological function among people with PTSD. Given the complex web of interactions among HPA, adrenergic, and immunologic systems, phasic enhancement of immune activity could be triggered by CRF, norepinephrine, or by cytokines such as IL-6 (Crofford et al., 1997) or any combination of the above (Ader, Cohen, & Felten, 1995; Leonard & Song, 1996; Zakowski, McAllister, Deal, & Baum, 1992; Ziegler, Ruiz-Ramon, & Shapiro, 1993).

Such findings are consistent with a chronic pattern of tonic immunosuppression, punctuated by stress-induced phasic episodes of acute enhancement of immunological activity. In the case of moderate-to-severe PTSD, it is possible that phasic episodes are of sufficient frequency and intensity to obscure the underlying tonic immunosuppression, thereby presenting a cross-sectional picture of enhanced immunological activity as has been found in several studies cited previously. One possible mechanism could be stress-enhanced inflammatory cytokine production superimposed on a tonic state of relative glucocorticoid deficiency. This is consistent with the phenomenology of a number of clinical states marked by episodic stress-induced increased incidence or exacerbation of symptoms. The list of medical conditions exacerbated by acute stress includes rheumatoid arthritis (Potter & Zautra, 1997), Type I diabetes (American Diabetes Association, 1997; Ionescu-Tirgoviste, Simion, Mariana, Dan, & Iulian, 1987), fibromyalgia and chronic fatigue syndrome (Crofford & Demitrack, 1996; Crofford, Jacobson, & Young, 1999), irritable bowel syndrome (Anton & Shanahan, 1998), temporomandibular disorders (Korszun, Papadopoulos, Demitrack, Engleberg, & Crofford, 1998), tension headaches, dysmenorrhea, irritable bladder syndrome (see Crofford et al., 1999), and multiple chemical sensitivity (Rowat, 1998).

Comparison of Medical Problems Associated With Chronic Stress Syndrome and PTSD

Both chronic stress syndrome and PTSD appear to be associated with a number of medical illnesses. Although PTSD research on this question is at an early stage, current evidence (shown in Table 7.2) indicates a remarkable consistency in the medical consequences of these two pathological states. This is most apparent in studies concerning cardiovascular abnormalities. The few clinical abnormalities related to opioid, thyroid, reproductive, metabolic, and immunological function also suggest how PTSD could lead to medical problems.

HOW DOES THE ALLOSTATIC LOAD MODEL ENHANCE OUR UNDERSTANDING OF THE ETIOLOGICAL SIGNIFICANCE OF SUCH ABNORMALITIES?

Although many specific PTSD-related biological abnormalities and associated disease entities are shown in Tables 7.1 and 7.2, they are all consequences of tonic and phasic alterations in the human mediators of the stress response. More generally, using the terminology of allostasis, which broadens the discussion beyond "stress" per se, these PTSD abnormalities reflect an imbalance in various systems that usually help the body to adapt to a variety of challenges, be they related to lifestyle (diet, exercise, smoking, alcohol) or to stressful life events. Dysregulation of HPA, adrenergic, metabolic, and immune mechanisms produces secondary abnormalities through a cascade of downstream mechanisms that all play crucial roles in the maintenance of homeostasis and health. This is the essence of the organizing concepts of allostatic states and allostatic load.

The psychobiological demands of chronic PTSD result in allostatic states of sustained activity that enable the organism to achieve a new steady state through which to maintain vital functions. "The price of this accommodation to stress can be *allostatic load*, which is the wear and tear that results from chronic overactivity or underactivity of allostatic systems" (McEwen, 1998). This allostatic state promotes pathophysiological changes over time. It is these changes that increase vulnerability to medical illness among individuals with PTSD.

McEwen (1998) has identified four types of allostatic states that result in allostatic load and, in turn, increase the risk for medical illness. We review each one and show that all four types of allostatic load are present in PTSD. Type 1 allostatic load (Figure 7.1) is "repeated 'hits' from multiple stressors," such as repeated surges of blood pressure that can trigger

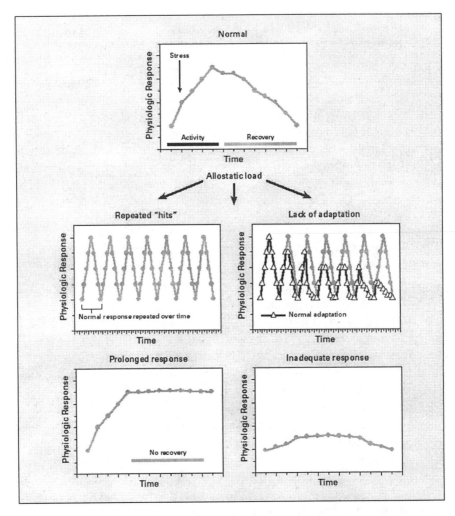

Figure 7.1. Four types of allostatic load. The top panel illustrates the normal allostatic response, in which a response is initiated by a stressor, sustained for an appropriate interval, and then turned off. The remaining panels illustrate four conditions that lead to allostatic load; repeated "hits" from multiple stressors; lack of adaptation; prolonged response due to delayed shutdown; and inadequate response that leads to compensatory hyperactivity of other mediators (e.g., inadequate secretion of glucocorticoids, resulting in increased concentrations of cytokines that are normally counterregulated by glucocorticoids). From "Protective and Damaging Effects of Stress Mediators," by B. S. McEwen, 1998, *New England Journal of Medicine, 338,* p. 174. Copyright 1998 by the Massachusetts Medical Society. Reprinted with permission.

myocardial infarction or atherosclerosis in susceptible individuals (Muller, Tofler, & Stone, 1989). As discussed previously, a number of phasic abnormalities in PTSD appear to exemplify this type of allostatic load. Most notably, they include cardiovascular and adrenergic hyperreactivity to environmental demands that are experienced as stressful. In addition, traumatic reminders, intrusive recollections, and traumamimetic stimuli can all elicit cardiovascular hyperreactivity among individuals with PTSD. Other hyperreactive mechanisms in PTSD appear to include glucocorticoid receptor supersensitivity and enhanced immune response to acutely stressful situations. As shown in Table 7.2, these may contribute to exacerbation of chronic disease states, allergic conditions, and autoimmune diseases.

Allostasis is not only an outgrowth of past experiences but may be based in part on the expectation of future events. Although realistic anticipation is certainly adaptive, problems may arise if expectations are not well calibrated to external reality. Thus, abnormalities may occur in the accuracy of stress and threat appraisal rather than with responsivity to reality per se. Problems in signal detection may take one of two possible forms; either the individual fails to recognize important stressors to which he or she must respond (i.e., false negatives) or the individual misinterprets harmless stimuli as threats to survival (i.e., false positives). False positives are common in PTSD. Most often, affected individuals misperceive danger during conditions of safety. This general tendency to perceive false positive threat signals produces a response bias toward hyperreactivity. In other words, the threat-averse, hypervigilant person with PTSD is more likely to experience danger in nondangerous situations and, therefore, elicit stress responses unnecessarily. Pathophysiologic manifestations of hypervigilance may include glucocorticoid enhanced negative feedback responsivity, startle response hyperreactivity and possibly CRF activation, stress-induced analgesia, and cytokine mediated mobilization of the immune system. In short, Type 1 allostatic load is a common occurrence in PTSD.

Type 2 allostatic load (Figure 7.1), "lack of adaptation," results from a progressive allostatic state in which the organism loses its capacity to habituate or adapt to repeated stressors. Failure to habituate—that is, to dampen physiological responses to the same stressor over time—results in excessive and potentially deleterious overexposure to the various components of the stress response. An experimental example of Type 2 allostatic load in PTSD is seen in resistance to extinction of the acoustic startle response (Shalev et al., 1992). Type 2 allostatic load might also result from sensitization or kindling of limbic nuclei as proposed by Post and associates (Post, Weiss, Li, Leverich, & Pert, 1999; Post, Weiss, & Smith, 1995) in which repeated exposure to stressful or traumatic stimuli produces a progressive enhancement (rather than habituation) of the stress response among affected individuals. It may also be relevant to episodic flare-ups of chronic illness under stressful circumstances (e.g., irritable bowel syndrome, rheumatoid arthritis).

Allostatic load Type 3, "prolonged response," is the result of an allostatic state reflecting the failure to shut off the allostatic response when it is no longer needed. Prolonged phasic elevations in cardiovascular, HPA, and immunologic activity are all applicable here and would very likely increase the risk for pathological states in those systems.

Whereas allostatic load Type 2 is a pathological phasic response, allostatic load Type 3 is primarily a tonic abnormality. This includes tonic elevations of blood pressure and heart rate that constitute a risk for cardiovascular disease. Prolonged HPA hyperactivity promotes immunosuppression, with all the previously described potential complications of such a state, including reduced disease resistance, cancer susceptibility and autoimmune problems. Chronically elevated HPA activity will also produce endocrine (thyroid, gonadotropic, and growth hormone), metabolic, and opioid system dysregulation as previously described.

Allostatic load Type 4, "inadequate response," is a more chronic state in which key components of the stress system have lost their capacity to mount an adequate response. This can result from depleted resources, irreversible consequences of prolonged suppression, or other mechanisms. An example offered elsewhere might also apply to PTSD: An inadequate HPA response is unable to terminate the mobilization of lymphocytes and NK cells during an acute inflammatory episode (McEwen, 1998). Under such conditions, the apparent clinical problem of excessive immunologic activity is really caused by an insufficient HPA response, which normally contains the immune response. Another example of allostatic load Type 4 is hypocortisolism, which predisposes individuals to several stress-related medical disorders such as chronic fatigue syndrome, fibromyalgia, somatoform disorders, idiopathic pain syndromes, rheumatoid arthritis, and asthma. Whether any or all of these syndromes will prove to be associated with PTSD remains to be seen.

Psychological, behavioral, and social factors observed in PTSD that promote its association with medical illness (see Schnurr & Jankowski, 1999; Seeman & McEwen, 1996) can also be understood in terms of allostatic load. These factors constitute the lifestyle of individuals with PTSD, and they contribute to the physiological responses that constitute allostasis. Maladaptive behavioral responses to stressors, such as smoking and ethanol consumption, ingestion of high fat diets, and lack of exercise, all intensify allostatic states and exacerbate allostatic load (see McEwen, 1998; Schnurr & Jankowski, 1999). As noted by Schnurr and Jankowski (1999), the heuristic value of applying the allostatic load model to PTSD is "its multivariate, longitudinal perspective and an emphasis on the cumulative and interactive effects" (p. 301) of a large number of chronic, disease-enhancing elements that produce clinically significant "wear and tear" on individuals with this disorder.

HOW MIGHT THE ALLOSTATIC LOAD MODEL HELP US APPROACH RESILIENCE, PREVENTION, AND TREATMENT?

Allostatic load provides a conceptually coherent and parsimonious model with which to understand how the many diverse abnormalities associated with PTSD increase the risk for medical illness. It places the pathophysiological focus on the stress response as a whole, rather than on a specific dysregulation in a psychobiological system. Whether it is a tonic or phasic abnormality, the wear and tear on the system maintaining vital functions comes at a price that increases vulnerability to a large variety of medical disorders.

Allostasis, stability through change, does not necessarily imply a change for the worse. Changing behavior to promote regular exercise, judicious diet, stress reduction, psychological wellness, loving relationships, social support, and a sense of control over one's life, all have a salutary impact on health (McEwen, 1998; Seeman & McEwen, 1996). Dienstbier's (1989) concept of physiological toughening through aerobic exercises and other salubrious activities is also relevant here. Such measures provide an extra margin of safety with which to buffer the potentially deleterious impact of traumatic stress. We refer to allostatic change in such positive directions as *allostatic support* to differentiate it from the pathophysiological changes denoted by allostatic load.

We define allostatic support as any nonhomeostatic, biopsychosocial strategy that will oppose allostatic load. Individuals endowed with a healthy titer of inherited or acquired allostatic support are resilient. Conscious individual or societal efforts to increase allostatic support are likely to foster prevention of adverse health consequences. Efforts to reduce allostatic load by enhancing allostatic support constitute treatment.

Resilience, prevention, and treatment of PTSD might result from enhancing allostatic support in any of the psychobiological systems discussed previously (see Friedman, 2002). Such approaches should be effective whether allostatic load (constitutionally) preceded the onset of PTSD or occurred after an individual acquired the disorder. We believe that two of the most promising lines of research would focus on reducing hyperreactivity and normalizing dysregulated HPA function. A third approach might focus on increasing anabolic factors, such as GH, IGF-1, testosterone, or neurotrophins in the brain, to promote allostatic support.

Allostatic load Type 2 (Figure 7.1) is hyperreactivity that is sustained because of a failure of habituation or resistance to extinction. Because most people exposed to traumatic stress do not develop PTSD (Kessler, Sonnega, Bromet, Hughes, & Nelson, 1995) it may be inferred that most people are resilient because they are equipped with inherited or acquired allostatic support mechanisms that effectively buffer the intense stress response triggered by exposure to a traumatic event, or that allow it to habituate subsequently. Theoretically, a preventive strategy (especially desirable for people entering potentially traumatizing professions such as the military, police work, and so forth) might consist of confidential screening procedures by which to identify deficiencies in one or more allostatic support capacities. Individuals wishing to overcome such deficits might request special psychophysiological training or physiological toughening designed to mobilize and enhance their capacity for habituation and extinction of excessive stress reactions (Dienstbier, 1989; Shalev, 1999). We expect that this type of voluntary preventive approach could attenuate the potentially deleterious effects of hyperreactivity, by fostering resilience and preventing the subsequent development of PTSD.

A second example emphasizes efforts to reduce allostatic load, or promote allostatic support, with respect to HPA dysregulation. This might be achieved with pharmacological agents that reduce CRF activity, such as CRF antagonists. It might also be achieved with prophylactic administration of cortisol, as in a study on septic shock in which modest cortisol doses reduced the incidence of PTSD (Schelling et al., 1999).

A third approach might be with medications that enhance NPY's capacity to inhibit both CRF and catecholamine activity. An experiment with American special forces military personnel exposed to an extremely stressful training experience showed that individuals who were best able to mobilize NPY tolerated the experience better than those with lower NPY levels (Morgan et al., 2000). This suggests that the capacity to efficiently mobilize NPY may be a marker of resilience against PTSD. It also suggests that people in dangerous professions who lack such a capacity might benefit from pretraumatic NPY administration (prevention) or posttraumatic NPY treatment to forestall the later development of PTSD.

Other examples of allostatic support will undoubtedly become apparent as we learn more about the pathophysiology of PTSD. In coming years, we expect that new ways to promote allostatic support will emerge that will foster resilience, prevent PTSD, and provide effective treatment (Friedman, 2002).

CONCLUSIONS AND FUTURE DIRECTIONS

PTSD is a major public health problem. We have proposed in this chapter that in addition to psychiatric morbidity, the complex pathophysiology of PTSD makes it a risk factor for a wide spectrum of medical disorders.

Research has just begun to demonstrate that the medical morbidity of PTSD may be at least as significant as its deleterious psychiatric consequences. Furthermore, individuals with PTSD are more likely to seek treatment from primary and specialty medical practitioners than from mental health professionals. A major reason they seek such treatment is because PTSD-related dysregulation of HPA, LC/NE, opioid, endocrine, metabolic, and immune systems can produce clinically significant medical illness.

We hope that the theoretical context and specific information presented in this chapter will promote better recognition of the wide array of medical and psychiatric sequelae among individuals who have PTSD.

REFERENCES

Ader, R., Cohen, N., & Felten, D. (1995). Psychoneuroimmunology: Interactions between the nervous system and the immune system. *Lancet, 345*, 99–103.

American Diabetes Association. (1997). *American Diabetes Association complete guide to diabetes.* Alexandria, VA: Author.

Anton, P. A., & Shanahan, F. (1998). Neuroimmunomodulation in inflammatory bowel disease: How far from "bench" to "bedside?" *Annals of the New York Academy of Sciences: Vol. 851* (pp. 723–734). New York: New York Academy of Sciences.

Aston-Jones, G., Valentino, R. J., Van Bockstaele, E. J., & Meyerson, A. T. (1994). Locus coeruleus, stress, and PTSD: Neurobiological and clinical parallels. In M. M. Murburg (Ed.), *Catecholamine function in posttraumatic stress disorder: Emerging concepts* (pp. 17–62). Washington, DC: American Psychiatric Press.

Baker, D. G., West, S. A., Nicholson, W. E., Ekhator, N. N., Kasckow, J. W., Hill, K. K., et al. (1999). Serial CSF corticotropin-releasing hormone levels and adrenocortical activity in combat veterans with posttraumatic stress disorder. *American Journal of Psychiatry, 156*, 585–588.

Baker, D. G., West, S. A., Orth, D. N., Hill, K. K., Nicholson, W. E., Ekhator, N. N., et al. (1997). Cerebrospinal fluid and plasma β-endorphin in combat veterans with post-traumatic stress disorder. *Psychoneuroendocrinology, 22*, 517–529.

Benedikt, R. A., & Kolb, L. C. (1986). Preliminary findings on chronic pain and posttraumatic stress disorder. *American Journal of Psychiatry, 143*, 908–910.

Bergman, B., & Brismar, B. (1991). A 5-year follow-up study of 117 battered women. *American Journal of Public Health, 81*, 1486–1489.

Blanchard, E. B., Kolb, L. C., Prins, A., Gates, S., & McCoy, G. C. (1991). Changes in plasma norepinephrine to combat-related stimuli among Vietnam veterans with posttraumatic stress disorder. *Journal of Nervous and Mental Disease, 179*, 371–373.

Boscarino, J. A. (1997). Diseases among men 20 years after exposure to severe stress: Implications for clinical research and medical care. *Psychosomatic Medicine, 59,* 605–614.

Boscarino, J. A., & Chang, J. (1999). Electrocardiogram abnormalities among men with stress-related psychiatric disorders: Implications for coronary heart disease and clinical research. *Annals of Behavioral Medicine, 21,* 227–234.

Bremner, J. D., Innis, R. B., Ng, C. K., Staib, L. H., Salomon, R. M., Bronen, R. A., et al. (1997). Positron emission tomography measurement of cerebral metabolic correlates of yohimbine administration in combat-related posttraumatic stress disorder. *Archives of General Psychiatry, 54,* 364–374.

Bremner, J. D., Licinio, J., Darnell, A., Krystal, J. H., Owens, M. J., Southwick, S. M., et al. (1997). Elevated CSF corticotropin-releasing factor concentrations in post-traumatic stress disorder. *American Journal of Psychiatry, 154,* 624–629.

Britton, K. T., Southerland, S., Van Uden, E., Kirby, D., Rivier, J., & Koob, G. (1997). Anxiolytic activity of NPY receptor agonists in the conflict test. *Psychopharmacology, 132,* 6–13.

Buckley, T. C., & Kaloupek, D. G. (2001). A meta-analytic examination of basal cardiovascular activity in PTSD. *Psychosomatic Medicine, 63,* 585–594.

Burges Watson, I. P., Muller, H. K., Jones, I. H., & Bradley, A. J. (1993). Cell-mediated immunity in combat veterans with posttraumatic stress disorder. *Medical Journal of Australia, 159,* 513–516.

Cannon, W. B. (1932). *The wisdom of the body.* New York: Norton.

Carmichael, S. L., & Shaw, G. M. (2000). Maternal life event stress and congenital anomalies. *Epidemiology, 11,* 30–35.

Chrousos, G. P. (1998). Stressors, stress, and neuroendocrine integration of the adaptive response: The 1997 Hans Selye Memorial Lecture. *Annals of the New York Academy of Sciences: Vol. 851* (pp. 311–335). New York: New York Academy of Sciences.

Colmers, W., & Bleakman, D. (1994). Effects of neuropeptide Y on the electrical properties of neurons. *Trends in Neuroscience, 17,* 373–379.

Corder, R., Castagne, V., Rivet, J. M., Mormede, P., & Gaillard, R. C. (1992). Central and peripheral effects of repeated stress and high NaCl diet on neuropeptide Y. *Physiology and Behavior, 52,* 205–210.

Crofford, L. J., & Demitrack, M. A. (1996). Evidence that abnormalities of central neurohormonal systems are key to understanding fibromyalgia and chronic fatigue syndrome. *Rheumatic Disease Clinics of North America, 22,* 267–284.

Crofford, L. J., Jacobson, J., & Young, E. (1999). Modeling the involvement of the hypothalamic–pituitary–adrenal and hypothalamic–pituitary–gonadal axes in autoimmune and stress-related rheumatic syndromes in women. *Journal of Women's Health, 8,* 203–215.

Crofford, L. J., Kalogeras, K. T., Mastorakos, G., Magiakou, M. A., Wells, J., Kanik, K. S., et al. (1997). Circadian relationships between interleukin (IL)-6 and hypothalamic–pituitary–adrenal axis hormones: Failure of IL-6 to cause sustained hypercortisolism in patients with early untreated rheumatoid arthritis. *Journal of Clinical Endocrinology and Metabolism, 82,* 1279–1283.

Dhabhar, F., & McEwen, B. S. (1997). Acute stress enhances while chronic stress suppresses cell-mediated immunity: A potential role for leukocyte trafficking. *Brain Behavior and Immunology, 11,* 286–306.

Dienstbier, R. A. (1989). Arousal and physiological toughness: Implications for mental and physical health. *Psychological Review, 96,* 81–100.

Everson, S. A., Lynch, J. W., Chesney, M. A., Kaplan, G. A., Goldberg, D. E., Shade, S. B., et al. (1997). Interaction of workplace demands and cardiovascular reactivity in progression of carotid atherosclerosis: Population based study. *British Medical Journal, 314,* 553–558.

Falger, P. R. J., Op den Velde, W., Hovens, J. E. J. M., Schouten, E. G. W., De Groen, J. H. M., & Van Duijn, H. (1992). Current posttraumatic stress disorder and cardiovascular disease risk factors in Dutch Resistance veterans from World War II. *Psychotherapy and Psychosomatics, 57,* 164–171.

Friedman, M. J. (1981). Post-Vietnam syndrome: Recognition and management. *Psychosomatics, 22,* 931–943.

Friedman, M. J. (Ed.). (1999). Progress in the psychobiology of post-traumatic stress disorder. *Seminars in Clinical Neuropsychiatry, 4,* 229–316.

Friedman, M. J. (2002). Future pharmacotherapy for PTSD: Prevention and treatment. *Psychiatric Clinics of North America, 25,* 427–442.

Friedman, M. J., Charney, D. S., & Deutch, A. Y. (1995). *Neurobiological and clinical consequences of stress: From normal adaptation to post-traumatic stress disorder.* Philadelphia: Lippincott-Raven.

Friedman, M. J., McDonagh-Coyle, A., Jalowiec, J. E., Wang, S., Fournier, D. A., & McHugo, G. (2001, December). Neurohormonal findings during treatment of women with PTSD due to CSA. In M. J. Friedman (Chair), *PTSD-CSA treatment: Psychological, physiological, and hormonal responses.* Symposium conducted at the meeting of the International Society for Traumatic Stress Studies, New Orleans, LA.

Friedman, M. J., & Schnurr, P. P. (1995). The relationship between trauma, PTSD, and physical health. In M. J. Friedman, D. S. Charney, & A.Y. Deutch (Eds.), *Neurobiological and clinical consequences of stress: From normal adaptation to PTSD* (pp. 507–524). Philadelphia: Lippincott-Raven.

Heim, C., Ehlert, U., & Hellhammer, D. H. (2000). The potential role of hypocortisolism in the pathophysiology of stress related bodily disorders. *Psychoneuroendocrinology, 25,* 1–35.

Heim, C., Newport, D. J., Bonsall, R., Miller, A. H., & Nemeroff, C. B. (2001). Altered pituitary–adrenal axis responses to provocative challenge tests in adult survivors of childhood abuse. *American Journal of Psychiatry, 158,* 575–581.

Hoffman, L., Burges Watson, I. P., Wilson, G., & Montgomery, J. (1989). Low plasma β-endorphin in post-traumatic stress disorder. *Australian and New Zealand Journal of Psychiatry, 23,* 268–273.

Ionescu-Tirgoviste, C., Simion, P., Mariana, C., Dan, C. M., & Iulian, M. (1987). The signification of stress in the aetiopathogenesis of type-sub-2 diabetes mellitus. *Stress Medicine, 3,* 277–284.

Kardiner, A. (1941). *The traumatic neuroses of war.* New York: Hoeber.

Kask, A., Rago, L., & Harro, J. (1996). Anxiogenic-like effect of the neuropeptide Y Y1 receptor antagonist BIBP3226: Antagonism with diazepam. *European Journal of Pharmacology, 317,* R3–R4.

Keane, T. M., Kolb, L. C., Kaloupek, D. G., Orr, S. P., Blanchard, E. B., Thomas, R. G., et al. (1998). Utility of psychophysiological measurement in the diagnosis of posttraumatic stress disorder: Results from a Department of Veterans Affairs cooperative study. *Journal of Consulting and Clinical Psychology, 66,* 914–923.

Kessler, R. C., Sonnega, A., Bromet, E., Hughes, M., & Nelson, C. B. (1995). Posttraumatic stress disorder in the National Comorbidity Survey. *Archives of General Psychiatry, 52,* 1048–1060.

Korszun, A., Papadopoulos, E., Demitrack, M. A., Engleberg, C., & Crofford, L. (1998). The relationship between temporomandibular disorders and stress-associated syndromes. *Oral Surgery, Oral Medicine, Oral Pathology, 86,* 416–420.

Laudenslager, M. L., Aasal, R., Adler, L., Berger, C. L., Montgomery, P. T., Sandberg, E., et al. (1998). Elevated cytotoxicity in combat veterans with long-term post-traumatic stress disorder: Preliminary observations. *Brain, Behavior, and Immunity, 12,* 74–79.

Leonard, B. E., & Song, C. (1996). Stress and the immune system in the etiology of anxiety and depression. *Pharmacology, Biochemistry, and Behavior, 54,* 299–303.

Lerer, B., Gur, E., Bleich, A., & Newman, M. (1994). Peripheral adrenergic receptors in PTSD. In M. M. Murburg (Ed.), *Catecholamine function in posttraumatic stress disorder: Emerging concepts—Progress in psychiatry, No. 42* (pp. 257–276). Washington, DC: American Psychiatric Press.

Mason, J. W., Giller, E. L., Jr., Kosten, T. R., & Wahby, V. S. (1990). Serum testosterone levels in posttraumatic stress disorder patients. *Journal of Traumatic Stress, 3,* 449–457.

Mason, J. W., Wang, S., Yehuda, R., Bremner, J. D., Riney, S. J., & Lubin, H. (1995). Some approaches to the study of the clinical implications of thyroid alterations in post-traumatic stress disorder. In M. J. Friedman, D. S. Charney, & A. Y. Deutch (Eds.), *Neurobiological and clinical consequences of stress: From normal adaptation to post-traumatic stress disorder* (pp. 367–380). Philadelphia: Lippincott-Raven.

McEwen, B. S. (1998). Protective and damaging effects of stress mediators. *New England Journal of Medicine, 338,* 171–179.

McEwen, B. S., & Stellar, E. (1993). Stress and the individual: Mechanisms leading to disease. *Archives of Internal Medicine, 153,* 2093–2101.

McFall, M. E., Murburg, M. M., Ko, G. N., & Veith, R. C. (1990). Autonomic responses to stress in Vietnam combat veterans with posttraumatic stress disorder. *Biological Psychiatry, 27,* 1165–1175.

Mellman, T. A., Kulick-Bell, R., Ashlock, L. E., & Nolan, B. (1995). Sleep events in combat-related posttraumatic stress disorder. *American Journal of Psychiatry, 152,* 110–115.

Morgan, C. A., Wang, S., Southwick, S. M., Rasmusson, A. M., Hazlett, G., Hauger, R. L., et al. (2000). Plasma NPY in humans experiencing acute uncontrollable stress. *Biological Psychiatry, 109,* 290–298.

Mulchahey, J. J., Ekhator, N. N., Zhang, H., Kasckow, J. W., Baker, D. G., & Geracioti, T. D. (2001). Cerebrospinal fluid and plasma testosterone levels in post-traumatic stress disorder and tobacco dependence. *Psychoneuroendocrinology, 26,* 273–285.

Muller, J. E., Tofler, G., & Stone, P. (1989). Circadian variation and triggers of onset of acute cardiovascular disease. *Circulation, 79,* 733–743.

Pernow, J. (1988). Co-release and functional interactions of neuropeptide Y and noradrenaline in peripheral sympathetic vascular control. *Acta Physiologica Scandinavia,* (Suppl. 568), 1–56.

Perry, B. D. (1994). Neurobiological sequelae of childhood trauma: PTSD in children. In M. M. Murburg (Ed.), *Catecholamine function in post-traumatic stress disorder: Emerging concepts* (pp. 233–255). Washington, DC: American Psychiatric Press.

Perry, B. D., Giller, E. L., & Southwick, S. M. (1987). Altered platelet alpha2 adrenergic binding sites in post-traumatic stress disorder. *American Journal of Psychiatry, 144,* 1511–1512.

Perry, S. W., Cella, D. F., Falkenberg, J., Heidrich, G., & Goodwin, C. (1987). Pain perception in burn patients with stress disorders. *Journal of Pain and Symptom Management, 2,* 29–33.

Pitman, R. K., Orr, S. P., Forgue, D. F., de Jong, J., & Clairborn, J. M. (1987). Psychophysiological assessment of posttraumatic stress disorder imagery in Vietnam combat veterans. *Archives of General Psychiatry, 44,* 970–975.

Pitman, R. K., Orr, S. P., Shalev, A. Y., Metzger, L. J., & Mellman, T. A. (1999). Psychophysiological alterations in post-traumatic stress disorder. *Seminars in Clinical Neuropsychiatry, 4,* 234–241.

Pitman, R. K., van der Kolk, B. A., Orr, S. P., & Greenberg, M. S. (1990). Naloxone-reversible analgesic response to combat-related stimuli in post-traumatic stress disorder. *Archives of General Psychiatry, 47,* 541–544.

Post, R. M., Weiss, S. R. B., Li, H., Leverich, G. S., & Pert, A. (1999). Sensitization components of post-traumatic stress disorder: Implications for therapeutics. *Seminars in Clinical Neuropsychiatry, 4,* 282–294.

Post, R. M., Weiss, S. R. B., & Smith, M. A. (1995). Sensitization and kindling: Implications for the evolving neural substrate of PTSD. In M. J. Friedman, D. S. Charney, & A. Y. Deutch (Eds.), *Neurobiological and clinical consequences of stress: From normal adaptation to post-traumatic stress disorder* (pp. 203–224). Philadelphia: Lippincott-Raven.

Potter, P. T., & Zautra, A. J. (1997). Stressful life events' effects on rheumatoid arthritis disease activity. *Journal of Consulting and Clinical Psychology, 65,* 319–323.

Rapaport, M. H. (1987). Chronic pain and post-traumatic stress disorder. *American Journal of Psychiatry, 144,* 120.

Rasmusson, A. M., & Friedman, M. J. (2002). The neurobiology of PTSD in women. In R. Kimerling, P. C. Ouimette & J. Wolfe (Eds.), *Gender and PTSD* (pp. 43–75). New York: Guilford Press.

Rasmusson, A. M., Hauger, R. L., Morgan, C. A., Bremner, J. D., Charney, D. S., & Southwick, S. M. (2000). Low baseline and yohimbine-stimulated plasma neuropeptide Y (NPY) in combat-related PTSD. *Biological Psychiatry, 47,* 526–539.

Rasmusson, A. M., Lipschitz, D. S., Wang, S., Hu, S., Vojvoda, D., Bremner, J. D., Southwick, S. M., et al. (2001). Increased pituitary and adrenal reactivity in premenopausal women with PTSD. *Biological Psychiatry.*

Ross, R. J., Ball, W. A., Sullivan, K. A., & Caroff, S. N. (1989). Sleep disturbance as the hallmark of post-traumatic stress disorder. *American Journal of Psychiatry, 146,* 697–707.

Rowat, S. C. (1998). Integrated defense system overlaps as a disease model—with examples for multiple chemical sensitivity. *Environmental Health Perspective, 106*(Suppl. 1), 85–109.

Sabioncello, A., Kocijan-Hercigonja, D., Rabatic, S., Tomasic, J., Jeren, T., Matijevic, L., et al. (2000). Immune, endocrine, and psychological responses in civilians displaced by war. *Psychosomatic Medicine, 62,* 502–508.

Sausen, K. P., Moore, J. L., Ambrose, M. R., Wells, A. F., & Mitchell, R. E. (2001). The relationship between PTSD and osteopenia [Abstract No. 1234]. *Psychosomatic Medicine, 63,* 144.

Schelling, G., Stoll, C., Kapfhammer, H. P., Rothenhausler, H. B., Krauseneck, T., Durst, K., et al. (1999). The effect of stress doses of hydrocortisone during septic shock on posttraumatic stress disorder and health-related quality of life in survivors. *Critical Care Medicine, 27,* 2678–2683.

Schneiderman, N. (1977). Animal models relating behavioral stress and cardiovascular pathology. In T. M. Dembroski, S. M. Weiss, J. L. Shields, S. G. Haynes, & M. Feinleib (Eds.), *Coronary-prone behavior* (pp. 155–182). New York: Springer-Verlag.

Schneiderman, N. (1987). Psychophysiologic factors in atherogenesis and coronary artery disease. *Circulation, 76,* 41–47.

Schnurr, P. P., & Jankowski, M. K. (1999). Physical health and post-traumatic stress disorder: Review and synthesis. *Seminars in Clinical Neuropsychiatry, 4,* 295–304.

Schnurr, P. P., Spiro, A., III, & Paris, A. H. (2000). Physician-diagnosed medical disorders in relation to PTSD symptoms in older male military veterans. *Health Psychology, 19,* 91–97.

Seeman, T. E., & McEwen, B. S. (1996). Impact of social environment characteristics on neuroendocrine regulation. *Psychosomatic Medicine, 58*, 459–471.

Selye, H. (1956). *The stress of life*. New York: McGraw-Hill.

Seng, J. S., Oakley, D. J., Sampselle, C. M., Killion, C., Graham-Bermann, S., & Liberzon, I. (2001). Posttraumatic stress disorder and pregnancy complications. *Obstetrics and Gynecology, 97*, 17–22.

Shalev, A. Y. (1999). Psychophysiological expression of risk factors for PTSD. In R. Yehuda (Ed.), *Risk factors for posttraumatic stress disorder* (pp. 143–161). Washington, DC: American Psychiatric Press.

Shalev, A. Y., Bleich, A., & Ursano, R. J. (1990). Posttraumatic stress disorder: Somatic comorbidity and effort tolerance. *Psychosomatics, 31*, 197–203.

Shalev, A. Y., Orr, S. P., Peri, T., Schreiber, S., & Pitman, R. K. (1992). Physiological responses to loud tones in Israeli patients with posttraumatic stress disorder. *Archives of General Psychiatry, 49*, 870–875.

Shalev, A. Y., Peri, T., Canetti, L., & Schreiber, S. (1996). Predictors of PTSD in injured trauma survivors: A prospective study. *American Journal of Psychiatry, 153*, 219–225.

Shapiro, A. P. (1988). Psychological factors in hypertension: An overview. *American Heart Journal, 116*, 632–637.

Smith, M. A., Davidson, J. R., Ritchie, J. C., Kudler, H., Lipper, S., Chappell, P., et al. (1989). The corticotropin-releasing hormone test in patients with posttraumatic stress disorder. *Biological Psychiatry, 26*, 349–355.

Southwick, S. M., Krystal, J. H., Morgan, C. A., Johnson, D. R., Nagy, L. M., Nicolaou, A. L., et al. (1993). Abnormal noradrenergic function in posttraumatic stress disorder. *Archives of General Psychiatry, 50*, 266–274.

Southwick, S. M., Paige, S. R., Morgan, C. A., Bremner, J. D., Krystal, J. H., & Charney, D. S. (1999). Adrenergic and serotonergic abnormalities in PTSD: Catecholamines and serotonin. *Seminars in Clinical Neuropsychiatry, 4*, 242–248.

Spivak, B., Shohat, B., Mester, R., Avraham, S., Gil-As, I., Bleich, A., et al. (1997). Elevated levels of serum interleukin-1β in combat-related posttraumatic stress disorder. *Biological Psychiatry, 42*, 345–348.

Sterling, P., & Eyer, J. (1988). Allostasis: A new paradigm to explain arousal pathology. In S. Fisher & J. Reason (Eds.), *Handbook of life stress, cognition, and health* (pp. 629–649). New York: John Wiley.

Wang, S., & Mason, J. (1999). Elevations of serum T3 levels and their association with symptoms in World War II veterans with combat-related posttraumatic stress disorder: Replication of findings in Vietnam combat veterans. *Psychosomatic Medicine, 61*, 131–138.

Yehuda, R. (1997). Sensitization of the hypothalamic–pituitary–adrenal axis in posttraumatic stress disorder. *Annals of the New York Academy of Sciences: Vol. 821* (pp. 57–75). New York: New York Academy of Sciences.

Yehuda, R. (1999). Linking the neuroendocrinology of post-traumatic stress disorder with recent neuroanatomic findings. *Seminars in Clinical Neuropsychiatry, 4,* 256–265.

Yehuda, R., Levengood, R. A., Schmeidler, J., Wilson, S., Guo, L. S., & Gerber, D. (1996). Increased pituitary activation following metyrapone administration in post-traumatic stress disorder. *Psychoneuroendrocrinology, 21,* 1–16.

Yehuda, R., & McFarlane, A. C. (Eds.). (1997). *Annals of the New York Academy of Sciences: Vol. 821. Psychobiology of posttraumatic stress disorder* (pp. 1–550). New York: New York Academy of Sciences.

Zakowski, S. G., McAllister, C. G., Deal, M., & Baum, A. (1992). Stress, reactivity, and immune function in healthy men. *Health Psychology, 11,* 223–232.

Ziegler, M. G., Ruiz-Ramon, P., & Shapiro, M. (1993). Abnormal stress responses in patients with diseases affecting the sympathetic nervous system. *Psychosomatic Medicine, 55,* 339–346.

Zubovic, I., Mikac, G., Biukovic, M., Skrobic, M., & Rajkovaca, Z. (1993). The frequency of thyrotoxicosis in war time period. *Medicinski Preglad, 46,* 85–86.

IV

ATTENTIONAL AND BEHAVIORAL MECHANISMS LINKING TRAUMA AND HEALTH

8

SOMATIZATION AND MULTIPLE IDIOPATHIC PHYSICAL SYMPTOMS: RELATIONSHIP TO TRAUMATIC EVENTS AND POSTTRAUMATIC STRESS DISORDER

CHARLES C. ENGEL, JR.

Physical symptom syndromes following war and other traumatic events have gone by an array of colorful labels over the past 150 years, and our medical and societal penchant for relabeling these syndromes continues to this day (see Table 8.1; Hyams, Wignall, & Roswell, 1996; Shorter, 1992; Schnurr & Green, chap. 1, this volume). Yet after many years of research, debate, and medical efforts, we are still far from a thorough etiologic or therapeutic understanding of these syndromes. The mainstream tradition in medicine has been to conceptualize medically unexplained (or, in the standard medical lexicon, idiopathic) symptoms as *psychogenic*. These

This chapter was authored or coauthored by an employee of the United States government as part of official duty and is considered to be in the public domain. The views expressed in this chapter are those of the author and do not necessarily represent the official policy or position of the Uniformed Services University of the Health Sciences, Walter Reed Army Medical Center, Department of the Army, Department of Defense, or the United States government.

TABLE 8.1

Historical War Syndromes Since the United States Civil War and the Symptoms Common to All of Them (Hyams, Wignall, & Roswell, 1996)

War	Syndrome	Common overlapping symptoms
Civil War	DeCosta's syndrome Irritable heart	1. Fatigue or exhaustion 2. Headache or other chronic pain
WW I	Effort syndrome Soldier's heart Shell shock Neurocirculatory asthenia	3. Disturbed sleep 4. Forgetful, poor concentration 5. Dizziness
WW II	Battle fatigue	
Vietnam War	Agent Orange Posttraumatic stress disorder	
Gulf War	Gulf War syndrome	

"conversion symptoms" were so named because patients who experienced idiopathic symptoms were viewed as having converted psychological concerns and conflicts into less stigmatized physical symptoms. This dynamic process of converting psychological problems into physical illness came to be known as *somatization*. Today, idiopathic symptom syndromes still occur in association with traumatic and other stressful events, but scientific formulations of somatization are more phenomenological and based less on speculative etiological mechanisms.

The purpose of this chapter is to review the literature linking traumatic events and PTSD to somatization. I discuss and unify common diagnostic labels and case definitions under the operational umbrella of *multiple idiopathic physical symptoms* or MIPS. I explore the scientific literature examining the relationship of MIPS to various traumatic events, dissociation and the dissociative disorders, and PTSD. Although this literature remains small, nascent, and in need of longitudinal studies, it suggests that traumatic events may lead to MIPS and that PTSD may be a mediator of that effect: If a traumatic event is associated with subsequent PTSD, the likelihood of MIPS is increased.

In chapter 2 of this book, Green and Kimerling review the relationships among trauma, PTSD, and health status. Care has been taken here to narrow the scope to MIPS to avoid redundancy, but this is a difficult task given the strong and consistent correlations usually noted between MIPS and self-reported health status. MIPS occur in roughly a third of the general population and among primary care patients (Kroenke & Price, 1993; Kroenke et al., 1994), and therefore influence population health status more than disease per se. When a study measures health status and MIPS, the two findings often mirror one another, and in many studies the two constructs are not easily parsed.

MULTIPLE IDIOPATHIC PHYSICAL SYMPTOMS

Somatization is most commonly operationalized as a pattern of symptoms for which medical assistance is sought without an adequate medical cause identified after appropriate medical assessment (Lipowski, 1988). Instead of somatization, a term that implies psychogenicity, the trend is toward more phenomenological labels such as "medically unexplained symptoms," "unexplained physical symptoms," or "functional somatic symptoms" (Engel & Katon, 1999; Wessely, Nimnuan, & Sharpe, 1999). "Multiple idiopathic physical symptoms" is used in this chapter because it captures three cardinal characteristics of somatization: (a) its subjective and medically unexplained nature; (b) its physical (rather than only emotional) manifestations; and (c) its existence as a pattern resulting in decreased functioning (i.e., more than one symptom that is intermittently relapsing or else persistent). Somatization cannot be completely displaced as a term in this chapter, however, because many applicable research findings rely heavily on that concept.

MIPS are best conceptualized as resulting from a four-step process, moving from symptoms to disrupted functioning that is poorly explained medically. First, a person experiences symptoms. The experience of symptoms may or may not represent the effect of an underlying illness or disease. Physical symptoms are sometimes produced by mental disorder (for example, PTSD, panic disorder, or depression), psychosocial distress, or physical illness. Second, the symptomatic person assesses or appraises the symptoms. Symptom appraisal occurs through the lens of past experiences, knowledge, biases, context, and beliefs. Key aspects of symptom appraisal include conclusions regarding possible causes, seriousness, prognosis, and appropriate treatment. Psychosocial distress or mental disorders such as depression and anxiety disorders, including PTSD, may also influence an individual's appraisal of symptoms. For example, an individual with depression may develop more pessimistic or catastrophic symptom appraisals than someone who is not depressed. Third, the person responds behaviorally on the basis of the symptom appraisal. For example, he or she may seek health care, avoid activities or roles, or his or her functioning may be reduced.

The fourth step is social: If care is sought, the provider proffers an explanation. In the case of MIPS, the provider concludes the symptom is medically unexplained. This may lead to contentious differences in provider and patient appraisals. These differences can adversely impact the provider–patient relationship, resulting in modest tension, serious frustration, or mutual rejection and total disruption of care. Note that the degree to which the symptom is truly unexplained can vary widely. Kroenke (2001) argued from empirical data that it is unnecessary to determine that physical symptoms are medically unexplained, because the relationship of symptoms to psychosocial distress and disability is more a function of duration and number of symptoms than of the presence or absence of a medical explanation. However, for conceptual clarity and to prevent the confusing mixtures of different but related constructs (e.g., symptoms resulting from disease, general health status), this chapter will emphasize studies that specifically investigate physical symptom syndromes that are idiopathic.

This four-part model suggests that physical factors (e.g., coexisting disease or injury), cognitive factors (e.g., community or individual beliefs regarding a trauma), behavioral factors (e.g., patterns of health care use), and health service experience (e.g., iatrogenic harm, satisfaction with care, and differing provider and patient explanations for symptoms) may impact the onset, course, and duration of MIPS and related distress and disability. Another implication of this model is the potential for substantial heterogeneity, unexplained variance, and measurement uncertainty. For example, clinicians often view MIPS as a psychosocial component of illness, but MIPS may also have biomedical origins (e.g., subclinical disease states) that are missed because of imperfect biomedical diagnostic tools. In short, the frequent clinical convention of equating unexplained physical symptoms with a psychogenic pathogenesis is a pragmatic oversimplification at best.

One study of Veterans Affairs clinicians demonstrates another consequence of the medical uncertainty associated with MIPS. In the study, clinician beliefs regarding etiology and treatment of Gulf War syndrome (a nonmedical term often used for MIPS occurring in veterans of the 1991 Gulf War) divided along specialty lines: mental health providers tended to view veterans' MIPS as a physical illness requiring medical therapies whereas internists viewed the syndrome as a psychological illness requiring psychological treatment (Richardson et al., 2001).

DIAGNOSTIC LABELS AND CASE DEFINITIONS

Wessely and colleagues (1999) have suggested that the precise diagnosis a physician makes for patients with MIPS depends more on his or her specialty than actual differences among these syndromes. Table 8.2 displays some common examples of syndromes involving MIPS. The table illustrates how clinicians of all specialties encounter MIPS, and how different specialties describe MIPS using many different names. These syndromes seldom offer clinicians and patients much more than a label, and an individual often meets criteria for more than one of these syndromes concurrently (Aaron & Buchwald, 2001). The prognosis varies widely within any given syndrome, and the predictors of outcome are similar for different syndromes (Wessely et al., 1999). The relatively small differences in prognosis between syndromes may be due to differences in specific case criteria with regard to

TABLE 8.2
Common Syndromes Involving Multiple Idiopathic Physical Symptoms
(MIPS) and the Medical Specialties That Manage Them
(Engel, Kroenke, & Katon, 1994)

Specialty	Clinical syndrome	Specialty	Clinical syndrome
Orthopedics	Low back pain Patellofemoral syndrome	Dentistry	Temporomandibular disorder
Gynecology	Chronic pelvic pain Premenstrual syndrome	Rheumatology	Fibromyalgia Myofascial syndrome Siliconosis
ENT	Idiopathic tinnitus	Internal Medicine	Chronic fatigue syndrome
Neurology	Idiopathic dizziness Chronic headache	Infectious Disease	Chronic Lyme Chronic Epstein-Barr virus Chronic brucellosis Chronic candidiasis
Urology	Chronic prostatitis Interstitial cystitis Urethral syndrome		
Anesthesiology	Chronic pain syndromes	Gastro-enterology	Irritable bowel syndrome Gastroesophogeal reflux
Cardiology	Atypical chest pain Idiopathic syncope Mitral valve prolapse	Physical Medicine	Mild closed head injury
Pulmonary	Hyperventilation syndrome	Occupational Medicine	Multiple chemical sensitivity Sick building syndrome
Endocrinology	Hypoglycemia	Military Medicine	Gulf War syndrome
		Psychiatry	Somatoform disorders

key prognostic determinants such as duration and number of symptoms (Kroenke & Jackson, 1998; Kroenke, Jackson, & Chamberlin, 1997) and to variation in functional state related to symptom location (e.g., lower-extremity joint pain impedes walking, whereas headache pain does not; Engel & Katon, 1999).

The many examples of labels for MIPS include repetitive stress injury, Gulf War syndrome, chronic whiplash, irritable bowel syndrome, chronic pain syndromes, chronic pelvic pain, sick building syndrome, and pseudo-seizures (Barsky & Borus, 1999). These syndromes are sometimes collectively referred to as "functional somatic syndromes or symptoms" on the basis of a diagnostic convention starting in the early 20th century calling for physicians to differentiate illnesses and symptoms accompanied by structural changes (i.e., associated clinically with diagnostic laboratory or radioimaging findings) from those accompanied only by decrements in bodily functioning (Barsky & Borus, 1999; Wessely et al., 1999).

Some of the labels used for MIPS suggest a level of biomedical or scientific certainty that has not been reached. Some communicate medical gravity (e.g., fibromyalgia or myalgic encephalomyelitis). Others rely on hypothesized but unproven mechanisms (e.g., chronic Lyme disease) or triggers (e.g., multiple chemical sensitivities). A few of the labels use a single defining symptom (e.g., chronic fatigue syndrome) or body region (e.g., temporomandibular disorder). The problem with labels based on a defining symptom or region is that these labels fail to adequately portray the wide variability always found in "associated symptoms." Are all of these "syndromes" truly different? The epidemiological evidence suggests that there is indeed some phenomenological heterogeneity across syndromes. Yet the similarities in risk factors, prognosis, and effective treatments across these syndromes are striking and justify the more parsimonious practice of calling them MIPS.

I will now briefly discuss a few of the better-studied MIPS labels and case definitions to facilitate an understanding of the relevant research literature.

Fibromyalgia Syndrome

Fibromyalgia syndrome (FMS) involves nonspecific symptoms with widespread musculoskeletal pain and tenderness serving as its defining feature. FMS has gone by many names in the past, including "muscular rheumatism," "fibrositis," "fibromyositis," and "psychogenic rheumatism." To date, however, no clear pathogenesis has been established. The American College of Rheumatology case criteria for fibromyalgia require (a) history of widespread pain involving all four quadrants of the body and the axial skeleton and (b) tenderness to digital palpation in at least 11 of 18 specifically identified body surface tender points (Wolfe et al., 1990).

Concurrent MIPS are nearly universal in FMS. Generally, patients describe associated symptoms of fatigue, headaches, tingling, dizziness, cognitive difficulties such as subjective worsening of memory and measurable decreases in concentration, multiple allergies, noncardiac chest pain, palpitations, upper and lower gastrointestinal symptoms, sleep problems, anxiety, and depression (Clauw, 1995).

The physician tests tender points by pressing on the patient's body at strategic points using her fingers and asking the patient to report pain or tenderness when it is experienced. Some offer tender points as evidence that fibromyalgia is more "objective" than other symptom syndromes. However, tender point testing depends on the patient's report of pain or tenderness and is quite subjective. Results of tender point testing are consistently related to emotional distress, somatic symptoms, illness behavior, and adverse childhood experiences (McBeth, Macfarlane, Benjamin, Morris, & Silman, 1999).

EXHIBIT 8.1
1994 Centers for Disease Control Case Criteria for Chronic Fatigue Syndrome (Fukuda et al., 1994)

1. Clinically evaluated, unexplained, and persistent or relapsing fatigue that is of new or definite onset; is not the result of ongoing exertion; is not alleviated by rest; and results in substantial reduction in previous levels of occupational, educational, social, or personal activities; *and*
2. Four or more of the following symptoms that persist or reoccur during six or more consecutive months of illness and do not predate the fatigue:
   - self-reported impairment in short term memory or concentration
   - sore throat
   - tender cervical or axillary nodes
   - muscle pain
   - multijoint pain without redness or swelling
   - headaches of a new pattern or severity
   - unrefreshed sleep
   - postexertional malaise lasting more than 24 hours

Chronic Fatigue Syndrome

Chronic fatigue syndrome (CFS) is the term used to describe another set of nonspecific symptoms with severe disabling fatigue as its central feature. As in FMS, there are many associated symptoms including cognitive (memory and concentration) symptoms, sleep problems, and musculoskeletal pain. Historically, the illness has gone by many names, including febricula, nervous exhaustion, neurasthenia, epidemic neuromyasthenia, benign myalgic encephalomyelitis, royal free disease, and chronic mononucleosis (Demitrack, 1998; Shafran, 1991). There have been attempts to change the name to "neuro-immune dysfunction syndrome" to reflect inconsistent alterations in immune function noted in some studies. To date, however, no clear or consistent pathogenesis is known (Demitrack, 1997; Demitrack & Greden, 1991; Schwartz, 1988; Wilson, Hickie, Lloyd, & Wakefield, 1994). In 1994, an international study group coordinated by the Centers for Disease Control and Prevention (CDC) established the most widely accepted case criteria for CFS (Fukuda et al., 1994; see Exhibit 8.1).

Somatization Spectrum (or Somatoform) Disorders

The central feature of the somatization spectrum disorders are MIPS that the clinician judges are caused, exacerbated, prolonged, or perpetuated by psychosocial mechanisms. If a medical cause is present, it only partially explains the full extent of the symptoms or related disability. The *Diagnostic and Statistical Manual of Mental Disorders* (American Psychiatric Association, 2000) designates this general category of illness as "somatoform disorders."

Case Criteria for Somatization Disorder
(American Psychiatric Association, 2000)

A. A history of many physical complaints beginning before age 30 years that occur over a period of several years and result in treatment being sought or significant impairment in social, occupational, or other important areas of functioning.

B. Each of the following criteria (individual symptoms occurring at any time during the course of the disturbance):
  1. Pain symptoms related to at least four different sites or functions.
  2. Two gastrointestinal symptoms other than pain.
  3. One sexual, genital, or reproductive symptom other than pain.
  4. One symptom or deficit suggesting a neurological condition not limited to pain.

C. Either (1) or (2):
  1. After appropriate investigation, each of the symptoms in Criterion B cannot be fully explained by a known general medical condition or the direct effects of a substance (e.g., a drug of abuse, a medication).
  2. When there is a related general medical condition, the physical complaints or resulting social or occupational impairment are in excess of what would be expected from the history, physical examination, or laboratory findings.

D. The symptoms are not intentionally produced or feigned.

Somatization disorder is a relatively unusual but extremely chronic and disabling disorder characterized by a pattern of MIPS starting before age 30 and persisting relatively unchanged over time, sometimes over many years (see Exhibit 8.2). Only 0.1–0.2% of adults in the United States have a large enough number of different MIPS to satisfy somatization disorder criteria (Swartz, Landerman, George, Blazer, & Escobar, 1991). A much larger proportion of individuals in the general population report MIPS, however, and MIPS occur along a continuum of severity (Katon, Lin, et al., 1991). This has led a number of investigators to test diagnostic cut points that involve fewer idiopathic symptoms and therefore less-ill individuals. Escobar and colleagues have developed criteria for an "abridged" form of MIPS characterized by 4 or more idiopathic symptoms for men and 6 or more for women (also known as the Somatic Symptom Index 4/6 or SSI-4/6; Escobar, Rubio-Stipec, Canino, & Karno, 1989). They found that the SSI-4/6 criteria were met by 4.4% of U.S. adults studied (Escobar et al., 1987; Swartz et al., 1991).

Following Escobar's use of a lower diagnostic threshold, a myriad of low threshold MIPS criteria have come into research and clinical use. These include undifferentiated somatoform disorder (American Psychiatric Association, 2000), multisomatoform disorder (Kroenke et al., 1997), Somatic Symptom Index 3/5 (Rief et al., 1991), and chronic multisymptom illness (Fukuda et al., 1998). An expanding body of research has reinforced the reliability and validity of low-threshold MIPS (Escobar et al., 1987; Escobar et al., 1989; Escobar, Waitzkin, Silver, Gara, & Holman, 1998; Rief et al., 1991; Swartz et al., 1991). Escobar and colleagues noted that the SSI-4/6 has shown robust associations suggesting construct validity in diverse samples such as primary care patients, the general population in Puerto Rico, disaster survivors, community women in the United States, and patients seen in medical specialty clinics for one of a wide range of MIPS that emphasize a central defining symptom such as tinnitus, chronic pelvic pain, and persistent dizziness (Escobar et al., 1998).

Other somatization spectrum disorders are relevant to discussions of somatization and MIPS. Conversion disorder is a medically unexplained sensory or motor deficit that mimics neurological disease or another general medical condition for which psychological factors are judged to play a role because the symptom was preceded by a psychological conflict or other stressors (American Psychiatric Association, 2000). By diagnostic convention, if the symptom involves pain, then pain disorder is diagnosed instead of conversion disorder.

Summary

MIPS are common in the general population and in primary care settings. Psychiatrists often assign a diagnosis such as somatization disorder, undifferentiated somatoform disorder, conversion disorder, or pain disorder to explain them. MIPS may also represent the physical manifestations of an anxiety or depressive disorder, including PTSD. In a significant proportion of individuals with MIPS there is no adequate psychosocial or biomedical explanation for the symptoms. MIPS falling in this latter group may be due to early disease, subclinical distress, or measurement error.

I will now use MIPS to focus on the empirical links between traumatic events and somatization, and between PTSD and somatization.

RELATIONSHIP OF CHILDHOOD MALTREATMENT TO MIPS

It has long been assumed that childhood trauma is a risk factor for developing conversion disorder. Roelofs, Keijsers, Hoogduin, Naring, and Moene (2002) compared 54 patients with conversion disorder to 50 patients with a mood disorder and measured childhood trauma using a structured interview. They found that patients with conversion disorder reported significantly higher rates of physical and sexual abuse, more types of physical abuse, more childhood incest experiences, and a longer duration of child abuse than the patients with a mood disorder.

Taylor and Jason (2002) studied chronic fatigue and chronic fatigue syndrome in a representative community-based sample of more than 18,000 adults living near Chicago and found that membership in the chronic fatigue group (versus control individuals without chronic fatigue or CFS) was significantly related to reports of childhood sexual abuse and total number of different childhood abuse events. The investigators concluded that a history of abuse, particularly during childhood, might play a role in the development and perpetuation of a wide range of disorders involving chronic fatigue. In another analysis of data from the same sample, Taylor and Jason (2001) found that individuals with idiopathic fatigue (a subsyndromal form of CFS) and individuals with CFS and a mental or medical disorder were more likely than healthy controls to report a history of childhood sexual abuse. Individuals with CFS and no mental or medical disorder did not differ from controls.

Mcnutt and colleagues (McNutt, Carlson, Persaud, & Postmus, 2002) assessed 557 women from two urban primary care settings using a modified PRIME-MD structured interview for MIPS and asked the women about seven forms of abuse. Approximately 10% of the women who did not report any type of abuse reported MIPS, compared with 26–78% of the women reporting abuse of different types. In a study of women seeking care in a gastroenterology clinic for either irritable bowel syndrome or inflammatory bowel disease, Walker and colleagues (Walker, Gelfand, Gelfand, Koss, & Katon, 1995) found that 40% of women reported childhood sexual abuse. The women with sexual abuse were more likely than women with less severe or no abuse to report medically unexplained physical symptoms. Other cross-sectional studies have reported relationships between childhood maltreatment and fibromyalgia (Boisset-Pioro, Esdaile, & Fitzcharles, 1995; Imbierowicz & Egle, 2003; Taylor, Trotter, & Csuka, 1995; Walker et al., 1997), idiopathic environmental intolerance (Bell, Baldwin, Russek, Schwartz, & Hardin, 1998), "fictitious epilepsy" (Meadow, 1984), dysuria complaints, chronic abdominal pain, and vaginal discharge complaints (Rimsza, Berg, & Locke, 1988).

Longitudinal studies, particularly if they are prospective, usually offer more compelling evidence in support of a putative causal link than cross-sectional research because longitudinal assessment allows elucidation of the temporal sequence (i.e., that trauma exposure preceded the onset of MIPS rather than vice versa) and reduces bias associated with respondent recall. Longitudinal studies investigating the relationship between child abuse and assault and MIPS have yielded relatively unimpressive results. Raphael, Widom, and Lange (2001) followed a cohort of individuals with documented childhood abuse and neglect from 1967–1971 and reassessed them from 1989–1995. The investigators found that retrospective self-reports of abuse were associated with unexplained pain at follow-up. However, compared with demographically matched controls without documented abuse or neglect, there was no relationship between abuse status and either explained or unexplained pain complaints at follow-up.

Future longitudinal studies, particularly prospective studies, are clearly needed to elucidate the relationship between abuse and MIPS. The assessment of childhood trauma in cross-sectional studies and most retrospective longitudinal studies is retrospective and potentially subject to recall bias. There is also a need for population-based studies, because most available studies of abuse and MIPS study women presenting for health care, and it is conceivable that abuse is a risk factor for health care use rather than for MIPS per se. There are few studies of the relationship between childhood trauma and MIPS among men, and these studies are also needed. The current literature is strongly suggestive of a link between childhood trauma and subsequent MIPS, but prospective population-based studies of men and women without MIPS are needed before convincing conclusions can be drawn.

MIPS AFTER COMMUNITY-BASED TRAUMAS

Community-based traumas occur if an extreme event affects one or more specific groups with common relational, organizational, national, or geographic bonds. Community-based traumas may involve torture, war, disasters, or acts of terrorism. Several studies have examined the relationship of community-based trauma to MIPS. Van Ommeren, Sharma, and colleagues (2001) identified past trauma, particularly recent loss, as predictors of attacks of medically unexplained fainting or dizziness during "epidemic" MIPS in a Bhutanese refugee community. In a separate study, Van Ommeren, de Jong, and colleagues (2001) reported a higher prevalence of persistent idiopathic pain disorder (56% vs. 29%) and conversion disorder (13% vs. 2%) among tortured Bhutanese refugees than among nontortured refugees.

A great deal of research relating MIPS to war was spurred by fears of a toxic exposure syndrome after the 1991 Gulf War. Disease-related mortality and hospitalization rates among Gulf War veterans are similar or lower than in comparable Gulf War era veterans who did not deploy to the region (Kang & Bullman, 2001; Kang, Bullman, Macfarlane, & Gray, 2002; Gray et al., 1996), but it is now well established that the prevalence of virtually all physical symptoms are elevated compared to various control groups, a pattern consistent with psychosocial distress (Black et al., 2000; Iowa Persian Gulf Study Group, 1997; Reid et al., 2001; Unwin et al., 1999; Voelker et al., 2002).

The findings for Gulf War veterans have led some to note that MIPS have occurred after every modern war (Hyams et al., 1996). To examine this assertion, Jones and coworkers (2002) used British Army war pension files that dated back to 1872. They used these files to obtain data on the nature of the illnesses servicemen reported over six wars including the two World Wars and the 1991 Gulf War. The war pension process remained largely unchanged over the period of study, facilitating comparisons of symptoms across different conflicts. Pension records of nearly 2,000 veterans were abstracted for symptom data, and the symptoms were factor analyzed, revealing three distinct symptom clusters: a "debility" syndrome (mainly fatigue, weakness, and problems completing tasks, without a prominent psychiatric component), a "somatic" syndrome for which both patients and doctors frequently invoked cardiac explanations because of the protean nature of associated chest discomfort, and a "neuropsychiatric" syndrome (headache, depression, anxiety, fatigue, and disturbed sleep). Although all three syndromes occurred following all wars studied, the debility syndrome occurred mainly in early conflicts (Boer War through WWI), the somatic syndrome mostly from WWI to WWII, and the neuropsychiatric cluster mainly in later conflicts (WWII and the Gulf War). The investigators concluded there is no single postwar syndrome common to all modern wars, and variations seemed determined by the nature of combat, contemporary medical knowledge, and prevailing patterns of health beliefs and fears. They posited that symptoms did not change so much as did the social and political climate of each war era, climate changes that influence how soldiers report the symptoms and how physicians interpret them.

Two studies of 1991 Gulf War veterans have found relationships between body handling and somatization or somatoform disorders (Labbate, Cardeña, Dimitreva, Roy, & Engel, 1998; McCarroll, Ursano, Fullerton, Liu, & Lundy, 2002). Labbate and colleagues evaluated 131 Gulf War veterans seeking care at a tertiary referral facility as part of a Department of Defense registry for Gulf War-related health concerns. All patients underwent extensive multispecialty medical evaluations and psychiatric assessment to include the structured psychiatric and PTSD interviews. Sixty-nine percent of the overall sample had Axis I psychiatric conditions, the most common of which were major depressive disorder and undifferentiated somatoform disorder. Those veterans reporting dead body handling were three times more likely to have somatoform disorder than were those veterans who did not report body handling.

McCarroll and colleagues (2002) studied 352 service-members working in a mortuary affairs unit during the 1991 Gulf War. Somatization was assessed pre- and postwar for each individual and soldiers were divided into four groups according to their postwar reports of Gulf War body handling (unexposed, observed bodies, duty-related proximity to bodies, or actual body handling). After controlling for demographics, depression level, volunteer status, "mutilation fears," and prewar body handling experience, significant pre–post increases in somatization were observed in the body handlers and duty-related proximity to bodies, but not the other two groups. This study used the Brief Symptom Inventory's somatization subscale as an outcome measure. This somatization measure and its parent measure, the Hopkins Symptom Checklist, are subject to criticism for the high correlation of all subscale scores with global distress (Cyr, Doxey, & Vigna, 1988). In spite of this limitation, the study merits mention because of its longitudinal design, use of prewar assessments, and careful statistical analysis. In another longitudinal study, Escobar, Canino, Rubio-Stipec, and Bravo (1992) prospectively examined the prevalence of MIPS among community respondents after a natural disaster in Puerto Rico. Exposure to the disaster was related to a higher prevalence of MIPS, particularly gastrointestinal symptoms such as abdominal pain, vomiting, nausea, excessive gas, and pseudoneurological symptoms such as amnesia, paralysis, fainting, and double vision.

Terrorist attacks represent a new form of community-based trauma for Americans, although the phenomenon of terrorism is anything but new. Following September 11, 2001, there have been many reports in the news media about ailments and symptoms among first responders and people in or around the World Trade Center (WTC; e.g., France, 2001). These symptoms have included coughing and other respiratory concerns, eye irritation, gastrointestinal symptoms, and fatigue, symptoms that may be well explained by exposures to dust and other irritants and the long hours of work, as well as the psychological trauma involved. However, even in the presence of clear medical explanation for symptoms, psychosocial factors may amplify the severity or impact of the symptoms. For example, a survey study done by the Centers for Disease Control in the aftermath of the WTC attack found that respondent report of increased severity of asthma symptoms since September 11 was significantly more likely to occur in respondents who (a) had two or more life stressors during the 12 months before the attacks, (b) experienced a peri-event panic attack, (c) had depression during the preceding month, or (d) had symptoms of PTSD related to the attacks during the month before the survey (Centers for Disease Control and Prevention, 2002). Two other studies, however, have failed to reveal new cases of fibromyalgia syndrome (FMS) following September 11 or exacerbations of existing FMS cases (Raphael, Natelson, Janal, & Nayak, 2002; Williams, Brown, Clauw, & Gendreau, 2003).

The anthrax attacks on postal workers, news media, and politicians in October 2001 have been followed by case studies and news media reports of enigmatic MIPS among the 22 survivors of clinical anthrax infection, those with possible anthrax exposure who received antibiotic prophylaxis, and even among some exposed to mail that was irradiated to decontaminate potential anthrax-contaminated mail (e.g., Cymet, Kerkvliet, Tan, & Gradon, 2002; France, 2002; Sun, 2002). However, systematic assessments for MIPS within these groups have not been completed.

DISSOCIATION AND MIPS

As noted, MIPS were previously thought of as psychological symptoms converted to physical symptoms because defense mechanisms such as repression or dissociation countered the conscious recall of traumatic experiences. Similarly, dissociation has long been viewed as a component or hallmark of PTSD. Therefore dissociation and the dissociative disorders represent potential links of interest among psychological trauma, PTSD, and MIPS.

There have been many anecdotal descriptions of trauma and dissociation in association with MIPS. For example, Morse, Suchman, and Frankel (1997) completed an ethnographic study of 10 women with somatization disorder and history of child abuse and found that patients frequently described dissociation related to the abuse experience, and then later as a more chronic problem. Van Ommeren, Sharma, and colleagues (2001) investigated Bhutanese refugees suffering from an epidemic of unexplained illness and found MIPS associated with both acute anxiety and dissociation. In a second study the same investigators found a higher prevalence of dissociative disorders (9% vs. 2%) among tortured refugees than among nontortured refugees (Van Ommeren, de Jong, et al., 2001). The tortured refugees also had elevations in persistent idiopathic pain disorder, conversion disorder, and dissociative disorders.

Another study compared patients with epilepsy with patients with pseudoseizures and found significant elevations in somatoform dissociation, but not psychological dissociation, among the pseudoseizure patients, even after adjusting for distress (Kuyk, Spinhoven, van Emde Boas, & van Dyck, 1999). A significantly greater proportion of the patients with pseudoseizures also reported past sexual trauma. The elevation in somatoform dissociation among the pseudoseizure group was no longer present in analyses that statistically controlled for sexual trauma and other variables, suggesting that somatoform dissociation may partially mediate the impact of past sexual trauma on subsequent risk, severity, or duration of pseudoseizures (Kuyk et al., 1999). A study of women attending clinical psychology services similarly found that sexual abuse was associated with the extent of somatization and that dissociation served as a complete mediator of the abuse–somatization link. The authors concluded that clinical efforts should target dissociation (Ross-Gower, Waller, Tyson, & Elliott, 1998).

Several studies of women with chronic idiopathic pelvic pain have suggested associations with adverse childhood experiences and a few of these have investigated the potential role of dissociation. Badura, Reiter, Altmaier, Rhomberg, and Elias (1997) studied women with pelvic pain using a structured interview assessing sexual and physical abuse and surveys to assess somatization and psychological dissociation and found significant positive associations between dissociation and somatization. Similarly, Walker and colleagues (1995) studied women with either irritable bowel syndrome or inflammatory bowel disease who were seeking care in a gastroenterology clinic and compared women reporting abuse histories with those not reporting abuse. MIPS, dissociation, and psychiatric comorbidity were elevated in the abused group. The investigators suggested that medically unexplained physical symptoms might be expressed as part of the adaptation to severe sexual trauma.

These cross-sectional studies provide preliminary evidence to suggest that MIPS may be linked to dissociative symptoms or dissociative disorders, although there are no available longitudinal studies to help sort out the temporal sequence of these variables. It remains largely undetermined whether dissociation is a cause, effect, or epiphenomenon of MIPS.

RELATIONSHIP OF PTSD TO MIPS

Somatization is associated with PTSD. Cross-sectional studies have found that somatization disorder occurs in 13–15% of PTSD patients (Boudewyns, Albrecht, Talbert, & Hyer, 1991; Escobar et al., 1983). Although these studies examine clinical samples with PTSD, the population prevalence of somatization disorder is only 0.1–0.2% (Swartz et al., 1991). In a population-based study of PTSD and other mental disorders using the Diagnostic Interview Schedule in nearly 3,000 people living in North Carolina, Davidson, Hughes, Blazer, and George (1991) found that somatization disorder was the mental disorder most strongly associated with PTSD, yielding an odds ratio of over 90.

Several studies of 1991 Gulf War veterans relating PTSD and MIPS suggest that although MIPS are related to PTSD, PTSD is likely to explain only a small proportion of the MIPS Gulf War veterans report (Baker, Mendenhall, Simbartl, Magan, & Steinberg, 1997; Engel, Liu, McCarthy, Miller, & Ursano, 2000; Wolfe et al., 1999). For example, 43% of veterans seeking care in the Department of Defense registry for concerned Gulf War veterans had at least one physician-diagnosed "Signs, Symptoms, and Ill-Defined Conditions" ICD–9 diagnosis, whereas only 5% were diagnosed with PTSD (Department of Defense, 1996; Engel et al., 2000).

Engel and coworkers (2000) studied more than 21,000 Gulf War veterans seeking Department of Defense health care for Gulf War-related health concerns and found that self-reported physical symptoms were related more strongly to physician-diagnosed PTSD than to physician-diagnosed physical conditions. All patients were given a 16-item symptom checklist. The patients diagnosed with PTSD reported an average of 6.7 physical symptoms, patients diagnosed with physical conditions reported an average of 4.3 symptoms, and those diagnosed as "healthy" reported an average of 1.2 symptoms. Multivariable analyses suggested that the estimated relationship between MIPS and PTSD was stronger than the relationship between MIPS and physician-diagnosed medical conditions.

De Vries and colleagues (de Vries, Soetekouw, van der Meer, & Bleijenberg, 2002) used a cross-sectional survey administered to Dutch veterans of a United Nations peacekeeping operation in Cambodia to study the relationship of PTSD to fatigue. They found that 1.3% of 1,698 veterans met survey criteria for "presumptive PTSD" and 17% met survey criteria for significant fatigue. Fully 50% of the individuals with presumptive PTSD were significantly fatigued compared with only 16% of the veterans without presumptive PTSD. Similarly, individuals reporting significant fatigue had significantly higher mean levels of reexperiencing, hyperarousal, and avoidance symptoms. In one of their two studies of Bhutanese refugees, Van Ommeren, de Jong, and colleagues (2001) found a higher prevalence of PTSD (74% vs. 15%) among tortured versus nontortured refugees to go with the previously described elevations in idiopathic pain, dissociative, and conversion disorders.

Taylor and Jason's previously described population study (2002) found that within the chronic fatigue group, childhood sexual abuse, childhood death threats, number of childhood abuse events, and number of lifetime events of abuse were associated with PTSD, whereas sexual abuse in adolescence or adulthood was associated with other anxiety disorders. Lipschitz, Winegar, Hartnick, Foote, and Southwick (1999) examined correlates of PTSD in adolescent psychiatric inpatients. Compared with psychiatric controls, boys with PTSD were significantly more likely to have comorbid somatization disorder and both boys and girls with PTSD reported significantly more dissociative symptoms.

There is a paucity of longitudinal studies investigating the relationship between PTSD and subsequent MIPS. In a prospective study of 1,007 individuals followed for 5 years, a baseline history of PTSD was associated with a twofold increase in the risk of subsequent pain and conversion symptoms, and PTSD was observed to significantly increase the risk of somatization symptoms beyond that expected by the presence of comorbid psychiatric disorders (Andreski, Chilcoat, & Breslau, 1998).

The body of research including cross-sectional and longitudinal studies shows that PTSD is related to MIPS. One interpretation of the evidence is that PTSD mediates the relationship between trauma and MIPS, a possibility that would be consistent with findings on PTSD and other health outcomes (see chaps. 1, 2, and 10, this volume). Further research is needed to test this possibility.

CONCLUSIONS AND FUTURE DIRECTIONS

To summarize, MIPS are defined as physical symptoms that a person attributes to a dangerous cause and as a result seeks medical advice. The physician, however, is unable to find an adequate medical explanation for the symptoms. MIPS may be linked to PTSD in several possible ways. First, the biological or physiological symptoms of PTSD, like the symptoms of anxiety, depression, and other mental disorders, may directly result in MIPS. Second, PTSD may negatively affect individuals' cognitive appraisals, yielding more pessimistic or catastrophic appraisals of MIPS than might occur in the absence of PTSD. Third, PTSD may compound or exacerbate deficits in functional status that result from MIPS, an outcome that may in turn result in increased rates of general medical-care use.

In this chapter I have reviewed data from studies of traumatized individuals, including those experiencing childhood maltreatment, war veterans, and torture victims. This body of research is still emerging, but the available evidence, based mainly on cross-sectional studies, suggests a modest link between trauma and MIPS, and PTSD may play the role of a mediator of the impact of psychological trauma on MIPS. After a traumatic experience, PTSD may increase the risk of MIPS for the affected individual, whereas the individual who does not develop PTSD may only experience a minimal increase in risk of MIPS. As indicated above, this mediating role for PTSD is consistent with the primary theme of this book, that a person's reaction to a traumatic event determines whether physical health will be affected (see chaps. 1, 2, and 10, this volume). The research addressing dissociative symptoms and dissociative disorders is particularly preliminary, and there is a lack of consensus regarding the reliability, accuracy, and validity of these constructs.

There are other limitations to the research linking traumatic experiences to MIPS. For example, MIPS are common among war veterans, but for most conflicts the conclusions one can draw are limited by well-known problems with ecological inference. In this instance, the potential ecological fallacy would be to overlook the possibility that temporal associations between war and MIPS that occur for an entire population of war veterans may be due to confounding at the individual level (e.g., low-level toxic exposures). More studies are therefore needed that link high levels of individual wartime trauma exposure to subsequent MIPS (for a detailed discussion of ecological fallacy, see Greenland & Robins, 1994). Research is also needed to investigate the impact of social context on affected individuals' interpretation of MIPS following trauma (Engel, Adkins, & Cowan, 2002). Examples of potentially important social factors include news media coverage, political debates, and scientific dialogues. These public discourses may significantly impact symptom appraisals among individuals and communities affected by trauma. These factors may help account for differences in MIPS and resulting health behaviors across different generations and traumatic events (Jones et al., 2002). Recent research showing an association between television viewing and PTSD symptoms after the terrorist attacks of September 11, 2001, suggests the importance of these factors for PTSD (Schlenger et al., 2002).

To obtain a full appreciation of the potential linkages among psychological trauma, PTSD, and MIPS, one must consider all applicable research literature rather than only those studies evaluating the somatization or somatoform disorders. Emphasizing a stringent test of MIPS that requires high symptom counts, as in, for example, somatization disorder, probably contributes to underestimates of the true population impact of MIPS if they are viewed along a severity continuum (Katon et al., 1991; Wessely et al., 1999).

To resolve these issues, there is a need for consensus regarding standard MIPS measures. These measures must be reliable, valid, minimally burdensome to respondents, and responsive to state-related changes in MIPS. To be compelling clinically, these measures must use "real life indicators" of MIPS (an excellent example is the somatic symptom questionnaire from the PRIME-MD Patient Health Questionnaire). The somatization subscales of the Brief Symptom Inventory or the Hopkins Symptom Checklist, for example, are so highly correlated with distress that they lose their meaning apart from more transparent measures of distress and offer clinicians and researchers little new information for the amount of burden on the respondent. Similarly, to have clinical and research utility, an efficient measure of MIPS must be sufficiently responsive to important clinical changes in symptoms. The DIS, the structured psychiatric interview used to assess somatization disorder and other mental disorders in the NIMH Epidemiologic Catchment Area Survey completed in the 1980s, polls individuals almost exclusively for lifetime presence or absence of symptoms. This use of trait-related (i.e., stable long-term) rather than state-related MIPS measures may fail to detect important changes in individual MIPS status following traumatic experiences or preventive or therapeutic interventions. Standardized measurement tools would also allow comparisons across different traumatic events and different intervention strategies.

There is a virtual absence of treatment research that is generalizable to individuals with MIPS following trauma or in association with PTSD. People with MIPS tend to receive their care in general medical and primary care settings rather than in specialty mental health clinics. Many general medical providers are reluctant to target subjective health complaints for intervention or to accept them as measurable and valid outcomes. Consequently, intervention research developed very slowly after the 1991 Gulf War (Donta et al., 2003; Engel et al., 2002; Guarino et al., 2001). Emerging evidence suggests that rehabilitative strategies targeting symptom-related disability yield modest improvements for patients with MIPS. Findings also highlight the need for more concerted efforts to evaluate primary care-based rehabilitative interventions for psychologically traumatized individuals with MIPS (Donta et al., 2003; Engel et al., 2002). Similarly, intervention studies targeting PTSD should strongly consider evaluating MIPS as at least a secondary clinical outcome. Assessment of MIPS as a traumatic outcome is critical for gaining a more complete understanding of the impact of early intervention following traumatic events. For example, much more is currently known about the impact of so-called *psychological debriefing* on general psychosocial distress and PTSD symptoms than is known about its impacts on MIPS and related changes in functional status.

Ultimately, the objective must be to intervene, either to prevent trauma, PTSD, or MIPS, or to shorten the course of these disorders and reduce the morbidity associated with these debilitating problems after they have occurred.

REFERENCES

Aaron, L. A., & Buchwald, D. (2001). A review of the evidence for overlap among unexplained clinical conditions. *Annals of Internal Medicine, 134,* 868–881.

American Psychiatric Association. (2000). *Diagnostic and statistical manual of mental disorders* (4th ed., text revision). Washington, DC: Author.

Andreski, P., Chilcoat, H., & Breslau, N. (1998). Post-traumatic stress disorder and somatization symptoms: A prospective study. *Psychiatry Research, 79,* 131–138.

Badura, A. S., Reiter, R. C., Altmaier, E. M., Rhomberg, A., & Elias, D. (1997). Dissociation, somatization, substance abuse, and coping in women with chronic pelvic pain. *Obstetrics and Gynecology, 90,* 405–410.

Baker, D. G., Mendenhall, C. L., Simbartl, L. A., Magan, L. K., & Steinberg, J. L. (1997). Relationship between posttraumatic stress disorder and self-reported physical symptoms in Persian Gulf War veterans. *Archives of Internal Medicine, 157,* 2076–2078.

Barsky, A. J., & Borus, J. F. (1999). Functional somatic syndromes. *Annals of Internal Medicine, 130,* 910–921.

Bell, I. R., Baldwin, C. M., Russek, L. G., Schwartz, G. E., & Hardin, E. E. (1998). Early life stress, negative paternal relationships, and chemical intolerance in middle-aged women: Support for a neural sensitization model. *Journal of Women's Health, 7,* 1135–1147.

Black, D. W., Doebbeling, B. N., Voelker, M. D., Clarke, W. R., Woolson, R. F., Barrett, D. H., et al. (2000). Multiple chemical sensitivity syndrome: Symptom prevalence and risk factors in a military population. *Archives of Internal Medicine, 160,* 1169–1176.

Boisset-Pioro, M. H., Esdaile, J. M., & Fitzcharles, M. A. (1995). Sexual and physical abuse in women with fibromyalgia syndrome. *Arthritis and Rheumatism, 38*, 235–241.

Boudewyns, P. A., Albrecht, J. W., Talbert, F. S., & Hyer, L. A. (1991). Comorbidity and treatment outcome of inpatients with chronic combat-related PTSD. *Hospital and Community Psychiatry, 42*, 847–849.

Centers for Disease Control and Prevention. (2002). Self-reported increase in asthma severity after the September 11 attacks on the World Trade Center—Manhattan, New York, 2001. *Morbidity and Mortality Weekly Report, 51*, 781–784.

Clauw, D. J. (1995). Fibromyalgia: More than just a musculoskeletal disease. *American Family Physician, 52*, 843–851, 853–854.

Cymet, T. C., Kerkvliet, G. J., Tan, J. H., & Gradon, J. D. (2002). Symptoms associated with anthrax exposure: Suspected "aborted" anthrax. *Journal of the American Osteopath Association, 102*, 41–43.

Cyr, J. J., Doxey, N. C. S., & Vigna, C. M. (1988). Factorial composition of the SCL-90-R. *Journal of Social Behavior and Personality, 3*, 245–252.

Davidson, J. R., Hughes, D., Blazer, D. G., & George, L. K. (1991). Post-traumatic stress disorder in the community: An epidemiological study. *Psychological Medicine, 21*, 713–721.

de Vries, M., Soetekouw, P. M., van der Meer, J. W., & Bleijenberg, G. (2002). The role of post-traumatic stress disorder symptoms in fatigued Cambodia veterans. *Military Medicine, 167*, 790–794.

Demitrack, M. (1997). Neuroendocrine correlates of chronic fatigue syndrome. *Journal of Psychiatric Research, 31*, 69–82.

Demitrack, M. (1998). Chronic fatigue syndrome and fibromyalgia. Dilemmas in diagnosis and clinical management. *Psychiatric Clinics of North America, 21*, 671–692.

Demitrack, M., & Greden, J. (1991). Chronic fatigue syndrome: The need for an integrative approach. *Biological Psychiatry, 30*, 747–752.

Department of Defense. (1996). *Comprehensive clinical evaluation program for Gulf War Veterans: CCEP report on 18,598 participants.* Washington, DC: Author.

Donta, S. T., Clauw, D. J., Engel, C. C., Jr., Guarino, P., Peduzzi, P., Williams, D. A., et al. (2003). Cognitive behavioral therapy and aerobic exercise for Gulf War veterans' illnesses: A randomized controlled trial. *Journal of the American Medical Association, 289*, 1396–1404.

Engel, C. C., Jr., Adkins, J. A., & Cowan, D. (2002). Caring for medically unexplained physical symptoms following toxic environmental exposures: Effects of contested causation. *Environmental Health Perspectives, 110*(Suppl. 4), 641–647.

Engel, C. C., Jr., & Katon, W. J. (1999). Population and need-based prevention of unexplained symptoms in the community. In *Strategies to protect the health of deployed U.S. forces: Medical surveillance, record keeping, and risk reduction* (pp. 173–212). Washington, DC: National Academy Press.

Engel, C. C., Jr., Kroenke, K., & Katon, W. J. (1994). Mental health services in Army primary care: The need for a collaborative health care agenda. *Military Medicine, 159*, 203–209.

Engel, C. C., Jr., Liu, X., McCarthy, B. D., Miller, R. F., & Ursano, R. (2000). Relationship of physical symptoms to posttraumatic stress disorder among veterans seeking care for Gulf War-related health concerns. *Psychosomatic Medicine, 62*, 739–745.

Escobar, J. I., Canino, G., Rubio-Stipec, M., & Bravo, M. (1992). Somatic symptoms after a natural disaster: A prospective study. *American Journal of Psychiatry, 149*, 965–967.

Escobar, J. I., Golding, J. M., Hough, R. L., Karno, M., Burnam, M. A., & Wells, K. B. (1987). Somatization in the community: Relationship to disability and use of services. *American Journal of Public Health, 77*, 837–840.

Escobar, J. I., Randolph, E. T., Puente, G., Spiwak, F., Asamen, J. K., Hill, M., et al. (1983). Post-traumatic stress disorder in Hispanic Vietnam veterans: Clinical phenomenology and sociocultural characteristics. *Journal of Nervous and Mental Disease, 171*, 585–596.

Escobar, J. I., Rubio-Stipec, M., Canino, G. J., & Karno, M. (1989). Somatic Symptom Index (SSI): A new and abridged somatization construct. *Journal of Nervous and Mental Disease, 177*, 140–146.

Escobar, J. I., Waitzkin, H., Silver, R. C., Gara, M., & Holman, A. (1998). Abridged somatization: A study in primary care. *Psychosomatic Medicine, 60*, 466–472.

France, D. (2001, November 5). Now, World Trade Center Syndrome? *Newsweek, 138*, 10.

France, D. (2002, February 11). *US probes effects of zapped mail. Congressional body to look into Capitol Hill health complaints.* Retrieved June 17, 2002, from http://www.msnbc.com/news/697725.asp

Fukuda, K., Nisenbaum, R., Stewart, G., Thompson, W. W., Robin, L., Washko, R. M., et al. (1998). Chronic multisymptom illness affecting Air Force veterans of the Gulf War. *Journal of the American Medical Association, 280*, 981–988.

Fukuda, K., Straus, S. E., Hickie, I., Sharpe, M. C., Dobbins, J. G., & Komaroff, A. (1994). The chronic fatigue syndrome: A comprehensive approach to its definition and study. International Chronic Fatigue Syndrome Study Group. *Annals of Internal Medicine, 121*, 953–959.

Gray, G. C., Coate, B. D., Anderson, C. M., Kang, H. K., Berg, S. W., Wignall, F. S., et al. (1996). The postwar hospitalization experience of U.S. veterans of the Persian Gulf War. *New England Journal of Medicine, 335*, 1505–1513.

Greenland, S., & Robins, J. (1994). Invited commentary: Ecologic studies—Biases, misconceptions, and counterexamples. *American Journal of Epidemiology, 139*, 747–760.

Guarino, P., Peduzzi, P., Donta, S. T., Engel, C. C., Jr., Clauw, D. J., Williams, D. A., et al. (2001). A multicenter two by two factorial trial of cognitive behavioral therapy and aerobic exercise for Gulf War veterans' illnesses: Design of a Veterans Affairs cooperative study (CSP #470). *Controlled Clinical Trials, 22*, 310–332.

Hyams, K. C., Wignall, F. S., & Roswell, R. (1996). War syndromes and their evaluation: From the U.S. Civil War to the Persian Gulf War. *Annals of Internal Medicine, 125*, 398–405.

Imbierowicz, K., & Egle, U. T. (2003). Childhood adversities in patients with fibromyalgia and somatoform pain disorder. *European Journal of Pain, 7*, 113–119.

Iowa Persian Gulf Study Group. (1997). Self-reported illness and health status among Gulf War veterans. A population-based study. *Journal of the American Medical Association, 277*, 238–245.

Jones, E., Hodgins-Vermaas, R., McCartney, H., Everitt, B., Beech, C., Poynter, D., et al. (2002). Post-combat syndromes from the Boer war to the Gulf war: A cluster analysis of their nature and attribution. *British Medical Journal, 324*, 321–324.

Kang, H. K., & Bullman, T. A. (2001). Mortality among US veterans of the Persian Gulf War: 7-year follow-up. *American Journal of Epidemiology, 154*, 399–405.

Kang, H. K., Bullman, T. A., Macfarlane, G. J., & Gray, G. C. (2002). Mortality among US and UK veterans of the Persian Gulf War: A review. *Occupational and Environmental Medicine, 59*, 794–799.

Katon, W., Lin, E., Von Korff, M., Russo, J., Lipscomb, P., & Bush, T. (1991). Somatization: A spectrum of severity. *American Journal of Psychiatry, 148*, 34–40.

Kroenke, K. (2001). Symptoms are sufficient: Refining our concept of somatization. *Advances in Mind–Body Medicine, 17*, 244–249.

Kroenke, K., & Jackson, J. L. (1998). Outcome in general medical patients presenting with common symptoms: A prospective study with a 2-week and a 3-month follow-up. *Family Practice, 15*, 398–403.

Kroenke, K., Jackson, J. L., & Chamberlin, J. (1997). Depressive and anxiety disorders in patients presenting with physical complaints: Clinical predictors and outcome. *American Journal of Medicine, 103*, 339–347.

Kroenke, K., & Price, R. K. (1993). Symptoms in the community. Prevalence, classification, and psychiatric comorbidity. *Archives of Internal Medicine, 153*, 2474–2480.

Kroenke, K., Spitzer, R. L., deGruy, F. V., III, Hahn, S. R., Linzer, M., Williams, J. B., et al. (1997). Multisomatoform disorder: An alternative to undifferentiated somatoform disorder for the somatizing patient in primary care. *Archives of General Psychiatry, 54*, 352–358.

Kroenke, K., Spitzer, R. L., Williams, J. B., Linzer, M., Hahn, S. R., deGruy, F. V., III, et al. (1994). Physical symptoms in primary care. Predictors of psychiatric disorders and functional impairment. *Archives of Family Medicine, 3*, 774–779.

Kuyk, J., Spinhoven, P., van Emde Boas, W., & van Dyck, R. (1999). Dissociation in temporal lobe epilepsy and pseudo-epileptic seizure patients. *Journal of Nervous and Mental Disease, 187*, 713–720.

Labbate, L. A., Cardeña, E., Dimitreva, J., Roy, M., & Engel, C. C., Jr. (1998). Psychiatric syndromes in Persian Gulf War veterans: An association of handling dead bodies with somatoform disorders. *Psychotherapy and Psychosomatics, 67*, 275–279.

Lipowski, Z. J. (1988). Somatization: The concept and its clinical application. *American Journal of Psychiatry, 145*, 1358–1368.

Lipschitz, D. S., Winegar, R. K., Hartnick, E., Foote, B., & Southwick, S. M. (1999). Posttraumatic stress disorder in hospitalized adolescents: Psychiatric comorbidity and clinical correlates. *Journal of the American Academy of Child and Adolescent Psychiatry, 38*, 385–392.

McBeth, J., Macfarlane, G. J., Benjamin, S., Morris, S., & Silman, A. J. (1999). The association between tender points, psychological distress, and adverse childhood experiences: A community-based study. *Arthritis and Rheumatism, 42*, 1397–1404.

McCarroll, J. E., Ursano, R. J., Fullerton, C. S., Liu, X., & Lundy, A. (2002). Somatic symptoms in Gulf War mortuary workers. *Psychosomatic Medicine, 64*, 29–33.

McNutt, L. A., Carlson, B. E., Persaud, M., & Postmus, J. (2002). Cumulative abuse experiences, physical health and health behaviors. *Annals of Epidemiology, 12*, 123–130.

Meadow, R. (1984). Fictitious epilepsy. *Lancet, 2*(8393), 25–28.

Morse, D. S., Suchman, A. L., & Frankel, R. M. (1997). The meaning of symptoms in 10 women with somatization disorder and a history of childhood abuse. *Archives of Family Medicine, 6*, 468–476.

Raphael, K. G., Natelson, B. H., Janal, M. N., & Nayak, S. (2002). A community-based survey of fibromyalgia-like pain complaints following the World Trade Center terrorist attacks. *Pain, 100*, 131–139.

Raphael, K. G., Widom, C. S., & Lange, G. (2001). Childhood victimization and pain in adulthood: A prospective investigation. *Pain, 92*, 283–293.

Reid, S., Hotopf, M., Hull, L., Ismail, K., Unwin, C., & Wessely, S. (2001). Multiple chemical sensitivity and chronic fatigue syndrome in British Gulf War veterans. *American Journal of Epidemiology, 153*, 604–609.

Richardson, R. D., Engel, C. C., Jr., McFall, M., McKnight, K., Boehnlein, J. K., & Hunt, S. C. (2001). Clinician attributions for symptoms and treatment of Gulf War-related health concerns. *Archives of Internal Medicine, 161*, 1289–1294.

Rief, W., Heuser, J., Mayrhuber, E., Stelzer, I., Hiller, W., & Fichter, M. M. (1991). The classification of multiple somatoform symptoms. *Journal of Nervous and Mental Disease, 184*, 680–687.

Rimsza, M. E., Berg, R. A., & Locke, C. (1988). Sexual abuse: Somatic and emotional reactions. *Child Abuse and Neglect, 12*, 201–208.

Roelofs, K., Keijsers, G. P., Hoogduin, K. A., Naring, G. W., & Moene, F. C. (2002). Childhood abuse in patients with conversion disorder. *American Journal of Psychiatry, 159*, 1908–1913.

Ross-Gower, J., Waller, G., Tyson, M., & Elliott, P. (1998). Reported sexual abuse and subsequent psychopathology among women attending psychology clinics: The mediating role of dissociation. *British Journal of Clinical Psychology, 37,* 313–326.

Schlenger, W. E., Caddell, J. M., Ebert, L., Jordan, B. K., Rourke, K. M., Wilson, D., et al. (2002). Psychological reactions to terrorist attacks: Findings from the National Study of Americans' Reactions to September 11. *Journal of the American Medical Association, 288,* 581–588.

Schwartz, M. (1988). The chronic fatigue syndrome: One entry or many? *New England Journal of Medicine, 319,* 1726–1728.

Shafran, S. D. (1991). The chronic fatigue syndrome. *American Journal of Medicine, 90,* 730–739.

Shorter, E. (1992). *From paralysis to fatigue: A history of psychosomatic illness in the modern era.* New York: Free Press.

Sun, L. H. (2002, April 20). Anthrax patients' ailments linger: Fatigue, memory loss afflict most survivors of October attacks. *The Washington Post,* p. A1.

Swartz, M., Landerman, R., George, L. K., Blazer, D. G., & Escobar, J. I. (1991). Somatization disorder. In L. N. Robins & D. A. Reiger (Eds.), *Psychiatric disorders in America: The Epidemiologic Catchment Area Study* (pp. 220–257). New York: Free Press.

Taylor, M. L., Trotter, D. R., & Csuka, M. E. (1995). The prevalence of sexual abuse in women with fibromyalgia. *Arthritis and Rheumatism, 38,* 229–234.

Taylor, R. R., & Jason, L. A. (2001). Sexual abuse, physical abuse, chronic fatigue, and chronic fatigue syndrome: A community-based study. *Journal of Nervous and Mental Disease, 189,* 709–715.

Taylor, R. R., & Jason, L. A. (2002). Chronic fatigue, abuse-related traumatization, and psychiatric disorders in a community-based sample. *Social Science and Medicine, 55,* 247–256.

Unwin, C., Blatchley, N., Coker, W., Ferry, S., Hotopf, M., Hull, L., et al. (1999). Health of UK servicemen who served in Persian Gulf War. *Lancet, 353,* 169–178.

Van Ommeren, M., de Jong, J., Sharma, B., Komproe, I., Thapa, S. B., & Cardeña, E. (2001). Psychiatric disorders among tortured Bhutanese refugees in Nepal. *Archives of General Psychiatry, 58,* 475–482.

Van Ommeren, M., Sharma, B., Komproe, I., Poudyal, B. N., Sharma, G. K., Cardena, E., et al. (2001). Trauma and loss as determinants of medically unexplained epidemic illness in a Bhutanese refugee camp. *Psychological Medicine, 31,* 1259–1267.

Voelker, M. D., Saag, K. G., Schwartz, D. A., Chrischilles, E., Clarke, W. R., Woolson, R. F., et al. (2002). Health-related quality of life in Gulf War era military personnel. *American Journal of Epidemiology, 155,* 899–907.

Walker, E. A., Gelfand, A. N., Gelfand, M. D., Koss, M. P., & Katon, W. J. (1995). Medical and psychiatric symptoms in female gastroenterology clinic patients with histories of sexual victimization. *General Hospital Psychiatry, 17,* 85–92.

Walker, E. A., Keegan, D., Gardner, G., Sullivan, M., Bernstein, D., & Katon, W. J. (1997). Psychosocial factors in fibromyalgia compared with rheumatoid arthritis: II. Sexual, physical, and emotional abuse and neglect. *Psychosomatic Medicine, 59,* 572–577.

Wessely, S., Nimnuan, C., & Sharpe, M. (1999). Functional somatic syndromes: One or many? *Lancet, 354,* 936–939.

Williams, D. A., Brown, S. C., Clauw, D. J., & Gendreau, R. M. (2003). Self-reported symptoms before and after September 11 in patients with fibromyalgia. *Journal of the American Medical Association, 289,* 1637–1638.

Wilson, A., Hickie, I., Lloyd, A., & Wakefield, D. (1994). The treatment of chronic fatigue syndrome: Science and speculation. *American Journal of Medicine, 96,* 544–550.

Wolfe, F., Smythe, H. A., Yunus, M. B., Bennett, R. M., Bombardier, C., Goldenberg, D. L., et al. (1990). The American College of Rheumatology 1990 criteria for the classification of fibromyalgia. Report of the Multicenter Criteria Committee. *Arthritis and Rheumatism, 33,* 160–172.

Wolfe, J., Proctor, S. P., Erickson, D. J., Heeren, T., Friedman, M. J., Huang, M. T., et al. (1999). Relationship of psychiatric status to Gulf War veterans' health problems. *Psychosomatic Medicine, 61,* 532–540.

9

TRAUMA, POSTTRAUMATIC STRESS DISORDER, AND HEALTH RISK BEHAVIORS

ALYSSA A. RHEINGOLD, RON ACIERNO, AND HEIDI S. RESNICK

The leading causes of morbidity and mortality in the United States are behavioral in nature. Health risk behaviors can be defined as those actions that increase an individual's risk for illness and health-related problems. For example, the most prominent contributors to mortality in the United States include tobacco use (an estimated 400,000 deaths per year), diet and activity patterns (300,000 deaths), alcohol use (100,000 deaths), sexual behavior (30,000 deaths), and illicit drug use (20,000 deaths; McGinnis & Foege, 1993). Exposure to traumatic events and its resulting psychopathology may lead to the development or maintenance of health risk behaviors through their short-term ability to reduce negative affect. Indeed, some of these behaviors may have immediate pharmacological or psychological benefits. Findings from several studies investigating the association of traumatization and health across a wide range of risk behaviors clearly indicate that reported trauma history is related to higher levels of multiple health risk behaviors, such as smoking, alcohol abuse, drug abuse, sexual risk behaviors, sedentary lifestyles, and obesity (Felitti et al., 1998; Springs & Friedrich, 1992; Walker et al., 1999). Greater frequency of exposure is associated with greater risk for engaging in each health risk behavior. In addition, there is a positive relationship between the number of trauma exposures and presence of diseases in adulthood (see Green & Kimerling, chap. 2, this volume), which may be mediated by health risk behaviors (Felitti et al., 1998; Walker et al., 1999).

In this chapter we outline research on trauma-related health risk behaviors, particularly in trauma victims who have posttraumatic stress disorder (PTSD). Where research is available, we first discuss each health risk behavior in terms of studies that consider its association with trauma exposure only. Then we examine the behavior in terms of its association with trauma and PTSD within studies that included assessment of both factors, allowing for consideration of possible mediating effects of PTSD in the association between trauma and health risk behaviors. Assessment strategies in health care services, as well as innovative interventions for health risk behaviors, are also discussed.

SUBSTANCE USE

In this section we discuss the most common health risk behavior, substance use. Substance use is particularly destructive because of the ready availability of most of these substances, and because of their addictive properties. The three behaviors we focus on are cigarette, alcohol, and drug use.

Cigarette Use

The mortality rate for people who smoke cigarettes is almost twice that for people who never smoked (Precott et al., 1998). Smoking contributes to more than 400,000 deaths each year from cancer (lung, esophagus, oral cavity, pancreas, kidney, and bladder), cardiovascular disease, lung disease, and burns (Jacobs et al., 1999). Moreover, smoking-related economic costs represent more than $138 billion per year in direct medical care expenditures, indirect medical costs, and the value of lost productivity for people who are ill, disabled, or die prematurely due to smoking (Rice, 1999).

Cigarette Use and Trauma

Several studies investigated the relationship between smoking and exposure to trauma. Walker and colleagues (1999) examined the relationship between smoking and childhood maltreatment in a sample of 1,225 women selected from a membership to an HMO (health maintenance organization). Women indicating exposure to maltreatment (childhood sexual abuse, physical abuse, emotional abuse, or neglect) via the Childhood Trauma Questionnaire (Bernstein & Fink, 1998) were significantly more likely to engage in smoking. Springs and Friedrich (1992) examined the relationship between sexual abuse and subsequent smoking in 511 women in a rural Midwestern community during a 2-year period. Sexual abuse was related to heavier smoking and earlier onset of smoking (1.6 years earlier).

In the Adverse Childhood Experiences (ACE) study, Felitti and colleagues (1998) considered the relationship between adverse childhood experiences (emotional, physical, and sexual abuse; having a battered mother, parental separation or divorce, and growing up with a substance-abusing, mentally ill, or incarcerated household member) and smoking. This study was a retrospective cohort survey of 9,215 adult patients at Kaiser Permanente's San Diego Health Appraisal Clinic. Comparing people who reported experiencing four or more categories of childhood exposure to those with no exposures revealed that the former group had a four- to twelvefold greater risk of smoking. Anda and colleagues (1999) further examined these relationships in the same sample and found that, compared with those reporting no adverse childhood experiences, people reporting five or more categories had substantially higher risks of ever smoking, of early smoking initiation, of current smoking, and of heavy smoking. Sexual abuse that occurred before age 14 and preceded the age of smoking initiation was associated with a fourfold greater risk in smoking initiation. These studies did not assess or control for trauma-related psychopathology.

Even though the majority of research has focused on cigarette use in traumatized adults, initial findings indicate that youths' health behaviors are affected by trauma as well (Cunningham, Rubin Stiffman, Dore, & Earls, 1994; Hernandez, 1992; Kaplan et al., 1998). For example, Hernandez (1992) noted that adolescents who were sexually abused were more likely to report cigarette use in a cross-sectional study of 3,179 adolescents in a rural Midwestern state. Kaplan and colleagues (1998) found similar results in a study of physical abuse survivors' smoking behaviors in a community sample of 99 physically abused and 99 nonabused Caucasian youths from middle-class Long Island, New York residences, in which smoking behaviors were reported more often by adolescents who were physically abused than by those who experienced no abuse.

The majority of research on trauma and smoking has been conducted with sexual trauma survivors rather than with those exposed to other potentially traumatic events. Further research is necessary to explore similarities and differences in smoking behaviors across trauma populations. In addition, the majority of these studies did not control for PTSD. It is unclear, based on these studies, whether trauma is directly related to smoking or has an impact through other influencing factors such as trauma-related psychopathology.

Cigarette Use and PTSD

The investigation of psychological effects of trauma, such as the development of PTSD and how it relates to cigarette use, is important in examining smoking behaviors within the trauma population. For example, Acierno, Kilpatrick, Resnick, Saunders, and Best (1996) examined the relationship among sexual and physical assault, psychopathology, and cigarette use in a national probability sample of 3,006 adult women. The odds of active smoking in women with a lifetime history of assault were 1.82 times those of women with no previous history of assault. Furthermore, they found that lifetime history of assault and lifetime depression were most strongly associated with current smoking status, compared with other possible risk factors such as recent assault, current and lifetime PTSD, and current depression. Lifetime history of PTSD best predicted actual number of cigarettes smoked.

Acierno and colleagues (2000) examined the impact of sexual assault, physical assault, and witnessed violence on the risk of adolescent smoking, as well as the effects of PTSD on smoking after controlling for each of the other variables in the model. In a national household probability sample of 4,023 adolescents ages 12 to 17, age, Caucasian ethnicity, and experiencing physical assault or witnessing violence elevated risk of current cigarette use for both genders, whereas sexual assault increased risk of smoking only for girls. PTSD was not associated with increased risk of smoking once other variables were controlled. These results contrast with previous research on adults in which PTSD served as a mediator (Acierno et al., 1996). However, Acierno and colleagues (2000) used multivariate analyses with PTSD entered in the last step. When trauma exposure, demographics, familial substance abuse, and depression were controlled, PTSD did not add unique variance. These related variables may have already "used up" shared variance when PTSD was entered into the equation.

Several studies investigated the relationship among smoking, trauma, and PTSD in veteran populations. In a sample of 921 American male military veterans, Schnurr and Spiro (1999) found a direct positive relationship between combat exposure and report of current smoking. They also found a direct positive relationship between PTSD symptoms and smoking. In path analysis, combat exposure had indirect and direct effects on smoking behaviors. PTSD mediated 16% of the effect of combat on smoking (P. P. Schnurr, personal communication, December 13, 2001). Rates of current smoking in Dutch Resistance veterans from World War II with current PTSD (57%) were significantly higher than rates of smoking in veterans without PTSD (34%; Falger et al., 1992). In their study of Israeli veterans with PTSD, Shalev, Bleich, and Ursano (1990) also found that rates of smoking in veterans with PTSD were significantly higher (66%) than those observed in veterans without PTSD (37%). Both figures were higher than smoking rates in the general U.S. population (20–30%; USDHHS, 1990). Shalev and colleagues (1990) also found that the PTSD group smoked significantly more cigarettes per day than the group without PTSD. Solomon's (1988) 3-year longitudinal data on smoking behaviors in Israeli soldiers also found that those soldiers with PTSD reported higher cigarette consumption than combat soldiers without a PTSD diagnosis. Beckham and colleagues (1997), however, found no differences in occurrence of smoking between Vietnam veterans with and without PTSD. They did find that for those veterans who smoked, combat veterans with PTSD reported a significantly higher rate of heavy smoking (greater than 25 cigarettes daily; Beckham et al., 1997). Furthermore, veterans with PTSD and heavy smoking status were more likely to report total health complaints, lifetime health complaints, health complaints in the past year, other negative health behaviors (such as alcohol use), and reported more PTSD symptoms (Beckham et al., 1997). For a more in-depth review of smoking behaviors in combat veterans with PTSD, see Beckham (1999).

Overall, research indicates a positive relationship among trauma, PTSD, and smoking behavior. All studies reveal that trauma exposure contributes to cigarette use and the majority found that PTSD is associated with smoking as well. Future research should be directed toward investigating the complexities of the connection among trauma, mental health sequelae, and smoking, as it may be that the combined effects of trauma and psychopathology are synergistic, leading to even greater use.

Alcohol Use

After heart disease and cancer, alcohol abuse and dependence is America's third largest health problem (McGinnis & Foege, 1993). It affects 20 million people, costs $176 billion, and is implicated in 200,000 deaths annually (Grant et al., 1994; McGinnis & Foege, 1993; Rice, 1999). Alcohol use has both direct and indirect impacts on health. Alcohol abuse and dependence contribute to certain malignancies and many diseases of the endocrine, cardiovascular, hematopoietic, gastrointestinal, and nervous systems (Lieber, 1998; Wetterling, Veltrup, Driessen, & John, 1999). Moreover, alcohol appears to play a facilitative role in deaths and injuries from accidents or violence. For example, Rivara and colleagues (1993) reported that almost half of emergency room trauma victims in their sample were using alcohol. Alcohol has been detected in at least one party in 63% of homicide incidents, 49% of unintentional injury fatalities, 35% of suicides, and 14.4% of natural deaths, according to data cited in Rutledge and Messick (1992).

Alcohol Use and Trauma

Research has indicated a positive relationship between exposure to assault and subsequent alcohol abuse (Kilpatrick, Acierno, Resnick, Saunders, & Best, 1997; Miller, Downs, & Testa, 1993; Springs & Friedrich, 1992; Walker et al., 1999; Winfield, George, Swartz, & Blazer, 1990). Combat exposure reported by veterans has also been found to be associated with increased prevalence of alcohol abuse (Kulka et al., 1990; Stewart, 1996). Furthermore, the level of trauma exposure may be specifically associated with a greater likelihood of abusive drinking (Kilpatrick & Resnick, 1993; Kulka et al., 1990).

In several retrospective studies, early childhood trauma has been found to be a significant risk factor for alcohol abuse in both adult men and women (Felitti et al., 1998; Kendler et al., 2000; Miller, Downs, et al., 1993; Pribor & Dinwiddie, 1992; Schaefer, Sobieraj, & Hollyfield, 1988; Springs & Friedrich, 1992; Walker et al., 1999). Miller, Downs, and Testa (1993) found a positive relationship between childhood traumatization and subsequent alcoholism in adult women, while controlling for effects of being in treatment, family background, and demographic factors. McCauley and colleagues (1997) conducted a cross-sectional survey study of 1,931 women from a community-based primary care setting to identify physical and psychological problems associated with childhood and adult physical or sexual abuse. Their results indicated that women who reported any abuse were more likely to have a history of alcohol abuse than women who reported never having experienced abuse. Women abused only as children did not differ on reports of current substance abuse from women who reported only abuse experienced during adulthood. Women who reported both childhood and recent adult abuse were at greatest risk for reporting drug or alcohol abuse. A study of 1,411 female adult twins (Kendler et al., 2000) found that women who reported experiencing child sexual abuse were at increased risk for developing alcohol problems. This relationship was maintained after controlling for background familial factors. In twin pairs discordant for child sexual abuse, the exposed twin was at consistently higher risk of illness.

Kilpatrick and colleagues (1997) studied the relationship between violent physical and sexual assaults and substance abuse in women in a 2-year longitudinal analysis of a national probability sample of 3,006 women. They found that violent assault was related to increased risk of alcohol abuse. Specifically, both lifetime and recent assault were associated with increased odds of alcohol abuse 2 years later, even with earlier substance use and assault history controlled. Moreover, those women who experienced an assault and displayed extreme emotional distress following the assault were at highest risk for developing alcohol problems. Alcohol abuse alone was not related to further trauma. These results coincided with findings reported by Winfield and colleagues (1990), who surveyed approximately 1,200 community women from the North Carolina site of the ECA study, and found that diagnoses of alcohol abuse and dependence were significantly higher in sexually assaulted women.

Several studies have been conducted examining the relationship between child victimization and alcohol use in youth populations. Hernandez (1992) found that adolescents who had been sexually abused were more likely to report alcohol use for themselves as well as for members of their immediate families. Hernandez also found that adolescents who reported extrafamilial sexual abuse reported more alcohol abuse and more alcohol related problems than those who experienced incest, indicating that different forms of abuse in childhood may affect differentially health risk behaviors in adolescents.

Hernandez, Lodico, and DiClemente (1993) further investigated effects of child abuse on risk-taking behaviors in 2,973 Black and White male adolescents in the 9th and 12th grade, of whom 412 reported being sexually or physically abused. Abuse history was related to drinking alcohol and drinking-related problems. Health risk behaviors, such as driving after drinking and drinking before having sex, were also related to prior sexual abuse.

Alcohol Use and PTSD

In the National Comorbidity Survey (NCS), a cross-sectional study of a representative U.S. national sample of 5,877 people age 15 to 54 years, Kessler, Sonnega, Bromet, Hughes, and Nelson (1995) found that individuals with PTSD were significantly more likely than individuals without PTSD to meet criteria for alcohol abuse or dependence. Kilpatrick and Resnick (1993) found similar results in their review of data from their large national probability study of violent assault victims, in which assault victims with PTSD were 3.2 times more likely than those without PTSD, and 13.7 times more likely than those not having experienced an assault, to report serious alcohol problems. Findings also indicated that women with a more severe history of adult sexual assault, such as completed rape, experienced dual diagnoses of PTSD and alcohol abuse at a higher rate than women with less severe history (Kilpatrick et al., 1989; Kilpatrick & Resnick, 1993; Ouimette, Wolfe, & Chrestman, 1996). Kilpatrick and colleagues (2000) found that adolescents who were victimized or witnessed violence were 1.5 to 3 times more likely than nonvictimized children to abuse alcohol. However, the diagnosis of PTSD was not associated with further risk of alcohol abuse. This may in part be due to the conservative manner in which its effects were tested, with PTSD entered last into the regression analysis.

PTSD symptoms reported by veterans have been found to be associated with increased prevalence of alcohol abuse (Kulka et al., 1990; Schnurr &

Spiro, 1999; Shalev et al., 1990; Solomon, 1988; Stewart, 1996). Schnurr and Spiro (1999) studied trauma, PTSD symptoms, and alcohol abuse in 921 male military veterans from the Normative Aging Study. A path analysis indicated that PTSD had a direct effect on alcohol problems. The National Vietnam Veterans Readjustment Study (NVVRS; Kulka et al., 1990) also examined the overlap between combat-related PTSD and alcohol abuse in Vietnam veterans. Seventy-four percent of the male veterans with PTSD and 29% of the female veterans with PTSD met criteria for alcohol abuse. These rates were significantly higher than rates for veterans without PTSD, and for civilians. Solomon (1988) found a higher rate of alcohol consumption in Israeli soldiers with PTSD compared to those without PTSD, a difference that remained significant over a 3-year follow-up.

Stewart (1996) critically reviewed studies on the relationship among trauma, PTSD, and alcohol abuse. Her review supported a strong relationship between the diagnosis of PTSD and alcoholism. Research findings suggested that trauma exposure may have an indirect effect on alcohol problems, through PTSD. Both longitudinal and cross-sectional data indicated that the relationship among alcohol, PTSD, and traumatization appears to be cyclical, with traumatization leading to PTSD, which may lead to initiation and exacerbation of alcohol use, which in turn leads to new traumatization (including injury) or even death. Various factors, theories, and possible mechanisms to account for these associations are highlighted later in this chapter (see Jacobsen, Southwick, & Kosten, 2001; Stewart, 1996 for extensive review).

Drug Use

In 2001, about 15.9 million Americans reported currently using illicit drugs (Substance Abuse and Mental Health Services Administration, 2002). Illicit drug use results in approximately 20,000 deaths per year and contributes to death due to overdose, suicide, homicide, motor vehicle injury, HIV infection, pneumonia, hepatitis, and endocarditis as well as to infant deaths (McGinnis & Foege, 1993). The relationship among drug use, trauma, and PTSD is quite complex. For example, the presence of a substance use disorder, PTSD, or a traumatizing event increases the risk of the other disorder or further traumatization to occur (Kilpatrick et al., 1997; Najavits, Weiss, & Liese, 1996).

Drug Use and Trauma

Clinical and epidemiological studies confirm that exposure to trauma increases the risk for drug use. In the Kilpatrick and colleagues (1997) study, assault led to increased drug use after previous substance use and assault history were controlled. Burnam and colleagues (1988) found that 18% of assault victims, but only 2% of matched controls, reported illicit drug use. Both illicit drug use and a diagnosis of drug abuse have also been significantly related to childhood maltreatment (Felitti et al., 1998; Kendler et al., 2000; Spatz Widom, Lunzt Weiler, & Cottler, 1999; Springs & Friedrich, 1992; Walker et al., 1999; Whitmire Johnsen & Harlow, 1996). Whitmire Johnsen and Harlow found greater hard drug use in college women who reported being abused during childhood than in college women who reported no abuse. This is especially noteworthy given the high-functioning samples they were comparing. Walker and colleagues (1992) also found a higher rate of lifetime diagnosis of drug abuse in women with severe childhood sexual abuse than in women without a history of childhood sexual abuse, in a sample of 100 women at an obstetrician–gynecologist private practice.

In a population-based sample of female adult twins, Kendler and colleagues (2000) found child sexual abuse to be significantly associated with an increased risk for the development of substance dependence during adulthood. Specifically, women who reported child sexual abuse were 2.6 times more likely to have a drug problem than women who reported no child sexual abuse history after controlling for background familial factors. This ratio increased to 6.6 for victims whose abuse included intercourse compared with women with no sexual abuse history.

Spatz Widom and colleagues (1999) examined childhood victimization and its increased risk of a diagnosis of drug abuse during adulthood using both prospective and retrospective data. They found differing results between the two methodologies. Their retrospective findings replicated other studies in that self-reported childhood victimization was related to drug abuse in adulthood. By contrast, prospective analysis indicated that history of a court-substantiated case of child abuse and neglect was not associated with an increased risk for lifetime drug problems. However, because most cases are not reported and not court substantiated (and hence, do not receive social services as court-referred cases would receive), this sample of victims is not necessarily representative. On the other hand, it does raise an important concern about retrospective data.

Kilpatrick and colleagues (2000) found that adolescents who were victimized or witnessed violence were 1.5 to 3 times more likely to use marijuana or hard drugs than nonvictimized children. Hernandez (1992) also found that adolescents who had been sexually abused were more likely to report all types of drug abuse problems and alcohol abuse problems for themselves as well as for members of their immediate families. In addition, Cunningham and colleagues (1994) found that, after controlling for gender and race, the odds were 1.4 times that adolescents who were physically abused would use intravenous drugs during adolescence compared with nonabused adolescents (5.13% vs. 1.34%).

Drug use also poses a direct health risk because it may increase one's risk of being assaulted. In a 2-year prospective longitudinal study, Kilpatrick and colleagues (1997) found that drug use was associated with increased risk of victimization. However, as mentioned previously, alcohol abuse was not associated with this increased risk. Women reporting drug use at baseline were almost twice as likely as women without drug use to experience an assault during the next 2 years, even after controlling for effects of demographic variables and previous lifetime assault. They also found that the risk of new victimization was greatest in women who used drugs and had been previously assaulted.

Drug Use and PTSD

Kulka and colleagues (1990) found that male combat veterans with current PTSD were six times more likely than combat veterans without PTSD to meet criteria for current drug abuse. Examining a different trauma population, Kilpatrick and Resnick (1993) found that violent assault victims with PTSD were 3.4 times more likely to have drug problems than assault victims without the disorder. Saladin, Brady, Dansky, and Kilpatrick (1995) compared patterns of PTSD symptoms in a sample of women (n = 28) seeking treatment for a substance use disorder (defined as having either an alcohol or drug abuse or dependence diagnosis) comorbid with PTSD, to symptom patterns of a sample of women (n = 28) with PTSD only. The PTSD-plus substance use disorder group evidenced significantly more symptoms in the avoidance and arousal clusters than the PTSD-only group. At the individual symptom level, the PTSD-plus substance use disorder group reported significantly more sleep disturbance than the PTSD-only group. Because this was a cross-sectional study, the causal relationship is unclear. It may be that those who have more severe PTSD rely more on substances to cope with their more distressing symptoms.

Saladin and colleagues (1995) also found individuals with alcohol-dependent PTSD exhibited significantly more arousal symptoms than those with cocaine-dependent PTSD. Again, there may be an interactive relationship wherein individuals experiencing more intense PTSD symptoms use drugs to cope with their intense distress, and the use of such drugs may exacerbate their symptoms. Specific drugs may also be chosen because of effects on specific symptoms (e.g., those with high arousal symptoms may use alcohol more frequently in an attempt to alleviate these symptoms). Brown, Stout, and Mueller (1996) further demonstrated the intertwined relationship between PTSD and substance abuse or dependence. They found that substance (alcohol or drug) dependent women who were diagnosed with PTSD relapsed more quickly than non-PTSD substance-dependent women after inpatient substance abuse treatment.

Kessler and colleagues' (1995) NCS data showed that PTSD was significantly associated with a diagnosis of drug abuse or dependence. In addition, they found that PTSD was more often the primary diagnosis. Considering these relationships in greater detail, Cottler, Compton, Mager, Spitznagel, and Janca (1992) evaluated the prevalence of PTSD among substance users in the general population by examining cross-sectional retrospective data from the St. Louis Epidemiologic Catchment Area study. Respondents were classified into one of four substance use categories: cocaine-opiate use, pill-hallucinogen use, marijuana use, and heavy alcohol use. These groups were compared with a nonuser group. Cocaine-opiate users were more than three times as likely to report a lifetime traumatic event as nonusers. Physical assault was the most prevalent event reported among cocaine-opiate users. Cocaine-opiate users, pill-hallucinogen users, and marijuana users were also more likely than nonusers to report any qualifying event. Overall, the odds of hard drug users' being assaulted were 5.06 times greater than those for nonusers, and for marijuana users, odds were 1.46 times those of nonusers. Among those exposed to traumatic events, cocaine-opiate users also were most likely to meet diagnostic criteria for PTSD. Their analyses showed that the onset of drug use preceded the onset of PTSD symptoms, suggesting a possible premorbid vulnerability to trauma victimization and PTSD in drug users. Interestingly, marijuana users were least likely to have PTSD.

Examining differences among 25 cocaine users with PTSD and 97 cocaine users without PTSD, Najavits and colleagues (1998) found that cocaine-dependent patients who met criteria for PTSD had significantly more psychopathology symptoms and co-occurring axis I and axis II disorders. This study was cross-sectional and therefore did not examine causation. Najavits and colleagues' findings are interesting in that the combination of cocaine use and PTSD symptoms was related to a higher degree of distress.

In summary, these studies suggest that both trauma exposure and PTSD increase the risk for drug use. Among those traumatized, those with PTSD may be more likely to use drugs. Furthermore, trauma victims who use drugs have more PTSD symptoms and distress, on average. The association between PTSD and drug use is clear; however, the majority of studies were cross-sectional in design and did not ask about which came first, therefore causation is difficult to distinguish. Notably, drug use places one at risk for future traumatization, which may directly affect one's health.

SEXUAL RISK BEHAVIORS

Some sexual behaviors, such as having unprotected intercourse or multiple sexual partners, increase risk of health problems and unintended pregnancies (McGinnis & Foege, 1993). Unprotected sexual intercourse resulted in almost 30,000 deaths in the United States in 1990, many of them attributable to AIDS (McGinnis & Foege, 1993). In addition to AIDS, sexual risk behaviors are also associated with other preventable diseases and disabilities (McKinzie, 2001). For example, pelvic inflammatory disease, a severe complication of lower genital tract infection, results from gonorrhea and chlamydia, two other sexually transmitted diseases (STDs; McKinzie, 2001). In addition, cervical cancer is related to early sexual activity and multiple sexual partners (Brinton et al., 1987). Not only do sexual risk behaviors have direct effects on health through infection, these behaviors can also lead to unintended pregnancies, which are also associated with medical problems (e.g., Sweeney, 1989).

The majority of research on trauma and sexual behaviors has examined the relationship between sexual risk behaviors and victimization. In a follow-up study of 389 adolescent and adult sexual assault victims, Holmes, Resnick, and Frampton (1998) found that of the assault victims who returned for a follow-up medical appointment (average 8 weeks after the assault) and had been sexually active since the assault, 73.3% reported engaging in sexual activity without consistent condom use following the assault. Harlow, Quina, Morokoff, Rose, and Grimly (1993) studied 430 sexually active college women and found that victimization by sexual or physical assault was a significant predictor both of partner-related risk (i.e., high number of partners, partner has engaged in HIV risky behavior) and of unprotected vaginal intercourse. Using the same sample, Whitmire Johnsen and Harlow (1996) concluded that college women who reported childhood sexual abuse were less assertive about using birth control and refusing unwanted sex, and were less effective in HIV prevention than nonabused college women. Specifically, abused women, compared with nonabused women, reported perceiving greater HIV risk, engaging more frequently in high-risk sexual behaviors, having a greater number of sexual partners, and having a lower sense of self-efficacy for AIDS prevention. In a retrospective study of abuse and sexual risk behaviors, Cunningham and colleagues (1994) found similar results in an adolescent and young adult sample of 602 youths. Youths with a history of physical or sexual abuse were more likely than nonabused youths to choose known risky partners in young adulthood and to have six or more sexual partners in a single year as young adults (Cunningham et al., 1994).

Brener, McMahon, Warren, and Douglas (1999) found similar results in a study of health risk behaviors in female college students. They found that 12% of women who had a prior history of rape had multiple sexual partners during the 3 months preceding their survey, but only 6% of women who had never been raped had multiple sexual partners during the same time period. Brener and colleagues (1999) also found that college women who had been raped were more likely to report use of alcohol or drugs the last time they had sexual intercourse (22%) compared with women who had never been raped (12%).

In a study of 186 women and men who were identified as at risk for acquiring or transmitting HIV infection (either because they had multiple sexual partners, were themselves HIV-infected, or had partners who were infected), Zierler and colleagues (1991) found that survivors of child sexual abuse were four times more likely to report working as a prostitute during their lifetime than those who reported no history of abuse. They also found that survivors of sexual abuse reported a 40% excess frequency of sex with someone they did not know, and were two times more likely to have multiple sexual partners on an average yearly basis compared with people who reported no sexual abuse. Felitti and colleagues (1998) found comparable results in the ACE study: The people who experienced four or more categories of childhood exposure to trauma, compared with those with no exposures, were 4 to 12 times more likely to report 50 or more sexual intercourse partners and sexually transmitted disease. Furthermore, Walker and colleagues' (1999) results indicated that women with childhood maltreatment histories were significantly more likely to frequently engage in sex with partners before knowing their sexual history. Similar findings by Springs and Friedrich (1992) indicated that victims of childhood sexual abuse were 2 years younger than nonabused women at age of first intercourse; had more sexual partners before 18 years of age; and had a higher total number of sexual partners. In addition, sexually abused women were twice as likely to have had a pregnancy prior to their 18th birthday.

Irwin and colleagues (1995) surveyed 1,104 women, most of whom were African American, recruited from public places such as shopping plazas and malls. They found that women who reported being raped in the past year were significantly more likely than others to report using crack cocaine, being homeless, having recent STDs, and engaging in HIV risk behaviors, including prostitution, intravenous drug use, and sex with intravenous drug users. Rape was also associated with a higher rate of HIV infection (23.3% vs. 13.4%), but was not a significant predictor of HIV after other HIV risk behavior variables were controlled. Victimization, therefore, is associated with sexual behaviors that increase risk of HIV and other STDs, and is associated with other behaviors (e.g., drug use) that increase risk of sexual behaviors and additional victimization. Moreover, sexual assault in the form of rape may lead to later unintended pregnancy and its accompanying medical complications. Dietz and colleagues (1999) analyzed the data from the ACE Study (described previously, Felitti et al., 1998) and found that frequent psychological abuse, frequent physical abuse of the mother by her partner, sexual abuse, peer sexual assault, and frequent direct physical abuse were strongly associated with unintended first pregnancies compared with other factors such as substance abuse of household family member and mental illness of household family member. The authors also found that women who experienced four or more types of abuse during their childhood were 1.5 times more likely to have an unintended first pregnancy during adulthood than women who did not experience any abuse. Likewise, Zierler and colleagues (1991) found that teenage pregnancy was 2.6 times more prevalent among female survivors of sexual abuse than among those reporting no history of abuse.

To account for increased sexual risk behaviors in trauma victims, Resnick, Acierno, and Kilpatrick (1997) postulated that victims of sexual assault may become anxious during consensual sexual activities as a result of previous learning experiences (i.e., traumas), and may therefore avoid adaptive behaviors necessary for risk reduction (e.g., communicating with partners about condom use). Victims may also use substances to ameliorate this anxiety. This maladaptive coping style may impair an individual's ability to take appropriate precautions to reduce the risk of HIV and other STDs, and may also reduce the likelihood of avoiding truly dangerous situations (Resnick et al., 1997). Miller (1999) theorized that sexual abuse and sexual risk behaviors may be mediated by deviant social network characteristics. Membership in deviant peer relationships would increase the probability of exposure to health risks such as syringe sharing and unprotected sex with high-risk partners. Additional research is needed to better understand the relationship among victimization, sexual risk behaviors, and health of victims. Further study of the interactions between the various health risk behaviors and the possible theoretical models of these behaviors is necessary for more efficacious prevention techniques of sexual risk behaviors. Although the majority of research has focused on victimization and sexual risk behaviors, no known studies have investigated the relationship between sexual risk behaviors and PTSD. PTSD may play an important role by mediating the trauma–risk behavior interaction.

EXERCISE, OBESITY, AND EATING DISORDERS

Additional health behaviors affected by exposure to traumatic events include diet and exercise. Dietary factors and sedentary activity patterns together account for at least 300,000 deaths in the United States each year (Allison, Fontaine, Manson, Stevens, & VanItallie, 1999; McGinnis & Foege, 1993). In a study of 100 obese adults, Felitti (1993) found that 25% of the participants reported a history of sexual abuse during childhood (versus 6% of a slender control group). In another study, Felitti and colleagues (1998) noted a 1.4- to 1.6-fold increased risk of severe obesity, indicated by a body mass index (BMI) greater than or equal to 35, and leisure time physical inactivity in adults who had been exposed to adverse childhood experiences. Similarly, Walker and colleagues' (1999) results indicated that women with childhood maltreatment histories were significantly less likely to exercise regularly, and significantly more likely to have a higher BMI. It seems, therefore, that childhood trauma is associated with both obesity and physical inactivity.

Trauma has also been examined in relationship to various eating disorders. Dansky, Brewerton, Kilpatrick, and O'Neil (1997) examined the relationship among assault, bulimia nervosa, and binge eating disorder in a nationally representative sample of 3,006 women. They found that lifetime prevalence of completed, forcible rape for respondents with bulimia nervosa was 26.6%, as compared with 11.5% for respondents with binge eating disorder and 13.3% for respondents without bulimia nervosa or binge eating disorder in a final model controlling for all variables entered. In addition, Kendler and colleagues (2000) found an increased risk for the development of bulimia nervosa in adult women who reported a history of child sexual abuse. The risk for developing bulimia nervosa increased from an odds ratio of 1.7 for any type of sexual abuse exposure to 5.6 for sexual abuse involving intercourse.

Researchers have begun to examine the association between PTSD and various eating related problems. In a sample of 605 male combat veterans, Schnurr, Spiro, and Paris (2000) found that PTSD symptoms were modestly correlated with BMI scores. Additionally, Shalev and colleagues (1990) found that both extreme obesity and low weight were present among veterans who had PTSD. Weight loss was reported by 16% of the participants with PTSD compared with 0% of those without PTSD. These findings suggest that extreme weight patterns may occur in individuals with PTSD after combat exposure. Dansky and colleagues (1997) noted that women with bulimia nervosa had significantly higher aggravated assault history (26.8%) and lifetime history of PTSD (36.9%) compared with respondents without bulimia nervosa or binge eating disorder (8.5%). Although the order of occurrence was not assessed, specific types of disordered eating like compensatory behaviors (e.g., purging) in bulimia nervosa were associated with higher rates of victimization. These results support the hypothesis that victimization may contribute to the development or maintenance of bulimia nervosa. Sexual trauma may not be a sole causal factor for eating disorders, but it appears to be a risk factor, especially for compensatory behaviors. Several recent reviews have been written that highlight the relationship between PTSD and eating disorders in more detail (Lating, O'Reiley, & Anderson, 2002; Mantero & Crippa, 2002; Molinari, 2001).

These initial studies on the relationship among eating behaviors, trauma, and PTSD indicated that trauma exposure and subsequent psychopathology may lead to extreme eating behaviors. Some trauma victims may become obese by means of overeating or physical inactivity, whereas others develop an eating disorder such as bulimia nervosa. However, there may even be an overlap between these groups. Future research is necessary to understand the relationship between different types of trauma, their resulting psychopathology, and specific eating behaviors.

LACK OF PREVENTATIVE HEALTH CARE AS A HEALTH RISK BEHAVIOR

Even though victims of trauma use the medical system more frequently than nonvictims, and have greater health care costs (see Walker, Newman, & Koss, chap. 3, this volume), they also may underutilize preventative medical care. Springs and Friedrich (1992) found that older sexually abused women scheduled Pap smears less frequently than did nonabused women. This is problematic because these women are at higher risk for cervical dysplasia at a later age. In addition, Holmes and colleagues (1998) found that only 31% of rape victims seen for an acute sexual assault medical examination returned for a scheduled 6-week follow-up evaluation that provided medical, psychologic, and advocacy services to rape victims. An important component of the follow-up appointment was to provide preventative interventions, including reassurance about examination findings and reproductive function, as well as to provide counseling about possible health risks. This would include risks that may be overestimated by the victim (such as HIV transmission) as well as risks for long-term medical problems that could be averted by early medical attention. Unfortunately, these services were greatly underutilized. All of these data indicate that the medical care system could be a very important point of contact from which trauma victims could be identified and offered proper treatment, not only for post-traumatic distress and PTSD but also to address health risk behaviors (Kamerow, Pincus, & Macdonald, 1986).

MECHANISMS FOR TRAUMA AND PTSD-RELATED HEALTH RISK BEHAVIORS

As evinced in the previous review of the literature, exposure to trauma appears to increase the risk for engaging in a variety of negative health behaviors ranging from substance abuse to risky sexual activity. PTSD also increases these risks. Models for interactions among these variables have been postulated (Golding, 1999; Resnick et al., 1997; Schnurr & Spiro, 1999); however, little research has been conducted thus far investigating the variables that may mediate the relationships among traumatization, PTSD, and health risk behaviors. Theoretical models examining mechanisms for trauma and PTSD related health risk behaviors primarily have focused on drug use, alcohol use, and smoking, with little attention given to mechanisms that play a role in sexual risk behaviors, eating and exercise behaviors, and lack of seeking preventative care.

What may account for the association among health risk behaviors of smoking, alcohol, and drug use with trauma exposure? Victims may increase use of substances to cope with PTSD symptoms or other mental health problems. It has been hypothesized that physiological arousal symptoms of PTSD may be characterized as true panic reactions that were experienced during initial exposure to a traumatic event, and that such reactions are reexperienced in response to reminders of the traumatic event (Falsetti, Resnick, Dansky, Lydiard, & Kilpatrick, 1995; Resnick et al., 1997). Postviolence use of alcohol and drugs is then theorized to be an attempt to decrease this arousal, as well as to decrease sleep disturbances and nightmares (Conger, 1951; Sher, 1987). It has also been proposed that use of alcohol and drugs may block cognitive symptoms such as intrusive memories (LaCoursiere, Godfrey, & Ruby, 1980), assist in reducing behavioral avoidance of stimuli associated with the trauma (Kovach, 1986), and reduce the depression-like dysphoria and guilt associated with PTSD symptoms so as to produce almost an alexithymic state (LaCoursiere et al., 1980). Volpicelli, Balaraman, Hahn, Wallace, and Bux (1999) described a model in which alcohol relieves symptoms of anxiety, irritability, and depression following a traumatic event through its effect on endorphin levels. Because alcohol use increases endorphin activity, drinking following trauma may be used to offset a hypothesized endorphin reduction and to avoid emotional distress. In addition, research indicates that nicotine facilitates release of important neurotransmitters (e.g., dopamine, serotonin) that modulate mood. Therefore, smoking also may be a coping mechanism following trauma exposure to reduce distress (Carmody, 1992).

Extremely high levels of negative affect produced by trauma exposure may motivate individuals to engage in behaviors that rapidly reduce negative emotions (Kilpatrick, Saunders, Veronen, Best, & Von, 1987). According to learning theory, the probability of the occurrence of this behavior in the future is increased if negative affect is indeed reduced (i.e., if the "coping response" is negatively reinforced). Moreover, because trauma exposure and psychopathology produce symptoms that are enduring or recurrent, coping responses such as substance use will be repeatedly used to minimize discomfort. However, although use or abuse of substances after trauma exposure may be a partially effective (albeit maladaptive and short-lived) coping strategy to reduce aversive emotions, after years of use, this strategy may result in medical illnesses such as emphysema, cardiovascular disease, or cancer (Felitti et al., 1998). Furthermore, with the development of substance dependence, physiological arousal resulting from substance withdrawal may exacerbate trauma-related symptoms. This may contribute to an attempt to self-medicate and subsequent relapse (Jacobsen et al., 2001). Extant research is consistent with these theories of alcohol and drug use for the reduction of physiological and emotional distress in trauma exposed individuals (for reviews see Jacobsen et al., 2001; Stewart, 1996; Volpicelli et al., 1999). Researchers also postulate that specific drugs may be chosen to alleviate specific PTSD symptoms. For example, McFall, MacKay, and Donovan (1992) found that reexperiencing and avoidance or numbing components of PTSD were more strongly associated with drug abuse, whereas physiological arousal symptoms were more highly correlated with alcohol abuse.

Trauma research has tended to focus on PTSD. However, PTSD has been associated with other mental health problems such as depression and panic disorder (Kessler et al., 1995), and the literature suggests that depression has been associated with various health risk behaviors, such as increased smoking and alcohol use (Breslau, Kilbey, & Andreski, 1993; Swendsen et al., 1998). The combination of PTSD and depression may further increase the risk for the development or maintenance of health risk behaviors. Considering these relationships, the causal mechanisms of health risk behaviors are likely multifactorial. Trauma researchers should not overlook non-PTSD psychopathology that may be associated with risk behaviors. Further research would also be useful to address the association between trauma exposure and lack of health promoting behaviors, including regular exercise and preventive medical care.

TRAUMA EXPOSURE ASSESSMENT AND INTERVENTION STRATEGIES FOR HEALTH CARE SETTINGS

Strategies to assess health risk behaviors and their causes might shed some light on the interaction among trauma exposure, health risk behaviors, and health outcomes. These approaches may be most fruitfully used in the medical health care system (the place in which victims most often present for services). In addition to assessment of health risk behaviors, identification of victims who are in need of preventative medical services (e.g., yearly exams), and victims who may be inappropriately using medical services (e.g., frequent visits to emergency rooms with symptoms of panic attacks) is important for proper medical treatment (Resnick et al., 1997).

Physicians need to be aware of the interaction among exposure to a trauma, resulting psychopathology, and health risk behaviors to make a proper assessment and provide the appropriate referral for treatment. In addition, clinicians should screen for trauma-related health risk behaviors. Even with research indicating a relationship between health risk behaviors and health outcomes, this screening is not performed on a regular basis. According to a survey of primary care physicians in two Maryland cities, only 41% of physicians routinely screen for alcohol problems and only 20% screen for other drug problems (Duszynski, Nieto, & Valente, 1995). Nonetheless, in their assessment of trauma-related health risk behaviors, clinicians should focus on cigarette use, alcohol consumption, drug use, sexual behaviors, exercise, and eating habits. There are several brief self-report assessment instruments available that may be helpful in efficiently screening for some of these risk behaviors, such as the CAGE questionnaire (Ewing, 1984) for screening drug- and alcohol-related problems. If trauma related health risk behaviors are identified, physicians should provide information about related health risks as well as possibly a referral to a mental health professional for treatment.

Prevention of and intervention for health risk behaviors that seem to be responses to adverse experiences first require the increased recognition of the frequency and severity of trauma by mental health professionals. An understanding of the behavioral coping devices that are commonly adopted to reduce emotional impact of victimization also needs to be gained by the health care or mental health provider. Importantly, attempts to eliminate a coping response, even if it is maladaptive, will routinely fail if alternate and equally effective replacement responses are not found. In addition, addressing both the health risk behaviors and trauma-related symptoms concurrently may be beneficial. For example, efficacy of smoking cessation and substance abuse treatments might be enhanced through concomitant attention to symptoms associated with trauma exposure, depression, or PTSD, if appropriate. An example of such an integrated treatment is provided by Najavits and colleagues (1996), who devised a group cognitive–behavioral therapy for women with PTSD and substance use disorder. It is unclear, however, what the most advantageous approach is for an integrated treatment of PTSD and health risk behaviors. Empirical research has not yet thoroughly examined whether addressing PTSD first and then treating the risk behavior, vice versa, or treating both problems conjointly would be most efficient and efficacious. Researchers are beginning to examine theoretical considerations regarding treatment for comorbid PTSD and substance abuse and question the optimal integration and order of administration of substance abuse and PTSD treatment components (Brady, 2001; Dansky, Brady, & Roberts, 1994).

Intervention for negative health behaviors may benefit from attempting to interrupt the trauma–health risk behavior cycle, potentially reducing both future trauma exposure (as in the case of substance use) and negative health behavior. Similarly, interventions for individuals who experience trauma should not be limited to attempts to reduce immediate and overt psychiatric symptomatology (e.g., anxiety, depression), but should also address development or exacerbation of health risk behaviors. They should address any concerns victims may have about the impact of the trauma on their health as well (Kilpatrick et al., 1997). Educating trauma victims on the relationship between trauma, PTSD symptoms, and the various health risk behaviors, as well as advice on how to break this cycle, is likely to increase their motivation to change. Motivational interviewing techniques may also be useful because they may foster a more supportive environment to address the problem behaviors as well as allow the individuals to increase their desire and motivation to change (Miller, 1989). Initial findings indicate promise for the use of motivational interviewing techniques as a component of intervention for various types of health risk behaviors (e.g., Miller, Benefield, & Tonigan, 1993; Saunders, Wilkinson, & Phillips, 1995). Miller and Rollnick (1991) provide a thorough overview of motivational interviewing theory and strategies.

Exposure-based treatments have been shown to be highly effective for the treatment of PTSD symptoms (Foa, Keane, & Friedman, 2000). Given the hypothesis of the association between physiological symptoms and increased risk for engaging in negative health behaviors, therapeutic exposure to physiological symptoms (Barlow & Craske, 1988) might be a useful strategy in conjunction with treatment of PTSD and risk reduction strategies targeting health risk behaviors. Exposure to physiological sensations, also termed interoceptive exposure, includes having clients engage in exercises, such as hyperventilation, to elicit physiological sensations of panic attacks. The goal of such exposures is to reduce anxiety and misinterpretations about danger of such sensations. If physiological cues precipitate some health risk behaviors, like cigarette smoking, in an attempt to decrease anxiety, then successful reduction of fear of physiological cues may reduce cues for risk behaviors. Current research is under way to investigate the treatment of PTSD and co-occurring panic attacks utilizing interoceptive exposure with imaginal exposure to trauma-related symptoms (Falsetti & Resnick, 2000).

Even though many authors have recommended the importance of addressing trauma-related symptomatology, health risk behaviors (e.g., drug and alcohol use), and their interaction, relatively little research has specifically addressed the treatment of co-occurring trauma-related psychopathology and health risk behaviors. There may be differences in treatment effectiveness for trauma victims with PTSD who engage in health risk behaviors compared with those who have PTSD without these behaviors (Najavits et al., 1998). In addition, there may be differences in the efficacy of standard approaches to change health risk behavior patterns among those who do, versus do not, have a history of trauma and related mental health problems such as PTSD.

CONCLUSIONS AND FUTURE DIRECTIONS

The impact of traumatic events such as crime victimization can be extremely stressful and sometimes crippling for the victim. Not only can traumatization affect the victim's emotional well-being, it also can indirectly and directly impact his or her perceptions about health and increase behaviors that put the victim at risk for future health problems. The studies reviewed in this chapter found that both trauma and PTSD are associated with a number of health risk behaviors including substance use, sexual risk behaviors, lack of exercise, obesity, eating disorders, and misuse of health care services. Assessment and treatment of these behaviors within this population is sorely lacking in general health care settings, in which many trauma victims present with other problems. Future research needs to examine in greater detail the interaction among trauma, PTSD, and health risk behaviors. In addition, future research needs to investigate the effectiveness of interventions for reducing health risk behaviors in trauma victims and for treating the combination of these behaviors with trauma-related psychopathology.

REFERENCES

Acierno, R., Kilpatrick, D. G., Resnick, H. S., Saunders, B. E., & Best, C. L. (1996). Violent assault, posttraumatic stress disorder, and depression: Risk factors for cigarette use among adult women. *Behavior Modification, 20*, 363–384.

Acierno, R., Kilpatrick, D. G., Resnick, H., Saunders, B. E., DeArellano, M., & Best, C. (2000). Assault, PTSD, family substance use, and depression as risk factors for cigarette use in youth: Findings from the National Survey of Adolescents. *Journal of Traumatic Stress, 13*, 381–396.

Allison, D. B., Fontaine, K. R., Manson, J. E., Stevens, J., & VanItallie, T. B. (1999). Annual deaths attributable to obesity in the United States. *Journal of the American Medical Association, 282*, 1530–1538.

Anda, R. F., Croft, J. B., Felitti, V. J., Nordenberg, D., Giles, W. H., Williamson, D. F., et al. (1999). Adverse childhood experiences and smoking during adolescence and adulthood. *Journal of the American Medical Association, 282*, 1652–1658.

Barlow, D. H., & Craske, M. G. (1988). The phenomenology of panic. In S. Rachman & J. D. Maser (Eds.), *Panic: Psychological perspectives* (pp. 11–35). Hillsdale, NJ: Erlbaum.

Beckham, J. C. (1999). Smoking and anxiety in combat veterans with chronic posttraumatic stress disorder: A review. *Journal of Psychoactive Drugs, 31*, 103–110.

Beckham, J. C., Kirby, A. C., Feldman, M. E., Hertzberg, M. A., Moore, S. D., Crawford, A. L., et al. (1997). Prevalence and correlates of heavy smoking in Vietnam veterans with chronic posttraumatic stress disorder. *Addictive Behaviors, 22,* 637–647.

Beckham, J. C., Roodman, A. A., Shipley, R. H., Hertzberg, M. A., Cunha, G. H., Kudler, H. S., et al. (1995). Smoking in Vietnam combat veterans with posttraumatic stress disorder. *Journal of Traumatic Stress, 8,* 461–472.

Bernstein, D. P., & Fink, L. (1998). *Childhood Trauma Questionnaire: A retrospective self-report.* San Antonio, TX: The Psychological Corporation.

Brady, K. T. (2001). Comorbid posttraumatic stress disorder and substance use disorders. *Psychiatric Annals, 31,* 313–319.

Brener, N. D., McMahon, P. M., Warren, C. W., & Douglas, K. A. (1999). Forced sexual intercourse and associated health-risk behaviors among female college students in the United States. *Journal of Consulting and Clinical Psychology, 67,* 252–259.

Breslau, N., Kilbey, M., & Andreski, P. (1993). Nicotine dependence and major depression: New evidence from a prospective investigation. *Archives of General Psychiatry, 50,* 31–35.

Brinton, L. A., Hamman, R. F., Huggins, G. R., Lehman, H. F., Levine, R. S., Mallin, K., et al. (1987). Sexual and reproductive risk factors for invasive squamous cell cervical cancer. *Journal of the National Cancer Institute, 79,* 23–30.

Brown, P. J., Stout, R. L., & Mueller, T. (1996). Posttraumatic stress disorder and substance abuse relapse among women: A pilot study. *Psychology of Addictive Behaviors, 10,* 124–128.

Burnam, M. A., Stein, J. A., Golding, J. M., Siegel, J. M., Sorenson, S. B., Forsythe, A. B., et al. (1988). Sexual assault and mental disorders in a community population. *Journal of Consulting and Clinical Psychology, 56,* 843–850.

Carmody, T. P. (1992). Affect regulation, nicotine addiction, and smoking cessation. *Journal of Psychoactive Drugs, 24,* 111–122.

Conger, J. J. (1951). The effects of alcohol on conflict behavior in the albino rat. *Quarterly Journal of Studies on Alcohol, 12,* 1–29.

Cottler, L. B., Compton, W. M., Mager, D., Spitznagel, E. L., & Janca, A. (1992). Posttraumatic stress disorder among substance users from the general population. *American Journal of Psychiatry, 149,* 664–670.

Cunningham, R. M., Rubin Stiffman, A., Dore, P., & Earls, F. (1994). The association of physical and sexual abuse with HIV risk behaviors in adolescence and young adulthood: Implications for public health. *Child Abuse and Neglect, 18,* 233–245.

Dansky, B. S., Brady, K. T., & Roberts, J. T. (1994). Post-traumatic stress disorder and substance abuse: Empirical findings and clinical issues. *Substance Abuse, 15,* 247–257.

Dansky, B. S., Brewerton, T. D., Kilpatrick, D. G., & O'Neil, P. M. (1997). The National Women's Study: Victimization and posttraumatic stress disorder to bulimia nervosa. *International Journal of Eating Disorders, 21,* 213–228.

Dietz, P. M, Spitz, A. M., Anda, R. F., Williamson, D. F., McMahon, P. M., Santelli, J. S., et al. (1999). Unintended pregnancy among adult women exposed to abuse or household dysfunction during their childhood. *Journal of the American Medical Association, 282*, 1359–1364.

Duszynski, K. R., Nieto, F. J., & Valente, C. M. (1995). Reported practices, attitudes, and confidence levels of primary care physicians regarding patients who abuse alcohol and other drugs. *Maryland Medical Journal, 44*, 439–446.

Ewing, J. A. (1984). Detecting alcoholism: The CAGE questionnaire. *Journal of the American Medical Association, 252*, 1905–1907.

Falger, P. R. J., Op den Velde, W., Hovens, J. E. J. M., Schouten, E. G. W., DeGroen, J. H. M., & Van Duijn, H. (1992). Current posttraumatic stress disorder and cardiovascular disease risk factors in Dutch resistance veterans from World War II. *Psychotherapy and Psychosomatics, 57*, 164–171.

Falsetti, S. A., & Resnick, H. S. (2000). Treatment of PTSD using cognitive and cognitive behavioral therapies. *Journal of Cognitive Psychotherapy, 14*, 261–285.

Falsetti, S. A., Resnick, H. S., Dansky, B. S., Lydiard, R. B., & Kilpatrick, D. G. (1995). The relationship of stress to panic disorder: Cause or effect? In C. M. Mazure (Ed.), *Does stress cause psychiatric illness?* (pp. 111–148). Washington, DC: American Psychiatric Press.

Felitti, V. J. (1993). Childhood sexual abuse, depression, and family dysfunction in adult obese patients: A case control study. *Southern Medical Journal, 86*, 732–736.

Felitti, V. J., Anda, R. F., Nordenberg, D., Williamson, D. F., Spitz, A. M., Edwards, V., et al. (1998). Relationship of childhood abuse and household dysfunction to many of the leading causes of death in adults. *American Journal of Preventive Medicine,14*, 245–258.

Foa, E. B., Keane, T. M., & Friedman, M. J. (Eds.). (2000). *Effective treatments for PTSD.* New York: Guilford.

Golding, J. M. (1999). Sexual-assault history and long-term physical health problems: Evidence from clinical and population epidemiology. *Current Directions in Psychological Science, 8*, 191–194.

Grant, B., Hartford, T., Dawson, D., Chou, P., Dufour, M., & Pickering, R. (1994). Prevalence of DSM–IV alcohol abuse and dependence: United States—1992. *Alcohol Health and Research World, 18*, 243–248.

Harlow, L. L., Quina, K., Morokoff, P. J., Rose, J. S., & Grimly, D. M. (1993). HIV risk in women: A multifaceted model. *Journal of Applied Behavioral Research, 1*, 3–38.

Hernandez, J. T. (1992). Substance abuse among sexually abused adolescents and their families. *Journal of Adolescent Health, 13*, 658–662.

Hernandez, J. T., Lodico, M., & DiClemente, R. J. (1993). The effects of child abuse and race on risk-taking in male adolescents. *Journal of the National Medical Association, 85*, 593–597.

Holmes, M. M., Resnick, H. S., & Frampton, D. (1998). Follow-up of sexual assault victims. *American Journal of Obstetrics and Gynecology, 179,* 336–342.

Irwin, K. L., Edlin, B. R., Wong, L., Faruque, S., McCoy, H. V., Word, C., et al. (1995). Urban rape survivors: Characteristics and prevalence of human immunodeficiency virus and other sexually transmitted infections. *Obstetrics and Gynecology, 85,* 330–336.

Jacobs, D. R., Jr., Adachi, H., Mulder, I., Kromhout, D., Menotti, A., Nissinen, A., et al. (1999). Cigarette smoking and mortality risk. *Archives of Internal Medicine, 159,* 733–740.

Jacobsen, L. K., Southwick, S. M., & Kosten, T. R. (2001). Substance use disorders in patients with posttraumatic stress disorder: A review of the literature. *American Journal of Psychiatry, 158,* 1184–1190.

Kamerow, D. B., Pincus, H. A., & Macdonald, D. I. (1986). Alcohol abuse, other drug abuse, and mental disorders in medical practice: Prevalence, costs, recognition, and treatment. *Journal of the American Medical Association, 255,* 2054–2057.

Kaplan, S. J., Pelcovitz, D., Salzinger, S., Weiner, M., Mandel, F. S., Lesser, M. L., et al. (1998). Adolescent physical abuse: Risk for adolescent psychiatric disorders. *American Journal of Psychiatry, 155,* 954–959.

Kendler, K. S., Bulik, C. M., Silberg, J., Hettema, J. M., Myers, J., & Prescott, C. A. (2000). Childhood sexual abuse and adult psychiatric and substance use disorders in women. *Archives of General Psychiatry, 57,* 953–959.

Kessler, R. C., Sonnega, A., Bromet, E., Hughes, M., & Nelson, C. B. (1995). Posttraumatic stress disorder in the National Comorbidity Survey. *Archives of General Psychiatry, 52,* 1048–1060.

Kilpatrick, D. G., Acierno, R., Resnick, H., Saunders, B. E., & Best, C. (1997). A two-year longitudinal analysis of the relationships among violent assault and substance use in women. *Journal of Consulting and Clinical Psychology, 65,* 834–847.

Kilpatrick, D. G., Acierno, R., Saunders, B. E., Resnick, H. S., Best, C. L., & Schnurr, P. P. (2000). Risk factors for adolescent substance abuse and dependence: Data from a national sample. *Journal of Consulting and Clinical Psychology, 68,* 19–30.

Kilpatrick, D. G., & Resnick, H. S. (1993). Posttraumatic stress disorder associated with exposure to criminal victimization in clinical and community population. In J. R. T. Davidson & E. B. Foa (Eds.), *Posttraumatic stress disorder: DSM–IV and beyond* (pp. 113–143). Washington, DC: American Psychiatric Press.

Kilpatrick, D. G., Saunders, B. E., Amick-McMullen, A., Best, C. L., Veronen, L. J., & Resnick, H. S. (1989). Victim and crime factors associated with the development of crime-related posttraumatic stress disorder. *Behavior Therapy, 20,* 199–214.

Kilpatrick, D. G., Saunders, B. E., Veronen, L. J., Best, C. L., & Von, J. M. (1987). Criminal victimization: Lifetime prevalence, reporting to police, and psychological impact. *Crime and Delinquency, 33,* 479–489.

Kovach, J. A. (1986). Incest as a treatment issue for alcoholic women. *Alcoholism Treatment Quarterly, 3*, 13–15.

Kulka, R. A., Schlenger, W. E., Fairbank, J. A., Hough, R. L., Jordan, B. K., Marmar, C. R., et al. (1990). *Trauma and the Vietnam War generation*. New York: Brunner/Mazel.

LaCoursiere, R. B., Godfrey, K. E., & Ruby, L. M. (1980). Traumatic neurosis in the etiology of alcoholism: Vietnam and other trauma. *American Journal of Psychiatry, 137*, 966–968.

Lating, J. M., O'Reiley, M. A., & Anderson, K. P. (2002). Eating disorders and posttraumatic stress: Phenomenological and treatment considerations using the two-factor model. *International Journal of Emergency Mental Health, 4*, 113–118.

Lieber, C. S. (1998). Hepatic and other medical disorders of alcoholics: From pathogenesis to treatment. *Journal of Studies of Alcohol, 59*, 9–25.

Mantero, M., & Crippa, L. (2002). Eating disorders and chronic post traumatic stress disorder: Issues of psychopathology and comorbidity. *European Eating Disorders Review, 10*, 1–16.

McCauley, J., Kern, D. E., Kolodner, K., Dill, L., Schroeder, A. F., DeChant, H. K., et al. (1997). Clinical characteristics of women with a history of childhood abuse: Unhealed wounds. *Journal of the American Medical Association, 277*, 1362–1368.

McFall, M. E., MacKay, P. W., & Donovan, D. M. (1992). Combat-related posttraumatic stress disorder and severity of substance abuse in Vietnam veterans. *Journal of Studies on Alcohol, 53*, 357–363.

McGinnis, J. M., & Foege, W. H. (1993). Actual causes of death in the United States. *Journal of the American Medical Association, 270*, 2207–2212.

McKinzie, J. (2001). Sexually transmitted diseases. *Emergency Medicine Clinics of North America, 19*, 723–743.

Miller, B. A., Downs, W. R., & Testa, M. (1993). Inter-relationships between victimization experiences and women's alcohol use. *Journal of Studies on Alcohol* (Suppl. 11), 109–117.

Miller, M. (1999). A model to explain the relationship between sexual abuse and HIV risk among women. *AIDS Care, 11*, 3–20.

Miller, W. R. (1989). Increasing motivation for change. In R. K. Hester & W. R. Miller (Eds.), *Handbook of alcoholism treatment approaches: Effective alternatives* (pp. 67–80). New York: Pergamon.

Miller, W. R., Benefield, R. G., & Tonigan, J. S. (1993). Enhancing motivation for change in problem drinking: A controlled comparison of two therapist styles. *Journal of Consulting and Clinical Psychology, 61*, 455–461.

Miller, W. R., & Rollnick, S. (1991). *Motivational interviewing: Preparing people to change addictive behavior*. New York: Guilford.

Molinari, E. (2001). Eating disorders and sexual abuse. *Eating and Weight Disorders, 6*, 68–80.

Najavits, L. M., Gastfriend, D. R., Barber, J. P., Reif, S., Muenz, L. R., Blaine, J., et al. (1998). Cocaine dependence with and without PTSD among subjects in the National Institute on Drug Abuse Collaborative Cocaine Treatment Study. *American Journal of Psychiatry, 155,* 214–219.

Najavits, L. M., Weiss, R. D., & Liese, B. S. (1996). Group cognitive-behavioral therapy for women with PTSD and substance use disorder. *Journal of Substance Abuse Treatment, 13,* 13–22.

Ouimette, P. C., Wolfe, J., & Chrestman, K. R. (1996). Characteristics of posttraumatic stress disorder–alcohol abuse comorbidity in women. *Journal of Substance Abuse, 8,* 335–346.

Precott, E., Osler, M., Anderson, P. K., Hein, H. O., Borch-Johnsen, K., Lange, P., et al. (1998). Mortality in women and men in relation to smoking. *International Journal of Epidemiology, 27,* 27–32.

Pribor, E. F., & Dinwiddie, S. H. (1992). Psychiatric correlates of incest in childhood. *American Journal of Psychiatry, 149,* 52–56.

Resnick, H. S., Acierno, R., & Kilpatrick, D. G. (1997). Health impact of interpersonal violence 2: Medical and mental health outcomes. *Behavioral Medicine, 23,* 65–87.

Rice, D. P. (1999). Economic costs of substance abuse, 1995. *Proceedings of the Association of American Physicians, 2,* 119–125.

Rivara, F. P., Jurkovich, G. J., Gurney, J. G., Seguin, D., Fligner, C. L., Ries, R., et al. (1993). The magnitude of acute and chronic alcohol abuse in trauma patients. *Archives of Surgery, 128,* 907–913.

Rutledge, R., & Messick, W. J. (1992). The association of trauma death and alcohol use in a rural state. *Journal of Trauma, 33,* 737–742.

Saladin, M. E., Brady, K. T, Dansky, B. S., & Kilpatrick, D. G. (1995). Understanding comorbidity between PTSD and substance use disorders: Two preliminary investigations. *Addictive Behaviors, 20,* 643–655.

Saunders, B., Wilkinson, C., & Phillips, M. (1995). The impact of a brief motivational intervention with opiate users attending a methadone programme. *Addiction, 90,* 415–424.

Schaefer, M. R., Sobieraj, K., & Hollyfield, R. L. (1988). Prevalence of childhood physical abuse in adult male veteran alcoholics. *Child Abuse and Neglect, 12,* 141–149.

Schnurr, P. P., & Spiro, A., III. (1999). Combat exposure, posttraumatic stress disorder symptoms, and health behaviors as predictors of self-reported physical health in older veterans. *Journal of Nervous and Mental Disease, 187,* 353–359.

Schnurr, P. P., Spiro, A., III, & Paris, A. H. (2000). Physician-diagnosed medical disorders in relation to PTSD symptoms in older male military veterans. *Health Psychology, 19,* 91–97.

Shalev, A., Bleich, A., & Ursano, R. J. (1990). Posttraumatic stress disorder: Somatic comorbidity and effort tolerance. *Psychosomatics, 31,* 197–203.

Sher, K. J. (1987). Stress response dampening. In H. T. Blane & K. E. Leonard (Eds.), *Psychological theories of drinking and alcoholism* (pp. 227–271). New York: Guilford.

Solomon, Z. (1988). Somatic complaints, stress reaction, and posttraumatic stress disorder: A three-year follow–up study. *Behavioral Medicine, 14,* 179–185.

Spatz Widom, C., Lunzt Weiler, B., & Cottler, L. B. (1999). Childhood victimization and drug abuse: A comparison of prospective and retrospective findings. *Journal of Consulting and Clinical Psychology, 67,* 867–880.

Springs, F. E., & Friedrich, W. N. (1992). Health risk behaviors and medical sequelae of childhood sexual abuse. *Mayo Clinical Procedures, 67,* 527–532.

Stewart, S. H. (1996). Alcohol abuse in individuals exposed to trauma: A critical review. *Psychological Bulletin, 120,* 83–112.

Substance Abuse and Mental Health Services Administration. (2002). *Results from the 2001 National Household Survey on Drug Abuse: Vol. 1. Summary of national findings* (Office of Applied Studies, NHSDA Series H-17, DHHS Publication No. SMA 02-3758). Rockville, MD: Author.

Sweeney, P. J. (1989). A comparison of low birth weight, perinatal mortality, and infant mortality between first and second birth to women 17 years old and younger. *American Journal of Obstetrics and Gynecology, 160,* 1361–1367.

Swendsen, J. D., Merikangas, K. R., Canino, G. J., Kessler, R. C., Rubio-Stipec, M., & Angst, J. (1998). The comorbidity of alcoholism with anxiety and depressive disorders in four geographic communities. *Comprehensive Psychiatry, 39,* 176–184.

U.S. Department of Health and Human Services. (1990). *Healthy people 2000: National health promotion and disease prevention objectives* (PHS Publication No. 91-50213). Washington, DC: Author.

Volpicelli, J., Balaraman, G., Hahn, J., Wallace, H., & Bux, D. (1999). The role of uncontrollable trauma in the development of PTSD and alcohol addiction. *Alcohol Research and Health, 23,* 256–262.

Walker, E. A., Gelfand, A., Katon, W. J., Koss, M. P., Von Korff, M., Bernstein, D., et al. (1999). Adult health status of women with histories of childhood abuse and neglect. *American Journal of Medicine, 107,* 332–339.

Walker, E. A., Katon, W. J., Hansom, J., Harrop-Griffiths, J., Holm, L., Jones, M. L., et al. (1992). Medical and psychiatric symptoms in women with children and sexual abuse. *Psychosomatic Medicine, 54,* 658–664.

Wetterling, T., Veltrup, C., Driessen, M., & John, U. (1999). Drinking pattern and alcohol-related medical disorders. *Alcohol and Alcoholism, 34,* 330–336.

Whitmire Johnsen, L., & Harlow, L. L. (1996). Childhood sexual abuse linked with adult substance use, victimization, and AIDS-risk. *AIDS Education and Prevention, 8,* 44–57.

Winfield, I., George, L. K., Swartz, M., & Blazer, D. G. (1990). Sexual assault and psychiatric disorders among a community sample of women. *American Journal of Psychiatry, 147,* 335–341.

Zierler, S., Feingold, L., Laufer, D., Velentgas, P., Kantrowitz-Gordon, I., & Mayer, K. (1991). Adult survivors of childhood sexual abuse and subsequent risk of HIV infection. *American Journal of Public Health, 81,* 572–575.

V

AN INTEGRATIVE MODEL AND ITS IMPLICATIONS FOR RESEARCH, PRACTICE, AND POLICY

10

UNDERSTANDING RELATIONSHIPS AMONG TRAUMA, POSTTRAUMATIC STRESS DISORDER, AND HEALTH OUTCOMES

PAULA P. SCHNURR AND BONNIE L. GREEN

Literature reviews have documented that exposure to trauma is related to adverse health outcomes across domains of self-reported health, morbidity, mortality, and utilization of health services (Friedman & Schnurr, 1995; Green & Kimerling, chap. 2, this volume; Resnick, Acierno, & Kilpatrick, 1997; Walker, Newman, & Koss, chap. 3, this volume). In this chapter we describe an integrative model that relates trauma to physical health through psychological, biological, behavioral, and attentional mechanisms. We use material presented in the preceding chapters to support the argument that posttraumatic stress disorder (PTSD) is the key mechanism through which trauma leads to poor health. We then discuss clinical, systems, and policy

This chapter was coauthored by an employee of the United States government as part of official duty and is considered to be in the public domain. Any views expressed herein do not necessarily represent the views of the United States government, and the author's participation in the work is not meant to serve as an official endorsement.

implications, and the chapter ends with a proposal for an agenda for basic and applied research.

A MODEL RELATING TRAUMA EXPOSURE TO PHYSICAL HEALTH

The question of mechanism is crucial to understanding the relationship between traumatic exposure and physical health. Knowing which factors lead to poor outcomes can facilitate detection of vulnerable individuals and implementation of preventive strategies to reduce risk. An understanding of mechanism also helps to make a plausible case for causality, which is important because the study of traumatic stress in humans is limited to correlational designs.

Figure 10.1 depicts a model that builds on one proposed by Schnurr and Jankowski (1999) to explain ways in which PTSD could lead to adverse health outcomes. We have expanded their model to include traumatic exposure to address the question of how a traumatic event *outside* the individual who experiences it leads to changes *within* the individual. The

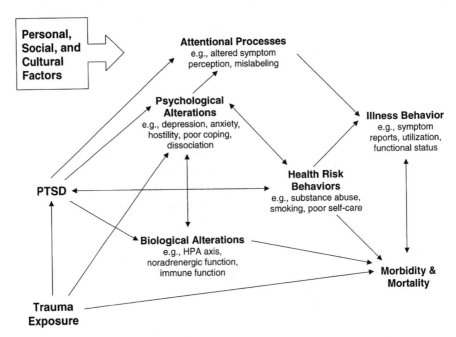

Figure 10.1. A model relating traumatic exposure and PTSD to physical health outcomes. From "Physical Health and Post-Traumatic Stress Disorder: Review and Synthesis," by P. P. Schnurr and M. K. Jankowski, 1999, *Seminars in Clinical Neuropsychiatry, 4,* p. 299. Copyright 1999 by W.B. Saunders Co. Adapted with permission.

model assumes that a distress reaction following traumatic exposure is essential for precipitating changes in health status or other aspects of a person's well-being. The only exception to this rule is the case of injury or illness incurred during the traumatic event. Although most trauma survivors are not injured or exposed to disease (e.g., Resnick, Kilpatrick, Dansky, Saunders, & Best, 1993; Kulka et al., 1990; White & Faustman, 1989), such trauma-related experiences obviously could affect health independent of distress. Even then, however, a distress response and its consequences are likely to accompany any threat to physical integrity, because trauma-related injury is associated with increased risk of developing PTSD (e.g., Green, Grace, Lindy, Gleser, & Leonard, 1990; Resnick et al., 1993; Schnurr, Ford, et al., 2000).

In our model, PTSD is proposed as the primary pathway through which trauma leads to poor health. Prior reviews have emphasized the role of PTSD as a mediator of the relationship between traumatic exposure and poor health (Friedman & Schnurr, 1995; Schnurr & Jankowski, 1999). The evidence presented by Green and Kimerling (chap. 2, this volume) is also highly consistent with the hypothesized mediational role of PTSD. Some studies have used regression procedures to demonstrate that the relationship between exposure and health is eliminated or substantially reduced when PTSD is added to a multivariate model (e.g., Kimerling, Clum, & Wolfe, 2000; Wagner, Wolfe, Rotnitsky, Proctor, & Erickson, 2000; Wolfe, Schnurr, Brown, & Furey, 1994). Other studies have used path analysis to show that the effects of exposure are primarily indirect, through PTSD (e.g., Ford et al., 2003; Schnurr & Spiro, 1999; Taft, Stern, King, & King, 1999). One study (Vedantham et al., 2001) divided trauma survivors into groups with and without PTSD and found particularly strong support for the importance of PTSD: Only the PTSD group had poorer health in comparison with traumatized and nontraumatized participants without PTSD.

Significant distress reactions other than PTSD also could mediate the relationship between trauma exposure and physical health. Support for this possibility comes from several sources. First of all, PTSD does not mediate all of the effect of traumatic exposure on health. For example, Taft and colleagues (1999) found that 42% of the effect of combat exposure on the number of health conditions reported by Vietnam veterans was direct: that is, not mediated through PTSD or other variables. Some internal mechanism is needed to explain findings like these. Second, although a few studies have found a mediational role for non-PTSD distress (e.g., Holman, Silver, & Waitzkin, 2000), this evidence is ambiguous because PTSD was not ruled out or included in the multivariate models. Third, the adverse health outcomes associated with depression (see Ford, chap. 4, this volume) indicate that an individual who develops depression following a traumatic event should be at increased risk of adverse health outcomes. Likewise, an individual who experiences a chronic stress reaction other than PTSD should be at increased risk, too (see Dougall & Baum, chap. 6; Friedman & McEwen, chap. 7, this volume). Generally speaking, however, studies of health outcomes in depression and chronic stress have not ruled out PTSD as a mediator.

Stronger evidence for the independent contribution of depression and other disorders comes from studies that take both PTSD and non-PTSD disorders into account (e.g., Beckham et al., 1998; Boscarino & Chang, 1999; Clum, Calhoun, & Kimerling, 2000; Schnurr, Friedman, Sengupta, Jankowski, & Holmes, 2000). Nevertheless, these same studies show that PTSD has an effect that is distinct from other disorders. In this chapter we discuss allostatic load (Friedman & McEwen, chap. 7, this volume; McEwen & Stellar, 1993) as an explanation for this distinctiveness. First we describe the mechanisms through which traumatic exposure and PTSD affect physical health.

Components of the Model

PTSD and other significant distress reactions that develop as a result of exposure to a traumatic event are assumed to influence physical health through psychological, biological, behavioral, and attentional mechanisms. Given the limited evidence available about the health effects of depression and disorders other than PTSD in trauma survivors, we focus primarily on PTSD in our discussion of these mechanisms, making reference to other disorders when possible.

Psychological Mechanisms

PTSD can substantially change numerous aspects of psychological functioning. Several of these changes have been linked to poor health in their own right. Depression was discussed previously in the context of distress reactions that could initiate processes affecting physical health. Depression is frequently comorbid with PTSD, occurring in about half of all PTSD cases (Kessler, Sonnega, Bromet, Hughes, & Nelson, 1995). Although a history of depression and other psychiatric disorders is a risk factor for developing PTSD, retrospective and prospective analyses have found the likelihood of an episode of depression to be significantly increased among trauma-exposed individuals who develop PTSD, relative to those who do not (Breslau, Davis, Peterson, & Schultz, 2000). Depression therefore may affect physical health not only as a primary reaction to trauma exposure but typically will do so as a consequence of PTSD. Ford's chapter (chap. 4, this volume) highlights several biological correlates of depression that could lead to cardiovascular disease: greater platelet activation, decreased heart rate variability, and greater likelihood of hypertension.

PTSD may be related to poor health through comorbid anxiety and panic (Schnurr & Jankowski, 1999), which are elevated in individuals with PTSD (Kessler et al., 1995; Kulka et al., 1990). Anxiety, in turn, is strongly related to cardiovascular morbidity and mortality (Hayward, 1995). Panic disorder is interesting because many panic attack symptoms involve the cardiovascular system. We discuss panic more fully later on because the effects of panic disorder on physical health are likely due to heightened symptom perception rather than biologically grounded disease processes (Jakubec & Taylor, 1999).

Dissociation is another psychological mechanism that may link trauma exposure to poor physical health outcomes, in part due to the strong relationship between dissociation and PTSD (Engel, chap. 8, this volume). A relatively high proportion of individuals with severe childhood abuse, or other extreme traumas like torture, report dissociation. Dissociation, in turn, has been linked with a number of somatoform-type illnesses, or multiple idiopathic physical symptoms (MIPS). Dissociation may serve to mediate the link between trauma and somatization (Ross-Gower, Waller, Tyson, & Elliott, 1998). Dissociation may also be implicated in attentional processes linking trauma with health outcomes.

As Aldwin and Yancura's chapter (chap. 5, this volume) indicates, PTSD is associated with the use of coping strategies that themselves have been linked to adverse health outcomes: less problem-focused and more emotion-focused strategies. Problem-focused or instrumental strategies are associated with more favorable health outcomes, whereas emotion-focused, and particularly avoidant strategies, are associated with poorer health outcomes. Most of these effects appear to be direct: for example, avoiding seeking medical attention for a health problem. However, some of the relationship between coping and health appears to be mediated through negative affect (a finding consistent with our model).

Hostility is another psychological correlate of PTSD that could lead to poor health (Schnurr & Jankowski, 1999). Hostility is associated with greater likelihood of cardiovascular disease (Goldstein & Niaura, 1995). Although behavioral factors such as smoking may play a role, a primary mechanism is assumed to be the tendency of hostile individuals to show greater sympathetically mediated cardiovascular responses to provocation stressors, and lesser parasympathetic response to the sympathetic activation (Williams, 1995).

Biological Mechanisms

Friedman and McEwen's chapter (chap. 7, this volume) describes the significant alterations of neurobiological systems in PTSD. At the core are alterations of the two primary systems of the stress response: the locus coeruleus/norepinephrine-sympathetic system (LC/NE) system and hypothalamic–pituitary–adrenal (HPA) systems. Individuals with PTSD have dysregulation of the HPA axis, resulting in higher or lower levels of cortisol, increased number of glucocorticoid receptors, and increased receptor sensitivity. Individuals with PTSD also have elevated basal adrenergic levels and adrenergic reactivity. Friedman and McEwen discuss how alterations of the HPA and LC/NE systems could affect the entire body. It is important to understand these primary alterations in light of the interactions among the immune, nervous, and endocrine systems (Schnurr & Jankowski, 1999). For example, Dougall and Baum (chap. 6, this volume) mention that cytokines, which are secreted by the immune system, affect the central and peripheral nervous systems, which in turn affect immune cells.

Friedman and McEwen's review indicates that the biological correlates of PTSD are similar to the biological correlates of chronic stress. Early research indicated potentially important differences between the two regarding cortisol levels (high in stress, low in PTSD) and glucocorticoid receptor sensitivity (low in stress, high in PTSD). More recent findings indicate elevated cortisol in PTSD (Rasmusson & Friedman, 2002), as well as marked individual differences and phasic alterations (Mason et al., 2001). Friedman and McEwen attempt to resolve the conflicting findings by suggesting that HPA axis function in PTSD can be characterized in terms of both tonic and phasic abnormalities. Mason and colleagues offered an interesting explanation: that cortisol levels reflect the balance between undifferentiated emotional arousal, or *engagement*, associated with higher cortisol levels, and *disengagement* defense mechanisms, associated with lower levels. If so, individuals with PTSD could appear relatively low or high depending on this balance.

The variable findings on the HPA axis in PTSD prevent firm conclusions as to whether the health effects of HPA axis alterations in PTSD are those associated with high or low cortisol. Because cortisol has immunosuppressive effects, the implications for the immune system are especially important. Low levels of cortisol in PTSD might lead to disorders associated with activation of immune-mediated inflammation—for example, rheumatoid arthritis (Chrousos, 1995). However, enhanced receptor sensitivity and high levels of cortisol in PTSD might lead to disorders involving decreased immune function, such as infectious disease, and suppression of immune-mediated inflammation (Schnurr & Jankowski, 1999).

The chapters by Dougall and Baum (chap. 6) and by Friedman and McEwen (chap. 7) show that the findings to date fail to resolve which of these alternatives is most likely. Dougall and Baum attempt to reconcile the findings by examining outcomes as a function of the timing of the traumatic stressor, given evidence that acute stressors are associated with enhanced immune function (and worsening of diseases like rheumatoid arthritis; Grady et al., 1991) and chronic stressors are associated with decreased immune function. However, there is evidence of both enhancement and suppression of the immune system in PTSD, as well as evidence that PTSD is associated with disorders that could result from enhancement (Boscarino, 1997; Schnurr, Spiro, & Paris, 2000) and suppression (Boscarino, 1997). Friedman and McEwen propose that PTSD is associated with a tonic state of immunosuppression and with phasic episodes of immune system enhancement. This is an interesting hypothesis that bears further examination. Friedman and McEwen's chapter also notes other pronounced biological changes associated with PTSD that are mostly similar to changes associated with chronic stress syndrome, so it appears safe to conclude that PTSD should be similar in its biological consequences to extreme levels of chronic stress, and perhaps may be distinct in terms of health effects of HPA axis dysregulation.

The preceding discussion illustrates several points of interaction between psychological and biological mechanisms. We wish to emphasize the interdependence and inseparability of these mechanisms. There are several plausible biological pathways through which the psychological correlates of PTSD could affect physical health, such as the balance between numbing and hyperarousal symptoms (Mason et al., 2001). The reverse should be true as well, that biological correlates of PTSD affect health through psychological pathways. Both in turn could affect behavior, although we propose that biological mechanisms affect behavior by eliciting responses perceived as distressing at some level.

Attentional Mechanisms

Traumatic exposure and PTSD are associated with illness behaviors such as reporting somatic symptoms (see Engel, chap. 8; Green & Kimerling, chap. 2, this volume) and seeking medical care (see Walker et al., chap. 3, this volume). Many explanations have been offered for why trauma in particular might increase negative health perceptions and illness behavior (e.g., Ford, 1997; Rodin, De Groot, & Spivak, 1998; van der Kolk, 1994). Pennebaker (2000) has proposed that the propensity to report somatic symptoms following traumatic exposure could result from four nonmutually exclusive sources. The first source is actual biological changes resulting from the exposure. The second source is the use of symptom reporting as a strategy to avoid thinking about trauma; the assumption here is that focusing on physical symptoms is less distressing than focusing on psychological distress. A third source, related to the use of avoidance, is mislabeling of autonomic and emotional consequences of trying to suppress thinking about trauma. The last source is secondary gain: Reporting symptoms can elicit help and comfort from others.

Another possibility is conditioning. Resnick and colleagues (1997) suggested that because physiological arousal is part of the initial "alarm" response to a traumatic event, arousal symptoms can trigger cognitions (such as threat to life or danger) that cause individuals to believe their symptoms require medical attention. Panic disorder is frequently comorbid with PTSD (Kessler et al., 1995; Kulka et al., 1990), and many trauma survivors interpret symptoms of a panic attack as indicating a medical emergency (Falsetti & Resnick, 1997). The effects of panic disorder on physical health, then, are likely due to increased sensitivity to symptoms, as well as behavioral factors (Jakubec & Taylor, 1999). Thus, panic and anxiety symptoms in trauma survivors may increase illness behavior directly through attentional mechanisms because the psychiatric symptoms are somatic in nature (e.g., rapid heartbeat, sweating, difficulty breathing).

Another important attentional mechanism is somatization, "a tendency to experience and communicate somatic distress and symptoms unaccounted for by pathological findings, to attribute them to physical illness, and to seek medical help for them" (Lipowski, 1988, p. 1358). Trauma and PTSD are associated with somatization and somatoform disorders, including MIPS (e.g., Andreski, Chilcoat, & Breslau, 1998; Engel, chap. 8, this volume; Labbate, Cardeña, Dimitreva, Roy, & Engel, 1998; van der Kolk et al., 1996).

Engel, in his chapter, argues against a simple cause–effect model for the association between traumatic exposure and somatization, and we agree. Individual, social/contextual, and triggering factors cause individuals to somatize (Green, Epstein, Krupnick, & Rowland, 1997). Green and colleagues present childhood trauma as one of a number of dispositional and experiential variables that could contribute to a tendency to somatize. Social and contextual factors include illness or somatization in family members, as well as a chaotic childhood environment, secondary gain, social support, and cultural influences. Precipitating factors include traumatic exposure and other acute life stressors, psychiatric illness, and personal or familial medical illness. Other factors like comorbid psychiatric disorders and dissociation may also mediate the relationship of trauma to somatization, as mentioned previously.

Attentional mechanisms can also involve decreased attention to medical problems or conditions. If a person is dissociating, he or she may be out of touch with physical pain or discomfort, through self-generated analgesia or anesthesia (Nijenhuis, Vanderlinden, & Spinhoven, 1998), such that real physical problems may go unnoticed and, by extension, untreated, exacerbating a medical condition or potentially rendering it more severe or dangerous—a situation that therapists who are trained to look for somatization may miss (Haven & Pearlman, in press). Haven (2002) described a patient with severe childhood trauma and current dissociation who did not experience pain associated with a malignant tumor that would have been painful to most people. The lack of pain cues postponed the identification of the tumor and the seeking of health care, and threatened his life.

Behavioral Mechanisms

Health risk behaviors account for a substantial proportion of deaths in the United States (McGinnis & Foege, 1993). Roughly speaking, poor health practices fall into two categories: substance use or abuse (smoking, alcohol, drugs, food) and failure to engage in preventive strategies (exercise, diet, safe sex, regular health care). The chapter by Rheingold, Acierno, and Resnick (chap. 9) documents that trauma exposure and PTSD are associated with both types (e.g., Felitti et al., 1998; Schnurr & Spiro, 1999; Walker et al., 1999). Although PTSD has substantial effects on physical health even if the effects of behaviors such as smoking are statistically controlled, these behaviors are an important part of the pathway from traumatic exposure to poor health.

Rheingold and colleagues discuss self-medication as a primary reason why trauma survivors engage in behaviors such as smoking and alcohol abuse, noting that this kind of coping strategy may backfire: for example, alcohol abuse may temporarily reduce distress but eventually lead to medical illness, and substance withdrawal may exacerbate symptoms of PTSD and other psychiatric disorders. Failure to decrease substance abuse, as well as failure to engage in preventive behaviors, likely results from factors that decrease motivation or the ability to maintain a behavior change regimen, such as low self-efficacy (e.g., DeVellis & DeVellis, 2001), lack of social support (e.g., Havassey, Hall, & Wasserman, 1991), and depression (e.g., Niaura et al., 2001). Failure to engage in preventive behaviors also may result from factors that impair the acquisition or use of necessary information, such as anxiety preventing the use of condoms in those with a history of sexual assault despite the fact that the individuals know of the importance of protected sex (e.g., Resnick et al., 1997).

Interaction Among Components

According to our proposed model, there are multiple pathways through which traumatic exposure could lead to poor health. As a way to understand how these many dimensions interact, Schnurr and Jankowski (1999) suggested the concept of allostatic load:

> The strain on the body produced by repeated up and downs of physiologic response, as well as the elevated activity of physiologic systems under challenge, and the changes in metabolism and wear and tear on a number of organs and tissues. (McEwen & Stellar, 1993, p. 2094)

Allostatic load is particularly useful for understanding the health outcomes associated with traumatic exposure because the construct emphasizes the cumulative and interactive effects of biological, psychological, and behavioral alterations, including those that alone would be insufficient to produce disease. For example, the elevated levels of arousal and hyperreactivity in PTSD may not by themselves cause cardiovascular disease, but may do so if coupled with behavioral risk factors that are also associated with PTSD. Schnurr and Jankowski also suggested that allostatic load might be greater in PTSD than in other disorders, due to the number and chronicity of factors that produce "wear and tear" in PTSD. This possibility has yet to be tested.

Friedman and McEwen's chapter in this book (chap. 7) provides further detail about allostatic load and offers a new and exciting parallel construct: allostatic support, defined as "any nonhomeostatic, biopsychosocial strategy that will oppose allostatic load" (p. 179). Allostatic support may reflect inherited protective tendencies, and also may reflect interventions designed to counter allostatic load. Allostatic support is related to the concept of "physiological toughening," proposed by Dienstbier (1989) to account for evidence that stressor exposure can lead to adaptive, rather than maladaptive, responding in both animals and humans. Physiological toughening may be a mechanism that promotes allostatic support.

If allostatic support works like allostatic load, then numerous small positive changes could add up to heightened resilience. One implication of Friedman and McEwen's proposal, then, is that interventions aimed at improving physical health in trauma survivors (or other populations) could be successful even if targeting multiple small improvements rather than major changes.

Other Considerations

Physical health is a multidimensional construct that is expressed on a continuum of increasing complexity, ranging from biological and physiological variables, symptoms, functional status, health perceptions, and finally, health-related quality of life (Wilson & Cleary, 1995). Given this complexity, physical health is influenced by many factors in addition to those depicted in Figure 10.1. We do not detail these factors, but we remind readers to consider that health also is affected by personal characteristics such as age, gender, and genetic makeup; social factors such as socioeconomic status, social support, and proximity to sources of preventive care; and ethnic and cultural background (Bird & Rieker, 1999; Fried, 2000; Grzywacz & Fuqua, 2000; Macera, Armstead, & Anderson, 2001; Wilson & Cleary, 1995). These factors interact; for example, Macera and colleagues suggested that adverse health outcomes in African Americans, relative to White Americans, might result from an interaction between racial stratification and discrimination on the one hand and socioeconomic status on the other. It would be helpful to know whether personal and sociocultural factors also interact with trauma and PTSD; for example, to what extent the likelihood of cardiovascular disease is increased in a genetically predisposed individual who also has PTSD. This and other questions for future research are discussed later in this chapter.

CLINICAL, SYSTEMS, AND POLICY IMPLICATIONS OF THE RELATIONSHIP BETWEEN TRAUMA AND HEALTH

The relationships among trauma, PTSD, and health suggest that it is important to make these links in clinical settings and practice. Green and Kimerling (chap. 2, this volume) began a discussion of the issues surrounding screening for trauma and for PTSD in primary care settings. We extend this discussion to include a range of clinical, training, and policy issues suggested by the links and pathways just proposed. Although we agree that primary prevention—that is, the prevention of trauma exposure in the first place—is a crucial aspect of reducing the burden of trauma-related problems on the health care system, as well as the suffering of exposed individuals, it is outside of the scope of the present discussion, and we refer the reader to other sources (e.g., Koss, 1993; Nadel, Spellman, Albarez-Canino, Lausell-Bryant, & Landsberg, 1996). The remaining discussion assumes that exposure has occurred, and considers ways in which the health care system and individual providers can ease psychological distress among victims, help to make the medical setting more "user friendly" for patients, decrease the artificial distinction between mental and physical health, increase the appropriate use of scarce health resources, and reduce the costs of trauma to the system at large.

Implications for Primary Care Settings

Identification

Before there can be an intervention to reduce the psychological and physical health consequences of traumatic exposure, those who have been exposed must be identified. Green and Kimerling (chap. 2, this volume) note that studies of the links between trauma and health have tended to recommend universal screening procedures. Whereas they suggest some of the drawbacks and limitations of screening, they also note that screening with enhanced treatment possibilities has proven beneficial to the patient, and possibly even cost-effective, for treatment of depression (e.g., Schoenbaum et al., 2001). Furthermore, knowing whether someone is a trauma survivor, and particularly whether he or she has a mental disorder, is important for appropriate assessment of the patient's medical and mental health status, potential needs, and for developing a treatment plan. Routine or intermittent screening, using short self-report screens in the context of collecting medical history information, is one easy and relatively inexpensive way to obtain such information, and numerous instruments are now available for this purpose.

Another approach is to key inquiries and discussions of trauma and distress to certain types of clinical encounters. For example, on the basis of qualitative studies, Miller (1992) characterized family practice visits as being of three types, which he called *routine*, *ceremony*, or *drama*. Although this classification was one suggested for determining when to involve family members or to obtain more information, it seems appropriate for trauma as well. Only drama visits trigger physician inquiries about what may be going on that is not apparent. Examples of these types of visits include a crisis in a chronic disease course, family discord, or the presentation of a complex syndrome with an hypothesized psychological component (e.g., chronic fatigue, lower-back pain). These visits revolve around uncertainty, conflict, physician–patient disagreement, nonadherence, or the delivery of bad news. At these times, the physician might ask questions that would help clarify the nature of the visit and the problem (What brings you here today? What worries you most about [presenting problem]? What do you hope that I can do for that?). There are also "quick checks" that can be woven into even the routine visit (Has anything changed at home? Do you feel safe at home? How is your family doing?) that give the patient an opening to report events that may be problematic (W. Miller, personal communication, October 2001). Regardless of how the information is obtained, there needs to be a plan for follow-through if trauma experiences or distress are uncovered.

In addition to screening for trauma exposure and PTSD, it is important for physicians to screen for health risk behaviors such as smoking, substance abuse, and failure to prevent negative health problems (Rheingold et al., chap. 9, this volume). This may be especially important if those behaviors are used as negative coping strategies to deal with trauma-related memories, triggers, affect, or symptoms (Aldwin & Yancura, chap. 5, this volume). These behaviors are dangerous and contribute to poor health whether or not they are related to trauma, but if they are coping strategies to deal with traumatic exposure, they may need to be addressed somewhat differently. As Rheingold and colleagues point out, eliminating a negative coping response without replacing it with a healthier one runs the risk of failing or of encouraging even more negative coping. It may help to explain to patients how they may be using these behaviors to cope, thus helping to support the importance of dealing with the problem behaviors and the need for mental health services.

Training of Caregivers in Primary Care Settings

Many trauma researchers have called for the training of nonpsychiatric physicians and other caregivers in the nature and consequences of trauma, and this approach appears to be a necessary, if not sufficient, condition for the improvement of services to survivors. The range of training needs for primary care providers is potentially wide. These needs encompass several areas, including *knowledge about mental health issues* (e.g., how trauma exposure relates to physical health, information about mental disorders, links between exposure and health risk behaviors, the potential of some medical procedures to be triggers for earlier traumatic experiences, screening strategies); *knowledge about interactions and communications with patients* (e.g., how to refer patients to specialty care, listening and being sensitive to survivors' needs for validation, providing education to trauma survivors, providing treatment [usually medication] to trauma survivors); and *knowledge about community issues* (e.g., legal reporting requirements, community resources for victims). Providers may not be able to address each issue with each patient. However, they do need to be aware of trauma reactions, as well as when and how to address them with particular patients, and to consider how some aspects of appropriate care for trauma patients could be incorporated into their practice at various levels (e.g., through education of staff, routine data collection, spreading responsibility for education, recognition, and referral among providers and staff).

Presently, there is very little training in medical schools about trauma and its effects, although mental disorders are routinely taught in medical school psychiatry courses. Psychiatry residents may get some training in trauma-related issues, especially sexual and physical abuse, but one survey showed that they felt their instruction about child abuse, the focus of the survey, was insufficient (Barnard-Thompson & Leichner, 1999). Their exposure to trauma-related courses and training opportunities may depend on the availability of local experts and the discretion of training directors. Nonphysician mental health programs may do somewhat better in introducing trauma content (Winkelspecht & Singg, 1998), but clinicians generally rate these training programs as not sufficient in preparing them for practice (Pope & Feldman-Summers, 1992; Winkelspecht & Singg, 1998). In a survey of nurses, dentists, dental hygienists, physicians, psychologists, and social workers, a third of participants reported having received no educational content on child, spouse, or elder abuse in their training programs (Tilden et al., 1994). Social workers, psychologists, and nurses reported the most training, dental personnel the least. Family practice residents receive training in mental disorders, including some training in counseling, but trauma is less emphasized. The exceptions to these generalizations are those related to detection and reporting of current sexual or physical abuse, which is also taught in emergency medicine and pediatric programs. Training in medical and nursing schools, as well as in graduate mental health programs, needs to include modules on the effects of trauma. Furthermore, innovative curricula for teaching students about patient communication need to be developed or improved. One study indicated that medical students do not necessarily receive training in communication skills during their obstetrician–gynecology rotations (Kleinman, Hage, Hoole, & Kowlowitz, 1996). This study also showed that having laywomen train medical students in the performance of a pelvic exam, an increasingly common medical school practice, significantly increased the students' interpersonal skills during an exam, suggesting the potential usefulness of involving patients in training professionals to communicate and respond sensitively to patients.

Interventions by Primary Care Providers

Once there has been an inquiry and a positive response to questions about current or past trauma exposure, the physician or caregiver has several options. One is to ask the patient whether he or she wants to discuss anything reported, or asking additional questions to get a clinical sense of their potential connection, psychologically or temporally, with the physical complaints for which the patient seeks treatment. A clear follow-up plan or procedure needs to be in place when significant trauma is recognized, especially if it is current. Another reasonable option is to schedule a follow-up visit to explore the impact of the trauma history more thoroughly. A nurse within a practice might be designated to follow up with patients and to explore options for those who need social services or mental health treatment. These procedures might result in referral to support services or education, a mental health consultation or referral, or treatment by the primary care physician for specific syndromes (i.e., PTSD or depression), usually with medication. In addition, caregivers who have been trained to understand the possible triggering effects of medical and diagnostic procedures for trauma survivors can prepare patients for these (Caulfield & Prins, 1999). Gynecologic procedures, dental procedures, and anesthesia are all situations in which patients with histories of abuse may experience heightened distress or even severe symptoms such as dissociation, and these can be avoided. Nurses and support staff can be trained to deal sensitively with traumatized female patients by recognizing some of the manifestations of fear and anxiety that may occur, for example, during pelvic exams (e.g., Robohm & Buttenheim, 1996), and by learning techniques to reduce anticipatory anxiety or fear.

If the provider suspects that the patient's symptoms are primarily due to *somatization*, certain management strategies may come into play. For example, care providers can help patients with somatization symptoms to understand that stress affects the body and one's physical health. Physicians may schedule more regular visits to discourage emergency care, and limit the use of diagnostic tests (Green et al., 1997). An important key to treating individuals with somatization disorder is a compassionate physician–patient relationship, with a physician who coordinates care and serves as a gatekeeper for consultation of medical specialists (Green et al., 1997). The general approach to treatment is long-term observation rather than diagnostic procedures. Acknowledging the patient's suffering, yet reassuring him or her that the symptoms most likely do not represent serious or disabling illness, may aid rapport and redirect the patient away from symptom complaints. It is also important to collect family and social histories, including mental disorders and substance abuse in family members, to help rule out bona fide medical conditions and enhance the detection of somatization.

Patient Education and Empowerment Strategies

To date, patient education and empowerment strategies have not been sufficiently explored, and few recommendations have been made for development of such strategies that are not physician driven. Yet, although physicians and other providers have a responsibility to educate and collaborate with their patients, not all do, for time reasons if nothing else. So it seems logical that patients take some of the responsibility themselves, and that appropriate materials and opportunities be developed for them, in and out of the doctor's office. Educational approaches have the potential to increase the patient's awareness of the interdependency of his or her mental and physical health. Patients can be helped to think about ways that they may take better care of themselves physically, with an eye toward improving their overall physical condition. Risk reduction education around behaviors that have negative health consequences are also important (Kilpatrick et al., 1997; Rheingold et al., chap. 9, this volume), and can be provided outside of the physician–patient relationship. Indeed, public health campaigns are already aimed at some of these behaviors, and trauma-focused materials could be developed as well. Patient-focused interventions might also be useful for the trauma-related patient–provider relationship problems of fear, discomfort, or overly dependent behavior. For example, Bassuk, Dawson, Perloff, and Weinreb (2001) have shown that poor women with PTSD, compared with women exposed to violence but without PTSD, were more concerned that they would not get good care, did not trust their doctors, found medical staff to be rude, and felt that staff did not understand their problems. Education about how trauma and PTSD affect relationships, and how they might affect interactions with caregivers, might help patients understand their role in their interactions with caregivers. Given increased access to, and use of, Web sites for medical information, the Internet should be considered a resource in the development of materials for patients as well.

Implications for Mental Health Professionals

For the clinician seeing patients in a mental health setting, more attention needs to be paid to physical manifestations of psychiatric illness and to helping patients understand the links between their psychological distress and their physical health (Caulfield & Prins, 1999). Patients can be given normative information about physical and psychiatric reactions, symptoms, disorders, and treatment. Patients with PTSD and other disorders can be helped to understand how these psychiatric problems affect their physical health (Green & Schnurr, 2000). The patient's physical health problems and visits to nonpsychiatric physicians should also be assessed and explored (Kilpatrick et al., 1997) to learn more about his or her general health history as well as to increase the patient's awareness of the interdependency of mental and physical health.

Integrated Care Models

In recent years there has been a move toward more integrated models of care: that is, including primary care and mental health providers in the same setting. These models seem particularly appropriate when considering the physical health consequences of traumatic stress. The strong links between trauma and physical health, and among trauma, mental disorders (especially PTSD), and health, suggest that integrated models are likely to be the most appropriate for many trauma survivors, and may improve their access to care. Closer alliances between health and mental health care providers, both professionally and geographically, are appropriate for many reasons. Blount (1998) described nine reasons to integrate primary and mental health behavioral care, of which four seem particularly pertinent to the present discussion. First, integrated care reflects the way that most patients experience and present their distress—that is, in an undifferentiated form. Most patients who present in primary care have problems that are psychological in some way (Kroenke & Mangelsdorff, 1989), with less than 20% of patient visits linked to discoverable organic causes. Second, for problems that are clearly psychological in origin, primary care is still the predominant focus of treatment. Most prefer to get their mental health treatment in primary care settings (Brody, Khaliq, & Thompson, 1997), by their primary care provider, with only 11% wanting to be referred out. Patients may also feel abandoned if they are referred to another facility or provider (Blount, 1998). Third, such an integrated setting, being closer to how the patient presents, is likely to increase adherence and thus produce better outcomes. For example, Katon and colleagues (1995) found that 74% of the people with major depression in their integrated treatment condition showed significant symptom reduction, whereas only 44% of the patients with physician treatment and referral showed significant improvement. Fourth, even primary care physicians trained in mental health cannot be expected to address the whole range of potential problems, and referrals are often not successful. Indeed, follow-through with referrals to mental health professionals is low, with estimates ranging from 10% to 50% (Glenn, 1987; Katon, 1995). Blount also points out that both parties are more satisfied under an integrated model, and that there does not tend to be an increase in costs. Thus, integrated services are likely to increase real access to care, leading to better quality and outcomes.

For these reasons, we encourage mental health practitioners to seek out partnerships with primary care physicians, including mutual education and active exchange of information and patient referrals. Blount (1998) pointed out that collaboration can take a variety of forms, from a courtesy report of involvement with the patient, at the low end, to actively working together on a regular basis in delivering services, at the high end. All forms are encouraged here. However, we hope that both groups, primary care providers and mental health professionals, will consider "on site" arrangements in which mental health practitioners actually spend time in the practice setting. Direct interventions by mental health professionals in primary care focused on specific disorders (primarily depression to date) have proved effective compared with usual care (e.g., Katon et al., 1996; Schulberg et al., 1996), particularly for major depression. Although some of the interventions that have been tested are relatively elaborate, even more modest interventions may improve access to care. For example, at Georgetown, two psychiatrists each spend one day per week at the family practice center run by Georgetown's Department of Family Medicine. The center serves a low-income population, many of whom are on Medicaid, and is a training site for the family medicine residents. The psychiatrists teach the family medicine residents about mental health issues, are available for consultation, and provide treatment. The study mentioned in Green and Kimerling's chapter (chap. 2), a treatment study for PTSD, screened for patients at this site. Although the rate of current PTSD screened (about 8%) was comparable to rates at public health clinics in the same county, all of the women who screened positive were already in mental health treatment for their PTSD, compared with almost none of those in the county clinics. Many factors vary among the sites, and the presence of psychiatry faculty at the setting indicates an interest in mental health issues on the part of this particular clinic to begin with. However, it seems likely that having mental health professionals on site, even though they may not be able to treat all of the practice's clients because of differences in insurance plans, contributed to the high proportion of women with PTSD being in treatment. Many practical suggestions for collaboration between mental health and medical professionals, and especially for integration of health and mental health services, including how to go about establishing these, are delineated in a recent book (Patterson, Peek, Heinrich, Bishoff, & Scherger, 2002).

It is also important to underline that there are a range of interventions that may be appropriate for those having trauma-related problems. Treatment interventions are costly, even if they are cost-effective, and might best be reserved for patients who do not respond to less-intensive approaches. They might also best be reserved for serious disorder, rather than subclinical symptoms (Von Korff, Gruman, Schaefer, Curry, & Wagner, 1997), or discomfort and fear associated with medical procedures. For these latter problems, some of the approaches mentioned previously may be appropriate, such as reassurance from the provider, patient pamphlets, educational or support groups for patients (e.g., Allen, Kelly, & Glodich, 1997), training of office staff, practice-based case management approaches, and so forth. Mental health providers, especially psychologists, are trained to conduct preventive behavioral interventions related to coping and health risk behaviors (Aldwin & Yancura, chap. 5, this volume; Rheingold et al., chap. 9, this volume). Triage may be an important additional function that the mental health professional can serve, and stepped-care models (Haaga, 2000; Katon et al., 1999) seem to make the best use of resources. These approaches will require thinking "outside of the box" and will challenge the skills of the mental health professional but would appear to be most likely to engage and help patients with prevention and mental health problems, including PTSD. Glenn (1987) has suggested criteria for the involvement of mental health professionals in a patient's care, and Blount (1998) has provided a process and a model for moving to this type of integrated treatment.

Implications for Public Policy and Systems Changes

Although individual providers and practices may make links on their own, and strive for more integrated care for their patients, unless whole systems are involved the options will continue to be somewhat limited. Access to care, as well as quality of life, may be improved in integrated models, and this may be sufficient motivation for patients and providers. However, costs are not likely to be reduced until larger systems are involved. As noted by Kilpatrick and colleagues (1997), not only changes in health care systems but more coordinated efforts across systems would improve access and outcomes. These systems include criminal justice and victim assistance, as well as the health and mental health systems. The sharing of information and services across these systems would be the ideal, but because they are supported by separate funding streams, such integration seems unlikely. Even so, some programs have overcome some of these obstacles. The Center for Mental Health in Washington, DC, provides comprehensive services to at-risk families with histories of violence and substance abuse that cut across generations. The Family Health Program, with integrated services, training, research, and advocacy aspects, was initially a federally funded demonstration project, but the funding has been taken over by Medicaid and local government.

Walker and colleagues (chap. 3, this volume) suggest how patients with trauma-related medical and psychological problems and conditions could be supported in the health care system in a way that seems logical for a large medical organization like an HMO. They discuss case management approaches and special tracks in the primary care clinic that enhance early recognition of anxiety and depression, which might otherwise appear as medically unexplained symptoms. This model focuses on stabilization of chronic problems, with the idea that initially high costs would be balanced out, in the long run, by lower costs once the presenting problems were stabilized and maintenance care had taken over. However, although this model has much to offer clinically, and it seems to address cost issues over the longer term, the authors point out that it is still not likely to be cost-effective in reality because of the high rates of turnover of patients in health plans. To Walker and colleagues, this dilemma suggests the importance of revisiting the issue of national health insurance. Unless health care is "portable," the investment made in one setting will not benefit another setting, so it will not be cost-effective for plans to focus on long-term gains.

Although these concerns require a commitment to changes in health care planning at the national level, it may be possible to implement some of them locally. The suggestions for integration of services seem likely to be helpful to patients and more satisfying for providers. As long as they do not increase costs, or the costs can be offset or otherwise absorbed, there is likely to be little opposition to them. Creative thinking is required for services that are not likely to be covered by health plans at all. For example, some of the training activities could potentially be donated, educational literature can be obtained on the Internet, graduate students could provide educational workshops and behavioral interventions as part of their training, videotapes are available or could be designed for patient education; the possibilities are endless. Although any one type of intervention may make only a small contribution, using the concept of allostatic support (Friedman & McEwen, chap. 7, this volume), it may be that even small interventions can begin to reverse the downward spiral that follows the wear and tear caused by PTSD and other mental disorders and symptoms. All of these possibilities require collaboration among health professionals with different training. The differences can enhance care for survivors if they are explored and incorporated into health settings rather than used to maintain barriers to more-integrated care.

AN AGENDA FOR RESEARCH

Although knowledge about the health consequences of traumatic exposure has grown substantially in recent years, more evidence is needed to document, understand, and treat these consequences. Given our view that a distress reaction is necessary to initiate the pathway from traumatic exposure to adverse physical health outcomes, we suggest that future research include measures of PTSD and not only measures of traumatic exposure. Another important issue is a need for studies that assess morbidity by physical exam or laboratory tests. Most research on the health effects of trauma and PTSD has used self-report methods. Although self-reports are useful and valid, they are not synonymous with more objective measures, which are needed to confirm the link between PTSD and disease processes. There is a need for studies of large, representative samples that permit wide generalization of findings; here we would add a need for international samples. Except for studies of torture victims or refugees (e.g., Hondius, Van Willigen, Kleijn, & Van der Ploeg, 2000), most research has focused on samples from North America or other developed countries. In low-income or developing countries, where physical health may be poorer to begin with, and where access to care may be more limited, the impact of trauma on health may be even more profound.

Many key questions remain unanswered. One is which physical disorders are, and are not, associated with PTSD. At present, a diverse range of disorders, involving multiple body systems, has been implicated. For example, one study found that PTSD was associated with increased incidence of arterial, dermatological, gastrointestinal, and musculoskeletal disorders (Schnurr, Spiro, et al., 2000). There are behavioral and neurobiological reasons why PTSD could result in medical problems across multiple body systems (see Friedman & McEwen, chap. 7; Rheingold et al., chap. 9, this volume), but the breadth of PTSD's effects needs confirmation. Understanding which disorders are associated with PTSD also would help to address another key question: the mechanisms through which PTSD leads to poor health. Better elaboration of biological pathways is needed, including evidence for allostatic load as an explanation for the health effects of PTSD. A useful strategy to enhance understanding of biological mechanisms is for investigators to include measures of health status in studies of neurobiological functioning.

Other questions concern the specificity of the effects of PTSD, versus disorders that are comorbid with PTSD. Research is needed to investigate the health consequences of significant distress reactions other than PTSD, and to distinguish the effects of PTSD from the effects of these other disorders. When possible, measures of PTSD and other types of distress should be used jointly, because this approach will enable investigators to address both issues. In particular, depression researchers are encouraged to include measures of PTSD in studies of depression and health to identify the unique contribution of depression. A related issue about the specificity of PTSD was raised in the preceding section: Does PTSD confer additional disease risk beyond genetic predisposition and other risk factors and, if so, are the results additive or interactive?

Next is the issue of treatment. It is necessary to know how interventions designed to reduce PTSD or other clinically significant posttraumatic distress reactions affect health. Pennebaker (e.g., 1997) has argued that writing about traumatic experiences can improve health, and although most of the supporting evidence comes from studies in which participants have written about nontraumatic stressors, the evidence is sufficient to recommend further investigation. Among published PTSD treatment outcome studies, we found only one that measured physical health. Malik and colleagues (1999), in a small, randomized, placebo-controlled pilot study of fluoxetine, found that treatment improved domains such as vitality, social functioning, and mental health, but not physical functioning or general health perceptions. Although these results are discouraging, larger studies are needed, including those with sufficiently long follow-up periods to observe changes in health.

It is also necessary to know how interventions designed to improve health status affect PTSD and other clinically significant distress reactions. A related question is whether trauma survivors need special health promotion interventions that target the ways in which their symptoms impede compliance with medical regimens or reduction of health risk behaviors. For example, Rheingold and colleagues (chap. 9, this volume) suggest that concurrent treatment of health risk behaviors and trauma symptoms might be beneficial, but note that research does not indicate whether concurrent treatment or sequential treatment (PTSD then behavior, or behavior then PTSD) is best.

A wide range of preventive, educational, and supportive interventions for trauma survivors need to be developed and tested for their efficacy in preventing or ameliorating trauma-related distress and their ability to improve physical health. Training for caregivers needs to be evaluated. System changes also need to be developed, implemented, and assessed; for example, such things as assigning a case manager to work with trauma patients who are having difficulty in the health care system, or offering education groups to all new patients with trauma histories. Recent quality improvement studies of depression (Wells et al., 2000) provide excellent models for these types of systems-level interventions and assessments. Once these interventions have been tested for their effectiveness, they will need to be tested for their cost-effectiveness as well (Schoenbaum et al., 2001; Simon et al., 2001).

More work is needed on the impact of trauma patients on the health care system, and the impact of the system on trauma patients at all levels

(Walker et al., chap. 3, this volume). Also, although there is no reason to expect that large systems will change in the near future, smaller research projects within HMOs or other closed systems such as the Department of Veterans Affairs can track the impact of new programs or alterations in clinical management of trauma survivors over time across all aspects of health care, to better understand effects on distress, health, and costs, as well as on patient and caregiver satisfaction.

SUMMARY

Since Selye (1956) first published his classic work, *The Stress of Life*, a great deal of research has investigated the relationship between stress and physical health. Most of this research has focused on stressors such as divorce, bereavement, and job loss, but some has examined the health effects associated with extreme stressors, including war, sexual victimization, disasters, and serious accidents. The evidence presented in this book shows that poor physical health should be recognized, along with mental health problems and impaired psychosocial functioning, as an outcome of traumatic exposure. PTSD and other clinically significant distress reactions are a key step in triggering the processes through which exposure affects health. These processes involve psychological, biological, behavioral, and attentional mechanisms that interact to strain the body's ability to adapt, thereby increasing the likelihood of disease and illness behavior. However, by addressing the physical health consequences of traumatic exposure in treatment and treatment systems, the burden on individuals and society may be reduced.

REFERENCES

Allen, J. G., Kelly, K. A., & Glodich, A. (1997). A psychoeducational program for patients with trauma-related disorders. *Bulletin of the Menninger Clinic, 61*, 222–239.

Andreski, P., Chilcoat, H., & Breslau, N. (1998). Post-traumatic stress disorder and somatization symptoms: A prospective study. *Psychiatry Research, 79*, 131–138.

Barnard-Thompson, K., & Leichner, P. (1999). Psychiatric residents' views on their training and experience regarding issues related to child abuse. *Canadian Journal of Psychiatry, 44*, 769–774.

Bassuk, E. L., Dawson, R., Perloff, J., & Weinreb, L. (2001). Post-traumatic stress disorder in extremely poor women: Implications for health care clinicians. *Journal of the American Medical Women's Association, 56*, 79–85.

Beckham, J. C., Moore, S. D., Feldman, M. E., Hertzberg, M. A., Kirby, A. C., & Fairbank, J. A. (1998). Health status, somatization, and severity of posttraumatic stress disorder in Vietnam combat veterans with posttraumatic stress disorder. *American Journal of Psychiatry, 155,* 1565–1569.

Bird, C. E., & Rieker, P. P. (1999). Gender matters: An integrated model for understanding men's and women's health. *Social Science and Medicine, 48,* 745–755.

Blount, A. (1998). Introduction to integrated primary care. In A. Blount (Ed.), *Integrated primary care: The future of medical and mental health collaboration* (pp. 1–43). New York: Norton.

Boscarino, J. A. (1997). Diseases among men 20 years after exposure to severe stress: Implications for clinical research and medical care. *Psychosomatic Medicine, 59,* 605–614.

Boscarino, J. A., & Chang, J. (1999). Electrocardiogram abnormalities among men with stress-related psychiatric disorders: Implications for coronary heart disease and clinical research. *Annals of Behavioral Medicine, 21,* 227–234.

Breslau, N., Davis, G. C., Peterson, E. L., & Schultz, L. R. (2000). A second look at comorbidity in victims of trauma: The posttraumatic stress disorder-major depression connection. *Biological Psychiatry, 48,* 902–909.

Brody, D. S., Khaliq, A. A., & Thompson, T. L., II. (1997). Patients' perspectives on the management of emotional distress in primary care settings. *Journal of General Internal Medicine, 12,* 403–406.

Caulfield, M. B., & Prins, A. (1999). The role of the mental health professional in addressing the physical complaints of trauma survivors. *National Center for PTSD Clinical Quarterly, 8*(2), 31.

Chrousos, G. P. (1995). The hypothalamic-pituitary-adrenal axis and immune-mediated inflammation. *New England Journal of Medicine, 332,* 1351–1362.

Clum, G. A., Calhoun, K. S., & Kimerling, R. (2000). Associations among symptoms of depression and posttraumatic stress disorder and self-reported health in sexually assaulted women. *Journal of Nervous and Mental Disease, 188,* 671–678.

DeVellis, B. M., & DeVellis, R. F. (2001). Self-efficacy and health. In A. Baum, T. A. Revenson, & J. E. Singer (Eds.), *Handbook of health psychology* (pp. 235–247). Mahwah, NJ: Erlbaum.

Dienstbier, R. A. (1989). Arousal and physiological toughness: Implications for physical and mental health. *Psychological Review, 96,* 84–100.

Falsetti, S. A., & Resnick, H. S. (1997). Frequency and severity of panic attack symptoms in a treatment seeking sample of trauma victims. *Journal of Traumatic Stress, 10,* 683–689.

Felitti, V. J., Anda, R. F., Nordenberg, D., Williamson, D. F., Spitz, A. M., Edwards, V., et al. (1998). Relationship of childhood abuse and household dysfunction to many of the leading causes of death in adults. *American Journal of Preventive Medicine, 14,* 245–258.

Ford, C. V. (1997). Somatic symptoms, somatization, and traumatic stress: An overview. *Nordisk Psykiatrisk Tidsskrift, 51,* 5–13.

Ford, J. D., Schnurr, P. P., Friedman, M. J., Green, B. L., Adams, G., & Jex, S. (2003). *Posttraumatic stress disorder symptoms, physical health outcomes, and health care utilization fifty years after exposure to a toxic gas.* Manuscript submitted for publication.

Fried, L. P. (2000). Epidemiology of aging. *Epidemiologic Reviews, 22,* 95–106.

Friedman, M. J., & Schnurr, P. P. (1995). The relationship between PTSD, trauma, and physical health. In M. J. Friedman, D. S. Charney, & A. Y. Deutch (Eds.), *Neurobiological and clinical consequences of stress: From normal adaptation to PTSD* (pp. 507–527). Philadelphia: Lippincott-Raven.

Glenn, M. L. (1987). *Collaborative health care: A family oriented approach.* New York: Praeger.

Goldstein, M. G., & Niaura, R. (1995). Cardiovascular death, part I: Coronary artery disease and sudden death. In A. Stoudemire (Ed.), *Psychological factors affecting medical conditions* (pp. 19–37). Washington, DC: American Psychiatric Press.

Grady, K. E., Reisine, S. T., Fifield, J., Lee, N. R., McVay, J., & Kelsey, M. E. (1991). The impact of Hurricane Hugo and the San Francisco earthquake on a sample of people with rheumatoid arthritis. *Arthritis Care and Research, 4,* 106–110.

Green, B. L., Epstein, S. A., Krupnick, J. L., & Rowland, J. H. (1997). Trauma and medical illness: Assessing trauma-related disorders in medical settings. In J. P. Wilson & T. M. Keane (Eds.), *Assessing psychological trauma and PTSD* (pp. 160–191). New York: Guilford.

Green, B. L., Grace, M. C., Lindy, J. D., Gleser, G. C., & Leonard, A. (1990). Risk factors for PTSD and other diagnoses in a general sample of Vietnam veterans. *American Journal of Psychiatry, 147,* 729–733.

Green, B. L., & Schnurr, P. P. (2000). Trauma and physical health. *National Center for PTSD Clinical Quarterly, 9*(1), 3–5.

Grzywacz, J. G., & Fuqua, J. (2000). The social ecology of health: Leverage points and linkages. *Behavioral Medicine, 26,* 101–115.

Haaga, D. (2000). Introduction to the special section on stepped care models in psychotherapy. *Journal of Consulting and Clinical Psychology, 68,* 547–548.

Havassey, B. E., Hall, S. M., & Wasserman, D. A. (1991). Social support and relapse: Commonalities among alcoholics, opiate users, and cigarette smokers. *Addictive Behaviors, 16,* 235–246.

Haven, T. (2002, November). Physical health and dissociation in relational trauma psychotherapies. In L. A. Pearlman (Chair), *Complex trauma and survivors' bodies.* Symposium conducted at the annual meeting of the International Society for Traumatic Stress Studies, Baltimore, MD.

Haven, T., & Pearlman, L. A. (in press). Minding the body: The intersection of dissociation and physical health in relational trauma psychotherapy. K. A. Kendall Tackett (Ed.), *Health consequences of abuse in the family: A clinical guide for evidence-based practice.* Washington, DC: American Psychological Association.

Hayward, C. (1995). Psychiatric illness and cardiovascular disease risk. *Epidemiology Review, 17,* 129–138.

Holman, E. A., Silver, R. C., & Waitzkin, H. (2000). Traumatic life events in primary care patients. *Archives of Family Medicine, 9,* 802–810.

Hondius, A. J. K., Van Willigen, L. H. M., Kleijn, W. C., & Van der Ploeg, H. M. (2000). Health problems among Latin-American and middle-eastern refugees in the Netherlands: Relations with violence exposure and ongoing sociopsychological strain. *Journal of Traumatic Stress, 13,* 619–634.

Jakubec, D. F., & Taylor, C. B. (1999). Medical aspects of panic disorder and its relationship to other medical conditions. In D. J. Nutt, J. C. Ballenger, & J. P. Lepine (Eds.), *Panic disorder: Clinical diagnosis, management, and mechanisms* (pp. 109–124). London: Martin Dunitz.

Katon, W. (1995). Collaborative care: Patient satisfaction, outcomes and medical cost-offset. *Family Systems Medicine, 13,* 351–365.

Katon, W., Robinson, P., Von Korff, M., Lin, E., Bush, T., Ludman, E., et al. (1996). A multifaceted intervention to improve treatment of depression in primary care. *Archives of General Psychiatry, 53,* 913–919.

Katon, W., Von Korff, M., Lin, E., Simon, G., Walker, E. A., Unutzer, J., et al. (1999). Stepped collaborative care for primary care patients with persistent symptoms of depression: A randomized trial. *Archives of General Psychiatry, 56,* 1109–1115.

Katon, W., Von Korff, M., Lin, E., Walker, E., Simon, G., Bush, T., et al. (1995). Collaborative management to achieve treatment guidelines: Impact on depression in primary care. *Journal of the American Medical Association, 273,* 1026–1031.

Kessler, D. C., Sonnega, A., Bromet, E., Hughes, M., & Nelson, C. B. (1995). Posttraumatic stress disorder in the National Comorbidity Survey. *Archives of General Psychiatry, 52,* 1048–1060.

Kilpatrick, D. G., Resnick, H. S., & Acierno, R. (1997). Health impact of interpersonal violence 3: Implications for clinical practice and public policy. *Behavioral Medicine, 23,* 65–78.

Kimerling, R., Clum, G. A., & Wolfe, J. (2000). Relationships among trauma exposure, chronic posttraumatic stress disorder symptoms, and self-reported health in women: Replication and extension. *Journal of Traumatic Stress, 13,* 115–128.

Kleinman, D. E., Hage, M. L., Hoole, A. J., & Kowlowitz, V. (1996). Pelvic examination instruction and experience: A comparison of laywoman-trained and physician-trained students. *Academic Medicine, 71,* 1239–1243.

Koss, M. (1993). Rape: Scope, impact, interventions, and public policy responses. *American Psychologist, 48,* 1062–1069.

Kroenke, K., & Mangelsdorff, A. D. (1989). Common symptoms in ambulatory care: Incidence, evaluation, therapy and outcome. *American Journal of Medicine, 86,* 262–266.

Kulka, R. A., Schlenger, W. E., Fairbank, J. A., Hough, R. L., Jordan, B. K., Marmar, C. R., et al. (1990). *Trauma and the Vietnam War generation*. New York: Brunner/Mazel.

Labbate, L. A., Cardeña, E., Dimitreva, J., Roy, M. J., & Engel, C. C., Jr. (1998). Psychiatric syndromes in Persian Gulf War veterans: An association of handling dead bodies with somatoform disorders. *Psychotherapy and Psychosomatics, 67,* 275–279.

Lipowski, Z. J. (1988). Somatization: The concept and its clinical application. *American Journal of Psychiatry, 145,* 1358–1368.

Macera, C. A., Armstead, C. A., & Anderson, N. B. (2001). Sociocultural influences on health. In A. Baum, T. A. Revenson, & J. E. Singer (Eds.), *Handbook of health psychology* (pp. 427–770). Mahwah, NJ: Erlbaum.

Malik, M. L., Connor, K. M., Sutherland, S. M., Smith, R. D., Davison, R. M., & Davidson, J. R. T. (1999). Quality of life and posttraumatic stress disorder: A pilot study assessing changes in SF-36 scores before and after treatment in a placebo-controlled trial of fluoxetine. *Journal of Traumatic Stress, 12,* 387–393.

Mason, J. W., Wang, S., Yehuda, R., Riney, S. J., Charney, D. S., & Southwick, S. M. (2001). Psychogenic lowering of urinary cortisol levels linked to increased emotional numbing, and a shame-depressive syndrome in combat-related post-traumatic stress disorder. *Psychosomatic Medicine, 63,* 387–401.

McEwen, B. S., & Stellar, E. (1993). Stress and the individual: Mechanisms leading to disease. *Archives of Internal Medicine, 153,* 2093–2101.

McGinnis, J. M., & Foege, W. H. (1993). Actual causes of death in the United States. *Journal of the American Medical Association, 270,* 2207–2212.

Miller, W. L. (1992). Routine, ceremony, or drama: An exploratory field study of the primary care clinical encounter. *Journal of Family Practice, 34,* 289–296.

Nadel, H., Spellman, M., Albarez-Canino, T., Lausell-Bryant, L., & Landsberg, G. (1996). The cycle of violence and victimization: A study of the school-based intervention of a multidisciplinary youth violence-prevention program. *American Journal of Preventive Medicine, 12,* 109–119.

Niaura, R., Britt, D. M., Shadel, W. G., Goldstein, M., Abrams, D., & Brown, R. (2001). Symptoms of depression and survival experience among three samples of smokers trying to quit. *Psychology of Addictive Behaviors, 15,* 13–17.

Nijenhuis, E. R. S., Vanderlinden, J., & Spinhoven, P. (1998). Animal defensive reactions as a model for trauma-induced dissociative reactions. *Journal of Traumatic Stress, 11,* 243–260.

Patterson, J., Peek, C. J., Heinrich, R. L., Bishoff, R. J., & Scherger, J. (2002). *Mental health professionals in medical settings: A primer.* New York: Norton.

Pennebaker, J. W. (1997). Writing about emotional experiences as a therapeutic process. *Psychological Science, 8,* 162–166.

Pennebaker, J. W. (2000). Psychological factors influencing the reporting of physical symptoms. In A. A. Stone, J. S. Turkkan, C. A. Bachrach, J. B. Jobe, H. S.

Kurtzman, & V. S. Cain (Eds.), *The science of self-report: Implications for research and practice* (pp. 299–315). Mahwah, NJ: Erlbaum.

Pope, K. S., & Feldman-Summers, S. (1992). National survey of psychologists' sexual and physical abuse history and their evaluation of training and competence in these areas. *Professional Psychology: Research and Practice, 23,* 353–361.

Rasmusson, A. M., & Friedman, M. J. (2002). The neurobiology of PTSD in women. In R. Kimerling, P. C. Ouimette, & J. Wolfe (Eds.), *Gender and PTSD* (pp. 43–75). New York: Guilford.

Resnick, H. S., Acierno, R., & Kilpatrick, D. G. (1997). Health impact of interpersonal violence 2: Medical and mental health outcomes. *Behavioral Medicine, 23,* 65–78.

Resnick, H. S., Kilpatrick, D. G., Dansky, B. S., Saunders, B. E., & Best, C. L. (1993). Prevalence of civilian trauma and posttraumatic stress disorder in a representative national sample of women. *Journal of Consulting and Clinical Psychology, 61,* 984–991.

Robohm, J. S., & Buttenheim, M. (1996). The gynecological care experience of adult survivors of childhood sexual abuse: A preliminary investigation. *Women and Health, 24,* 59–75.

Rodin, G. M., De Groot, J., & Spivak, H. (1998). Trauma, dissociation, and somatization. In J. D. Bremner & C. R. Marmar (Eds.), *Trauma, memory, and dissociation* (pp. 161–178). Washington, DC: American Psychiatric Press.

Ross-Gower, J., Waller, G., Tyson, M., & Elliott, P. (1998). Reported sexual abuse and subsequent psychopathology among women attending psychology clinics: The mediating role of dissociation. *British Journal of Clinical Psychology, 37,* 313–326.

Schnurr, P. P., Ford, J. D., Friedman, M. J., Green, B. L., Dain, B. J., & Sengupta, A. (2000). Predictors and outcomes of PTSD in World War II veterans exposed to mustard gas. *Journal of Consulting and Clinical Psychology, 68,* 258–268.

Schnurr, P. P., Friedman, M. J., Sengupta, A., Jankowski, M. K., & Holmes, T. (2000). PTSD and utilization of medical treatment services among male Vietnam veterans. *Journal of Nervous and Mental Disease, 188,* 496–504.

Schnurr, P. P., & Jankowski, M. K. (1999). Physical health and post-traumatic stress disorder: Review and synthesis. *Seminars in Clinical Neuropsychiatry, 4,* 295–304.

Schnurr, P. P., & Spiro, A., III. (1999). Combat exposure, posttraumatic stress disorder symptoms, and health behaviors as predictors of self-reported physical health in older veterans. *Journal of Nervous and Mental Disease, 187,* 353–359.

Schnurr, P. P., Spiro, A., III, & Paris, A. H. (2000). Physician-diagnosed medical disorders in relation to PTSD symptoms in older male military veterans. *Health Psychology, 19,* 91–97.

Schoenbaum, M., Unutzer, J., Sherbourne, C., Duan, N., Rubenstein, L. V., Miranda, J., et al. (2001). Cost-effectiveness of practice-initiated quality improvement for depression: Results of a randomized controlled trial. *Journal of the American Medical Association, 286,* 1325–1330.

Schulberg, H. C., Block, M. R., Madonia, M. J., Scott, C. P., Rodriguez, E., Imber, S. D., et al. (1996). Treating major depression in primary care practice. Eight-month clinical outcomes. *Archives of General Psychiatry, 53*, 913–919.

Selye, H. (1956). *The stress of life.* New York: McGraw-Hill.

Simon, G. E., Katon, W. J., Von Korff, M., Unutzer, J., Lin, E. H. B., Walker, E. A., et al. (2001). Cost-effectiveness of a collaborative care program for primary care patients with persistent depression. *American Journal of Psychiatry, 158*, 1638–1644.

Taft, C. T., Stern, A. S., King, L. A., & King, D. W. (1999). Modeling physical health and functional health status: The role of combat exposure, posttraumatic stress disorder, and personal resource attributes. *Journal of Traumatic Stress, 12*, 3–23.

Tilden, V. P., Schmidt, T. A., Limandri, B. J., Chiodo, G. T., Garland, M. J., & Loveless, P. A. (1994). Factors that influence clinicians' assessment and management of family violence. *American Journal of Public Health, 84*, 628–633.

van der Kolk, B. A. (1994). The body keeps the score: Memory and the evolving psychobiology of posttraumatic stress. *Harvard Review of Psychiatry, 1*, 263–265.

van der Kolk, B. A., Pelcovitz, D., Roth, S., Mandel, F. S., McFarlane, A., & Herman, J. L. (1996). Dissociation, somatization, and affect regulation: The complexity of adaptation to trauma. *American Journal of Psychiatry, 153*(Suppl.), 83–93.

Vedantham, K., Brunet, A., Boyer, R., Weiss, D. S., Metzler, T. J., & Marmar, C. R. (2001). Posttraumatic stress disorder, trauma exposure, and the current health of Canadian bus drivers. *Canadian Journal of Psychiatry, 46*, 149–155.

Von Korff, M., Gruman, J., Schaefer, J., Curry, S. J., & Wagner, E. H. (1997). Collaborative management of chronic illness. *Annals of Internal Medicine, 127*, 1097–1102.

Wagner, A. W., Wolfe, J., Rotnitsky, A., Proctor, S. P., & Erickson, D. J. (2000). An investigation of the impact of posttraumatic stress disorder on physical health. *Journal of Traumatic Stress, 13*, 41–55.

Walker, E. A., Gelfand, A., Katon, W. J., Koss, M. P., Von Korff, M., Bernstein, D., et al. (1999). Adult health status of women with histories of childhood abuse and neglect. *American Journal of Medicine, 107*, 332–339.

Wells, K. B., Sherbourne, C., Schoenbaum, M., Duan, N., Meredith, L., Unutzer, J., et al. (2000). Impact of disseminating quality improvement programs for depression in managed primary care: A randomized control trial. *Journal of the American Medical Association, 283*, 212–220.

White, P. A., & Faustman, W. O. (1989). Coexisting physical conditions among inpatients with post-traumatic stress disorder. *Military Medicine, 154*, 66–71.

Williams, R. B., Jr. (1995). Somatic consequences of stress. In M. J. Friedman, D. S. Charney, & A. Y. Deutch (Eds.), *Neurobiological and clinical consequences of stress: From normal adaptation to PTSD* (pp. 403–412). Philadelphia: Lippincott-Raven.

Wilson, I. B., & Cleary, P. D. (1995). Linking clinical variables with health-related quality of life. *Journal of the American Medical Association, 273,* 59–65.

Winkelspecht, S. M., & Singg, S. (1998). Therapists' self-reported training and success rates in treating clients with childhood sexual abuse. *Psychological Reports, 82,* 579–582.

Wolfe, J., Schnurr, P. P., Brown, P. J., & Furey, J. (1994). Posttraumatic stress disorder and war-zone exposure as correlates of perceived health in female Vietnam War veterans. *Journal of Consulting and Clinical Psychology, 62,* 1235–1240.

AUTHOR INDEX

Numbers in italics refer to listings in the reference sections.

282   AUTHOR INDEX

King, D. W., 25, 41, 249, 274
King, L. A., 25, 41, 249, 274
Kirby, A. C., 35, 238, 268
Kirby, D., 182
Kishino, Y., 139, 152
Klag, M. J., 89, 92, 93
Kleiger, R. E., 84, 95
Kleijn, W. C., 266, 271
Klein, T. W., 139, 151
Kleinman, D. E., 260, 271
Klimas, N., 151
Knapp, J. E., 138, 153
Knight, B. T., 96
Knight, R. G., 144, 154
Knook, L., 145, 150
Knopf, S., 152
Knudson, K. H., 17, 39
Ko, G. N., 168, 184
Kocijan-Hercigonja, D., 153, 186
Kolb, L. C., 166, 173, 181, 184
Kole-Snijders, A. M. J., 112, 122
Kolodner, K., 241
Komaroff, A., 144, 149, 211
Komproe, I., 10, 214
Koob, G., 182
Koolhaas, J. M., 107, 122
Koopman, C., 79, 97
Korszun, A., 174, 184
Korte, S. M., 122
Koss, M. P., 10, 13, 16, 38, 42, 54, 60,
       68, 67, 200, 214, 243, 257, 271,
       274
Koss, P. G., 54, 67
Kosten, T. R., 165, 184, 224, 240
Kotler, M., 92
Koumanis, J., 66
Kovach, J. A., 233, 241
Kowlowitz, V., 260, 271
Krauseneck, T., 186
Krieg, J. C., 119
Krikorian, R., 111, 122
Krinsley, K., 15, 36
Krishnan, K. R., 83, 96
Kroenke, K., 54, 67, 192, 193, 195, 198,
       211, 212, 262, 271
Kromhout, D., 94, 240
Kruesi, M. J., 149
Kruger, E., 46, 68
Krumholz, H. M., 95
Krupnick, J., 33, 37, 38, 74, 94, 254, 270
Krystal, J. H., 182, 187

Kucuk, O., 152
Kudler, H., 187, 238
Kuhns, J. B., 44, 69
Kuis, W., 145, 150
Kulick-Bell, R., 166, 185
Kulka, R. A., 5, 10, 17, 21, 38, 222, 223,
       224, 226, 241, 249, 251, 254,
       272
Kumar, M., 147
Kurata, T., 144, 153
Kutz, I., 148
Kuyk, J., 204, 212

L'Abate, L., 112, 120
Labbate, L. A., 202, 213, 254, 272
Lachman, M., 104, 118
LaCoursiere, R. B., 233, 241
Landerman, R., 198, 214
Landsberg, G., 257, 272
Lange, G., 200, 213
Lange, P., 242
LaPerriere, A., 140, 151, 152
Lardelli, P., 46, 65
Larson, D. B., 84, 91, 93
Larson, L., 153
Larson, M. G., 97
Larson, S. L., 81, 95
Lating, J. M., 231, 241
Laudenslager, M. L., 132, 134, 135, 137,
       151, 170, 184
Laudolt-Ritter, C., 119
Laue, L., 149
Laufer, D., 243
Lausell-Bryant, L., 257, 272
Lave, J. R., 30, 38
Lavelle, J., 39
Lazarus, R., 99, 101, 106, 121, 122
Lazenby, H. C., 65
Lebovits, B. Z., 78, 96
Lee, D. J., 141, 151
Lee, K. A., 103, 122
Lee, N. R., 150, 270
Leeka, J., 109, 121
Lefebvre, J. C., 117
Lehman, D. R., 104, 119, 120
Lehman, H. F., 238
Leichner, P., 259, 268
Leigh, H., 108, 121
Leischow, S. J., 94
Leitenberg, H., 112, 119

Victor, J., *154*
Vigna, C. M., 203, *210*
Vijan, S., 30, *41*
Visscher, B. R., 138, *153*
Vitaliano, P. P., *91*, 107, 108, *125*
Vlaeyen, J. W. S., *122*
Voelker, M. D., *35*, 201, 209, *214*
Vogt, T., 76, 97
Vojvoda, D., *186*
Volpicelli, J., 233, 234, *243*
Von, J. M., 233, *240*
Von Korff, M., *10*, 30, 38, *41*, 42, 51,
    57, 66, 68, *212*, *243*, 264, *271*,
    274
von Zerssen, S., *119*
Vrana, S. R., *35*

Waalen, J., 32, *41*
Wagner, A. W., 25, *41*, 249, *274*
Wagner, E. H., 264, *274*
Wahby, V. S., 165, *184*
Waitzkin, H., 27, *37*, 199, *211*, 249, *271*
Wakefield, D., 197, *215*
Walker, E. A., 7, *10*, 15, 18, 38, *42*, 54,
    55, 57, 58, 59, 61, 62, 68, 200,
    205, *214*, *215*, 217, 218, 222,
    225, 229, 231, *243*, 255, *271*,
    274
Walker, M. E., 44, *67*
Wallace, H., 233, *243*
Wallace, R. B., 78, 97
Waller, G., 204, *214*, 251, *273*
Walleus, H., *96*
Wang, H. J., 138, *153*
Wang, N. Y., 89, *92*, 93
Wang, S., 169, *183*, *184*, *185*, *186*, *187*,
    272
Wang, T., 131, *149*
Ward, C., 103, *125*
Ward, K., 108, *118*
Wardle, J., 86, 97
Warren, C. W., 228, *238*
Washko, R. M., *211*
Wasserman, D. A., 255, *270*
Wasserman, J., *118*
Wassertheil-Smoller, S., 78, 79, 97
Watkins, L. R., 136, *151*
Watson, D., 6, *10*
Watson, M., 111, *122*
Watson, R. R., 139, *154*

Weathers, F. W., 33, *42*, 61, 68
Weaver, M. J., *96*
Weihs, K. L., 111, *125*
Weiner, H., 137, *154*
Weiner, M., *240*
Weinreb, L., 261, *268*
Weinstein, M. C., 55, 66
Weinstein, P., 55, 68
Weintraub, J. K., 101, *119*
Weis, M., 84, 96
Weisberg, R. B., 26, *42*
Weiss, D. S., 28, *41*, *42*, *274*
Weiss, D. W., 132, 133, 148, *154*
Weiss, R. D., 224, *242*
Weiss, S. R. B., 177, *185*
Weiss, T. W., 57, 69
Weisse, C. S., 132, 138, *152*, *154*
Wells, A. F., 170, *186*
Wells, J., *182*
Wells, K., *42*, 211, 267, *274*
Wells, V. E., 76, 97
Wessely, S., 145, *148*, 193, 194, 195,
    208, *213*, *215*
West, S. A., *181*
Wetterling, T., 221, *243*
White, J., 44, 65
White, P. A., 249, *274*
Whiteside, T. T., 143, *154*
Whitmire Johnsen, L., 225, 228, *243*
Whitsel, E. A., *95*
Whittington, F. J., 139, 140, *153*
Widerlov, E., *96*
Widom, C. S., 44, 69, 200, *213*
Wiebe, J. S., 106, *123*
Wignall, F. S., 191, 192, *211*, *212*
Wiist, W. H., 32, *42*
Wilkinson, C., 236, *242*
Williams, C. S., *95*
Williams, D. A., 112, *119*, 203, *210*,
    211, *215*
Williams, J. B., *212*
Williams, P. G., 144, *154*
Williams, R. B., Jr., 88, *91*, 251, *274*
Williams, W., 57, 69
Williamson, D. F., 36, 66, 237, 239,
    269
Williamson, G. M., 6, 7, *10*, 138,
    153
Williger, D., *151*
Willis, L., 139, *155*
Wilson, A., 197, *215*

Wilson, D., *214*
Wilson, G., 169, *183*
Wilson, I. B., 6, *10*, 14, *42*, 256, *275*
Winde, P., 104, *125*
Winegar, R. K., 206, *213*
Winfield, I., 222, 223, *243*
Winkelspecht, S. M., 259, *275*
Winokur, G., 75, *92*
Winterbauer, N., 31, *39*
Wisner, D., 22, *42*
Wolde-Tsadik, G., 19, *39*
Wolf, A. M., 140, *155*
Wolf, C., *119*
Wolf, M. E., *152*
Wolfe, F., 196, *215*
Wolfe, J., 24, 25, 38, *41, 42*, 104, *125*,
    205, *215*, 223, 242, 249, 271,
    274, 275
Wong, L., *240*
Woodruff, W. J., 54, *67*
Woolson, R. F., *35*, 209, *214*
Word, C., *240*
Wortman, C. B., 104, *119, 120, 125*
Wright, K., *117*
Wulsin, L. R., 76, *97*
Wynings, C., *150*
Wynn, A., *94*

Xie, J. L., 109, *123*

Yamanishi, K., 144, *153*
Yanez, D., 55, 66
Yasko, J., 110, *121*
Yehuda, R., 136, 137, *155*, 163, 164,
    165, *184, 187, 188, 272*
Ying, Y. W., 30, *39*
Young, E., 174, *182*
Young, H. M., 107, *125*
Yuan, N., 33, *37*
Yunus, M. B., *215*

Zack, M. M., 14, *37*
Zakowski, S. G., 137, 138, *155*, 174,
    188
Zannino, L., 140, *147*
Zatzick, D., 22, 26, 28, *42*
Zautra, A. J., 110, *123, 125*, 143, *152*,
    174, *186*
Zayfert, C., 28, *42*
Zeber, J. E., 30, *41*
Zeidner, M., 104, 106, *125*
Zhang, H., *185*
Zhang, M., 30, *40, 42*
Zhao, S., *38*
Ziegler, M. G., 174, *188*
Zierler, S., 229, 230, *243*
Zilber, N., 75, *97*
Zoellner, L. A., 27, *42*
Zubovic, I., 173, *188*

SUBJECT INDEX

Access to care, 45
  public policy issues, 264–265
  utilization and, 45
Acquired immune deficiency syndrome/
    HIV, 19, 20, 23, 228, 229
  coping style and course of, 111
  immune response to trauma and,
    142
Adherence to medical treatment
  coping interventions to improve,
    117
  depression and, 87–88
Adrenergic system
  in PTSD, 167–168, 172
  in PTSD-mediated stress–health rela-
    tionship, 175
Adrenocorticotropic hormone, 159, 160,
    164
AIDS. *See* Acquired immune deficiency
    syndrome/HIV
Alcohol consumption
  associated medical disorders, 221
  depression and, 87
  health risk behavior, 217
  immune response to trauma and, 139
  mortality, 217, 221
  obstacles to treatment, 255
  PTSD and, 223–224, 227
  trauma exposure and, 222–223
Allergies, 108–109
Allostatic load model, 158–159, 253
  clinical significance, 179–180, 256
  in stress–health relationship, 171–
    172, 175–179, 255–256
Anger. *See* Hostility/anger
Angina, 74. See also Cardiovascular
    disease
Anxiety disorders, 26, 28, 251
  biological changes, 115
  hypertension and, 85–86
Assessment
  evaluating health status data in re-
    search, 14–15
  evaluating trauma experience re-
    search data, 15–16

family, 117
health risk behavior, 234–235, 258
hostility/anger, 88
immune function, 130–131
MIPS, 194–196, 208
process coping measures, 101, 103
See also Screening; Self-reported
    health
Atherosclerosis, 74. *See also* Cardiovascu-
    lar disease
Attentional processes, 253–255
Avoidant coping
  biological changes associated with,
    103, 109
  cardiovascular health and, 108,
    116
  disease outcomes and, 111, 115,
    116
  interventions to promote health,
    117

Back problems, 19
Behavioral factors in stress–health link-
    age, 8–9, 217–218
  allostatic load model, 178–179
  depression–cardiovascular disease, 82
  health care utilization and, 54
  integrative model, 255
  See also Health behavior
Biological factors in stress–health link-
    age, 8
  abnormalities in chronic stress, 160,
    171
  abnormalities in PTSD, 163–171,
    252, 253
  coping effects, 106–110
  depression–cardiovascular disease,
    82–83
  in integrative model, 251–253
  normal stress response, 159
Bone disorders, 170, 174
Bosnian refugees, 25, 27
Bulimia nervosa, 231
Bupropion, 86

physical health outcomes and,
105–110
problem-focused, 101, 102, 104–105,
109, 111–112, 113, 116, 251
process model, 101–103, 113–115
psychoanalytic conceptualization,
100
PTSD and strategy selection, 251
religious, 102
research needs, 116–117
response to trauma *vs.* response to
life event, 103–104
social support strategies, 102, 111,
113, 116
strategies, 101–102
in stress–health linkage, 8, 205, 251
Coronary artery disease, 74, 75–76. See
also Cardiovascular disease
Corticosteroids, 83
Corticotropin releasing factor, 83, 159,
160, 180
abnormalities in PTSD, 164
function, 164, 165
in PTSD-mediated stress–health relationship, 171–172, 174
Cortisol levels, 180, 252
coping and, 107–108
depression and, 83
immune system interactions, 136, 137
normal regulation, 165
in PTSD, 164–165
Cost of care
charges for care and, 49
claims data and, 49–50
context of analysis, 51–52
cost-effectiveness analysis, 50–51
data analysis, 47–48, 55–58
evidence of trauma exposure effects
on utilization, 58–63
indirect costs, 47–48
research design for analysis of, 53–55
research needs, 64–65
tobacco use, 218
trauma-related interventions, 264,
265
See also Economic analysis
Course of disease
coping skills in mediating, 111–112
MIPS, 194
Course of disease, trauma effects on, 19–
20, 34–35

Criminal victimization, health care utilization and, 60–61
Cytokines, 136, 170–171, 174, 252

Death, exposure to, 17
Debility syndrome, 202
Defenses
biological changes associated with,
107–108
in coping with trauma, 103
Dehydroepiandrosterone, 137, 160
Depression
assessment, 78–79
biology of, 82–84
cardiovascular disease linkage mechanism, 82–85
cardiovascular disease outcomes and,
8, 75–76, 79–80
cardiovascular disease prevention by
treatment of, 81–82, 90
as cardiovascular disease risk factor,
76–80, 81
coronary artery disease mortality
and, 75–76
health behaviors and, 61, 82, 86–87
hypertension and, 85–86
lipid metabolism and, 86
medical treatment adherence and,
87–88
as modifier of traditional risk factors
for cardiovascular disease,
85–87
PTSD comorbidity, 73–74, 250
relevance to PTSD studies, 73–74
research needs, 89, 90, 267
screening, 29–30
in stress–health linkage, 8, 28–29,
249–250, 250
stroke and, 80–81
tobacco use and, 220
Dexamethasone suppression test, 83
Diabetes, 163, 174
immune response to trauma and,
143, 144
Diet and nutrition
health risk behavior, 217, 230–232
immune response to trauma and,
139–140
Disclosure, in coping with trauma, 103,
110–111, 112

Dissociation
    MIPS and, 204–205, 207, 251,
        254–255
    in stress–health linkage, 251–252
Distress, 7
    biological changes associated with,
        108
Domestic and interpersonal violence
    health care utilization and, 61
    screening, 31–32, 33

Earthquake, 133–134
Eating disorders, 231–232
Economic analysis
    charges, analysis of, 49
    claims data, 49–50
    cost analysis, 47–48, 53–58
    cost-effectiveness, 50–51
    depression screening, 30
    early identification of disease, 63–64
    health care system trends, 46–47
    opportunity cost, 50
    research needs, 43–44
    role of, 43, 44
    stakeholder perspective in, 51–52
    time period used in, 52–53
    trauma research design issues, 53–55
    utilization research, 45–46, 53–58
Effectiveness and efficacy research, 64–65
Emotional functioning
    coping style, 101, 102, 104–105,
        109, 110–111, 113, 251
    expressivity as health outcome fac-
        tor, 106
Endocrine/neuroendocrine system
    coping effects, 106–108, 112, 115
    immune system interaction, 136–138
    PTSD and, 21, 173–174
    stress response, 159
Endorphins, 137
    in PTSD, 169
Epidemiology
    cardiovascular disease, 74
    depression–PTSD comorbidity, 73–74
    posttraumatic stress disorder, 4–5
    somatization disorders in PTSD, 205
    trauma exposure, 4
    trauma exposure–health linkage, 16
Epinephrine, 137, 159
    immune system interaction, 136

in PTSD, 167, 168
Epstein-Barr virus, 109, 143
Exercise. *See* Physical activity
Expectancy effects, 177
Exposure-based therapy, 236

Family assessment, 117
Fibromyalgia, 174
    childhood maltreatment and, 200
Fibromyalgia syndrome, 196

Gastrointestinal disorders, 17, 19, 21, 27
Glucocorticoids, 136–137
    in PTSD, 165–166
Gonadotropin-releasing hormone, 169
Growth hormone, 137
    abnormalities in PTSD, 170,
        173–174
Gulf War Syndrome, 194, 201–203,
    205–206

Hallucinogens, 227
Health behavior
    assessment, 234–235, 258
    in depression, 82, 86–87
    diet and exercise, 230–232
    as mediating immune response to
        trauma, 139–140
    patient education, 261
    preventive intervention, 235–236
    PTSD in mediating trauma–health
        risk behavior relationship, 218
    research needs, 237
    risk behavior conceptualization, 217
    sexual risk behaviors, 227–230
    in stress–health linkage mechanism,
        9, 217–218, 232–234
    trauma effects, 253–254
    See also Behavioral factors in stress–
        health linkage; Help-seeking be-
        havior; Substance abuse
Health Belief Model, 88
Health maintenance organizations, 48, 63
Hearing problems, 17, 19
Help-seeking behavior, 8
    environmental factors, 45
    personality factors, 44–45
    PTSD and, 181

Sertraline, 82, 87
Sexual assault
    associated health problems, 16, 54
    health care utilization and, 61, 62
    infectious disease transmission in, 54
    pregnancy related to, 54
    PTSD as mediator of trauma–health
        linkage, 25–26, 27
    somatoform dissociation and,
        204–205
    subsequent eating disorders and, 231
    subsequent sexual risk behavior,
        228–229
    substance use and, 218–219, 220,
        222–223, 225
Sexual behavior, health risk in, 217,
    227–230
Sexual dysfunction, 16, 18
Sexually transmitted disease, 228. *See also*
    Acquired immune deficiency
    syndrome/HIV
Skin disorders, 17, 54
Sleep dysfunction in PTSD, 166–167
Social support, 102, 111, 113, 116
    as mediator of immune response to
        trauma, 138
    trauma-related MIPS and, 207–208
Socioeconomic status, 89
Somatization, 8–9, 254
    clinical conceptualization, 191–192,
        193
    health care utilization and, 54
    primary care interventions, 260–261
    PTSD as mediator of trauma–health
        linkage, 27–28
    See also Multiple idiopathic physical
        symptoms
Somatization spectrum disorders,
    197–199
Specificity of coping in mediating disease
    outcomes, 110–111
Specificity of PTSD as mediator of
    trauma–health linkage, 27–29,
    266–267
Specificity of trauma–health linkage, 19
Sperm abnormalities, 19, 54
Startle response in PTSD, 166
Stress
    allostatic state responses, 177–178
    biological abnormalities in chronic
        exposure, 160

chronic, 131–132
    enhanced response, 177–178
    immune function response to, 131–
        132, 174
    normal biological response, 159–160
    prolonged response, 178
    recovery, 160
    threat appraisal problems, 177
    See also Coping; Mechanism of
        stress–health linkage; Trauma
        exposure
Stroke, 161
    depression and, 74, 80–81
Substance abuse, 109
    immune response and, 139
    mortality, 224
    obstacles to treatment, 255
    PTSD and, 226–227, 234
    risk of victimization and, 226
    stress–health linkage and, 233–234
    trauma exposure and, 139, 218–221,
        222–227
    See also Alcohol consumption; To-
        bacco use
Suicide, 23, 86, 221
Sympathetic nervous system, 160, 161
    in PTSD, 166, 172
    stress response, 159
Sympathoadrenal system, 83–85

Temporal orientation, 104
Temporomandibular disorders, 174
Terrorism, 203
Testosterone levels in PTSD, 169–170
Therapeutic relationship
    in MIPS, 193–194
    primary care interventions with
        trauma survivors, 261
    screening effectiveness and, 32
Threat appraisal, 177
Thyroid function, 173
Thyroid stimulating hormone, 169
Tobacco use
    assessment of, 90
    associated health care spending, 218
    depression and, 86–87, 220
    immune response and, 139
    mortality, 217, 218
    PTSD and, 220–221
    trauma exposure and, 139, 218–219

evidence of PTSD as mediator of trauma exposure–health linkage, 24–25, 28

evidence of PTSD–health linkage, 21–22

evidence of trauma–health linkage, 17–19

historical evidence of somatization, 201–202

immune function in PTSD patients, 134–135

MIPS and, 202–203, 207

mortality outcomes, 20

personality change in response to, 104

PTSD epidemiology, 4–5

subsequent eating disorders and, 231

tobacco use and, 220–221

Wound healing, 142

Yohimbine, 168

ABOUT THE EDITORS

Paula P. Schnurr, PhD, is deputy to the executive director of the Department of Veterans Affairs National Center for Post-Traumatic Stress Disorder and research professor of psychiatry at Dartmouth Medical School in Hanover, New Hampshire. She received her PhD in experimental psychology at Dartmouth College in 1984 and then completed a postdoctoral fellowship in the Department of Psychiatry at Dartmouth Medical School. Dr. Schnurr's administrative duties at the National Center involve the coordination of activities across the seven consortium sites, consultation on research and policy, and program development. She is president of the International Society for Traumatic Stress Studies, edits the *PTSD Research Quarterly*, and is the editor-elect of the *Journal of Traumatic Stress*.

Bonnie L. Green, PhD, is professor and director of research in the Department of Psychiatry at Georgetown University Medical School in Washington, DC. She received her PhD in experimental psychology at the University of Cincinnati in 1980 and served on the Department of Psychiatry faculty at the University of Cincinnati Medical School until 1990. She teaches psychiatry residents and conducts research on the consequences of traumatic events. Her current research addresses the mental health needs of low-income minority women with trauma in primary care settings. Dr. Green is past editor of the *Journal of Traumatic Stress* and past president of the International Society for Traumatic Stress Studies (ISTSS). She recently served as chief editor of *Trauma Interventions in War and Peace: Prevention, Practice, and Policy*, a book representing a collaboration between the ISTSS and the United Nations.